Clinical Documentation Improvement: Principles and Practice

Pamela Carroll Hess, MA, RHIA, CCS, CDIP, CPC

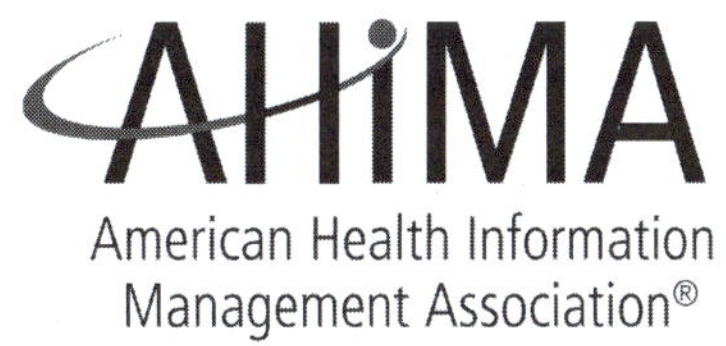

17 16 15   2 3

ISBN 978-1-58426-502-3
AHIMA Product No. AB121614

AHIMA Staff:
Chelsea Brotherton, MA, Assistant Editor
Melanie Endicott, MBA/HCM, RHIA, CDIP, CCS, CCS-P, FAHIMA, Technical Reviewer
Ashley Latta, Production Development Editor
Elizabeth Ranno, Vice President of Product and Planning
Lou Ann Wiedemann, MS, RHIA, CDIP, CHDA, CPEHR, FAHIMA, Technical Reviewer
Pamela Woolf, Director of Publications

For more information about AHIMA Press publications, including updates, visit http://www.ahima.org/publications/updates.aspx

American Health Information Management Association
233 North Michigan Avenue, 21st Floor
Chicago, Illinois 60601-5800
http://www.ahima.org

Brief Contents

Detailed Table of Contents

About the Author

Pamela Carroll Hess, MA, RHIA, CCS, CDIP, CPC is an AHIMA-approved ICD-10-CM trainer and is a health information management (HIM) professional with more than 30 years of healthcare experience in revenue cycle operations, electronic health record (EHR) applications, reimbursement, coding, billing, compliance, quality control, clinical documentation, and coding training. Ms. Hess has served in administrative, interim management, and consulting capacities within large academic and urban community hospitals. Her experience in the healthcare industry has focused on improving operational and financial performance in a variety of healthcare settings.

Ms. Hess has assisted her clients with regulatory issues related to accurate MS-DRG assignment, ICD-9, ICD-10, and CPT coding, claims and reimbursement reviews, fraud and abuse, corporate integrity agreements, Joint Commission accreditation, and payer billing guidelines. In addition, Ms. Hess has led numerous large clinical documentation improvement projects, clinical appeals department redesigns, middle revenue cycle reimbursement projects, claims assessment projects, and physician, clinician, and coder training programs for a wide variety of providers, including academic medical centers, community hospitals, and physician practices in the United States and abroad. She has designed and implemented monitoring and analytics information systems that identify and mitigate compliance risks and assist clients with reporting and corrective action plans. Ms. Hess is employed as a Director, CDI at **Him**agine Solutions Inc., the largest privately held HIM services organization in the country. Prior to joining **Him**agine, she led the CDI service line for Deloitte & Touche, LLC and Navigant Consulting, Inc. She is a President of the Arizona Health Information Management Association.

Acknowledgements

The author would like to acknowledge Nicolas A. Joye, BS, RHIT, CCS for his contributions to this textbook. Mr. Joye has experience in inpatient, outpatient, and professional fee coding using ICD-9-CM, ICD-10-CM/PCS, and CPT/HCPCS. He is a senior coder with MModal and an active member in the American Health Information Management Association (AHIMA) as well as the Arizona Health Information Management Association (AzHIMA).

AHIMA Press would like to acknowledge Ruthann Russo, PhD, JD, MPH, RHIT for her authorship on the original edition of this publication. AHIMA Press would also like to thank Sheila Graham, LPN, CCDS for her review and feedback on this text.

Introduction

The Importance of Clinical Documentation in Today's Healthcare Environment

Patient Care and Quality

Clinical documentation is a term used frequently and freely in the healthcare industry; however, it has escaped a consistent definition to date. For purposes of this book, clinical documentation is any manual or electronic notation (or recording) made by a physician or other healthcare clinician related to a patient's medical condition or treatment. Clinical documentation improvement (CDI) has evolved from the review of health records for completeness by the health information management (HIM) department, to a facility-wide activity that enhances the quality of the clinical record thus affecting patient care, reimbursement, severity, and quality scores. This book presents an objective and uniform set of clinical documentation principles that healthcare professionals can reliably apply throughout the industry.

Quality is another term the healthcare industry commonly uses that has escaped precise definition. Quality clinical documentation, as explained in chapter 1, meets the following seven criteria:

- Legible
- Reliable
- Precise
- Complete
- Consistent
- Clear
- Timely

Clinical documentation is the foundation of every patient health record. By creating records for the patients they treat, healthcare organizations are in essence, medical trustees for their patients' protected health information. Since the dawn of the Health Information Portability and Accountability Act (HIPAA), both patients and the organizations that treat them are beginning to appreciate the critical value of that information even more. The prime directive of the law is to ensure healthcare coverage for all, safeguard the privacy of clinical information, and reduce administrative costs for clinical record keeping. The next challenge for the healthcare industry is ensuring consistency in content and meaning of clinical information as it evolves from a manual to an electronic practice. Healthcare systems are digitally compiling all health information about one patient into a common location. The electronic health record has the potential of creating significant positive impact on healthcare quality—but *only* if the information in the record is itself of the highest possible quality.

High-quality clinical documentation and the need for a structure to support the function continuously is the premise for this book. High-quality clinical documentation is the goal of every CDI program. This book provides standardized criteria healthcare professionals can use to set goals and objectives for the CDI program. This book describes in detail the three necessary elements for a CDI program: implementation, operationalization, and continued maintenance. Part I addresses the fundamentals of clinical documentation including assessing the current quality of a healthcare organization's clinical documentation and deciding whether to move forward with a new program or adding improvements to the current program. Part II describes CDI program implementation from staffing the program through training and querying physicians, analyzing program data, and ensuring program compliance. Finally, part III recommends and explains a process for growing and refining a CDI program. The book ends, as it begins, with a focus on the patient, specifically addressing the possibility of involving patients in the CDI process.

The Users of Health Information

The vast and myriad uses and users of health information illustrate the importance of the health records that house that information. The record benefits the patient, but it can also benefit other patients when professionals in the healthcare industry use that information for research purposes. Furthermore, the health information derived from clinical documentation in the record drives the decision-making process of the healthcare industry for providers and payers alike. In fact, the information in a patient's record is the common ground shared by everyone who is involved in or touches the healthcare industry. Patients, the government, physicians, pharmaceutical firms, insurers, research organizations, healthcare systems, and other providers all need the information in patient health records to fulfill their responsibilities. It is important to define each of these health information users, how they individually benefit from the information, as well as how they contribute to the overall larger body of health information.

Patients

Without the patient, there is no health record. The primary purpose for maintaining a health record is to "accurately and adequately document a patient's life and health history, including past and present illness(es) and treatment(s), with emphasis on the events affecting the patient during the current episode of care" (Huffman 1994, 30). The health record is the primary reference tool for all physicians and clinicians treating the patient. Clinical documentation, which is the foundation of the patient's record, is the key factor in determining the quality of care provided to the patient.

It is also important for patients to know the quality of their health information depends on their responses to questions the physician and other clinicians ask them during a visit. Patients who are prepared to answer questions accurately about their symptoms provide clinicians with better raw material to work with in their own documentation.

To patients, information in the health record can be difficult to understand. Yet, patients who learn basic facts and become familiar with the record are more empowered than patients who are uninformed about their health information. The knowledgeable and proactive patient is also likely to respond to questions with greater accuracy.

HIPAA has raised awareness about patients' rights concerning their health information. As a result, more patients are likely to request copies of their records. HIPAA has also increased the popularity of the electronic health record. The act of reading, understanding, and asking questions about health information creates healthcare consumers who are better decision makers and participants in their own care. In addition, when patients are proactive participants in their healthcare planning, and they understand the importance of their health information, their providers are more likely to be accountable for the quality of information they document in the health record.

Physicians and Other Clinicians

The health record is the primary tool for clinicians to communicate with each other about a patient. As the next example shows, seven different clinicians treat a patient during an average acute care hospital stay. The typical hospital record includes entries made by the attending physician, specialists, house staff (for teaching hospitals), nurses, radiologists, pathologists, and therapists. The inaccurate or unreliable clinical documentation of one provider can create a domino effect that negatively affects the quality of care provided to the patient. While the importance of clinical documentation is clear to most physicians, they may not understand how important the quality of that documentation is. Medical school students, residents, and most clinicians do not receive thorough training in the principles of high-quality clinical documentation. Hospitals and healthcare systems need to fill that void by providing comprehensive and consistent training in clinical documentation as well as ongoing support through a structured CDI program.

Healthcare Provider Organizations

Clinical documentation reflects the quality of care, severity of illness, and treatment provided for each patient the organization treats. As a result, health records and the clinical documentation contained in them may be the most valuable asset of a healthcare organization. Individually, these records are the basis for payment for all services healthcare organizations provide. Each record is evidence that the patient actually received the care for which the organization billed. In aggregate, health records create a data set that healthcare organizations rely on for strategic and financial planning, budgeting, and internal research. A hospital's senior management team can detect trends in treatment and resource needs, staffing requirements, and disease patterns by reviewing the diagnostic data gleaned from the clinical documentation in patient records. In addition, hospitals can purchase data from other hospitals to run comparative analyses. The results of these analyses can help the management team determine future demand for services in their market so they can better prepare. The trustworthiness of management decisions in the healthcare industry is directly proportional to the quality of the clinical documentation in patient records.

Insurers

Insurers pay for care that subscribers received from a healthcare organization subject to policy limitations. However, because no plan pays for care an organization did not provide, most insurers regularly audit health record documentation. If the clinical documentation in the record does not support the bill for services, the insurer rejects the bill outright. Insurers also use clinical documentation in patient records to certify or preapprove services like magnetic resonance imaging (MRIs) or surgery. Inaccurate clinical documentation in this situation means a denial of service, thus the patient does not receive the necessary test or treatment.

Government and Regulatory Agencies

This category includes federal and state government agencies as well as organizations like the Joint Commission, Healthgrades, the LeapFrog Group, and other organizations that publish healthcare quality ratings. State and federal governments, when acting as an insurer for Medicare or Medicaid recipients, have the same interests and responses as the insurers. However, the government also plays a regulatory role in measuring and attempting to ensure a certain level of quality in healthcare. At the federal level, the Medicare quality indicators play an important role in comparative measurement among healthcare organizations. (CMS 2015) The Affordable Care Act has established new definitions and measures of quality care.

Accreditation organizations also produce measures healthcare consumers and insurers use to select healthcare providers. To some degree, all quality measurements rely on clinical documentation in patient records and the resulting coded data. Measures like Healthgrades rely entirely on data derived from clinical documentation in health records to assign quality ratings to hospital care, while a combination of data and original clinical documentation drives CMS's quality indicators. The bottom line is that quality measures that consumers use to make the best healthcare decisions are only as reliable as the clinical documentation quality.

Research Organizations and the Pharmaceutical Industry

Research organizations and the pharmaceutical industry sponsor a large percentage of clinical documentation research. Researchers rely on clinical documentation in two primary ways. First, the researchers scrutinize the health records of patients participating in research studies. Second, hospital- and academic-based researchers use the international classification of diseases (ICD) data derived from clinical documentation in patient health records to identify successful treatment trends and changes in disease patterns. Researchers may also use this data to support hypotheses and design new research studies. The validity of hypotheses and research studies is only as accurate as the clinical documentation in patient records.

The Need for High-Quality Clinical Documentation

This overview of the users and uses of health information demonstrates the crucial need for high-quality clinical documentation in patient records. The need starts with the individual patient and then impacts most healthcare consumers as well as industries. Current gaps in the clinical documentation process that this book attempts to fill include the lack of a consistent criteria set and the lack of a standardized training system for high-quality clinical documentation. In addition, the book presents suggestions for design, implementation, and continued renewal of a CDI program. It is imperative that healthcare providers and professionals standardize the way they measure clinical documentation quality for the benefit of patients, physicians, clinicians, and the entire healthcare industry.

REFERENCES

CMS. 2015. Quality Initiatives—General Information. http://www.cms.hhs.gov/QualityInitiativesGenInfo/15_MQMS.asp.

Huffman, E.K. 1994. *Health Information Management.* Berwyn, IL: Physicians Record Company.

Part I

Fundamentals of Clinical Documentation

Chapter 1

Criteria for High-Quality Clinical Documentation

⦿ The Need for High-Quality Clinical Documentation

High-quality clinical documentation is a necessary yet uncommon practice within today's healthcare communities. It is a practice all healthcare organizations and providers need and want, yet few are able to fully achieve. This chapter first presents the research that shows high-quality clinical documentation does not exist today in most healthcare organizations. Then, the chapter describes the theory of high-quality clinical documentation, followed by an explanation of seven criteria for high-quality clinical documentation. The chapter then includes peer-reviewed research results, as well as healthcare laws and regulatory guidelines that support the proposed theory and criteria.

Ultimately, it is the sharing and reinforcing of this information with physicians and clinicians in provider organizations that turns the theory into practice and impacts the quality of clinical documentation.

Lack of High-Quality Clinical Documentation

Research on clinical documentation by Brett M. Cascio from the Department of Orthopaedic Surgery at Johns Hopkins University in Baltimore, Maryland, and Yuri W. Novitsky from the University Hospital in Cleveland, Ohio, reveals the lack of adequate documentation throughout the healthcare industry (Cascio et al. 2005, 346; Novitsky et al. 2005, 627). The peer-reviewed academic literature also shows a relationship between documentation and quality of care, as well as support for concurrent clinical documentation improvement (CDI) programs.

Researchers identified the following reasons and causes of poor quality clinical documentation:

- Medical school and residency programs do not teach clinical documentation practices.
- The importance of physician clinical documentation is not a top priority for healthcare organizations.
- The information, especially in the inpatient setting, is complex.
- Multiple providers are needed when there are longer patient stays, resulting in additional clinical documentation with increased inconsistency between provider documentation.
- Unstructured or inconsistent processes for recording and collection of information are prevalent (Cascio et al. 2005; Novitsky et al. 2005).

The following is a brief synopsis of the peer-reviewed research published on the challenges associated with attaining high-quality clinical documentation.

Over the past two decades, researchers have found quality problems in physician documentation in many parts of the health record including progress notes, history and physical reports, problem lists, and operative notes. In addition, one study found significant discrepancies between orthopedic surgeon office notes and hospital notes for the same patient. An overview of the studies by type of documentation problem follows (Russo 2007).

Both Cascio and J.W. Bachman from the Mayo Clinic studied deficiencies in documenting history and physical exams. In the Cascio study, the researchers focused on clinical documentation specific to the clinical course of acute compartment syndrome. The term "compartment syndrome" refers to increased tissue pressure within a closed fascial space, resulting in tissue ischemia (Beers 2006).

In this study, researchers found inadequate documentation in 70 percent of the patient records. The researchers reviewed notes and consent forms for 30 consecutive patients with adequate follow-up who underwent a fasciotomy to treat compartment syndrome. The review included legibility, notation of time and date, and documentation of core physical examination and history findings, including pain, paresthesias, tenseness, pain on passive stretch, sensory deficit, motor deficit, pulses, compartment pressures, and diastolic blood pressure (Cascio et al. 2005, 346).

Here, the researchers found that thorough documentation contributes to the identification of subtle changes in the physical examination findings, which leads to increased quality of care to the patient. The researchers further note that a possible reason for the widespread lack of proper documentation is a lack of emphasis on careful documentation in medical schools, residency programs, and physician practices (Cascio et al. 2005, 346).

Bachman's research on the patient interview and documentation process revealed that physicians often omit questions, diagnoses, or other important information in the documentation of the patient's history and physical examination. According to Bachman, the researchers' review of the physician history-taking process revealed that it is often incomplete and time consuming. Here, the researchers performed a literature review to identify the importance of using a checklist while obtaining and documenting a patient's history. They compared the use of a checklist by a physician to an airplane pilot's checklist. Showing that just as a pilot would not take off without reviewing his checklist, a physician should not treat a patient without reviewing his checklist (Bachman 2003, 67).

Aaron E. Carroll with the Indiana University Department of Pediatrics found documentation discrepancies in 62 percent of the progress notes he and his research team reviewed. The team conducted a review of residents' progress notes over 40 random days in a four-month period in a neonatal intensive care unit (NICU). Using predetermined criteria, they assessed the reliability of medications, vascular lines, and patient weights. The researchers found progress note discrepancies in 28 percent of medication documentation, 34 percent of vascular lines documentation, and 13 percent of documented weights (Carroll et al. 2003).

In this study, patients with more medications or vascular lines, and longer lengths of stay, were significantly more likely to have higher rates of documentation error. The study concluded that daily progress notes written by resident physicians in the NICU often contained inaccuracies or omitted pertinent information (Carroll et al. 2003).

Carroll deduced that clinical documentation errors are common in healthcare settings where the patient stays are longer and more complicated. This finding supports the idea that inpatient acute care health record documentation should be a top priority when undertaking a CDI program. In addition, the researchers found that when the physicians did not provide documentation immediately after caring for a patient, the quality of the documentation in the patient's record was susceptible to neglect and data loss (Carroll et al. 2003).

This finding shows concurrent review and concurrent physician inquiry as the key activity of a clinical documentation program. In this study, physicians themselves also identified that they were not always able to access the information they were seeking in the patient's record to help treat the patient. These physicians attributed this problem to illegible handwriting, too little time, and disorganized charts.

Though an increasing number of facilities have an electronic health record (EHR) system, specific views of the data vary depending on the provider or user. Information accessible to one user type may not be visible to other users. The information technology (IT) department implementation team should ensure that each user can access data necessary for their job function. The copy and paste function has also created a problem for data integrity. For example, dates of service may not be valid and historical data may be misleading. Healthcare organizations should establish compliance guidance and well-thought-out policies regarding the copy-paste function in the EHR.

Two different research teams addressed problem list documentation quality: the team of Elizabeth Spencer from the University of Wisconsin and the team of Marlene Weitzel from the University of Texas. The Spencer team's research demonstrated that current smoking status, an important data element in measuring patient quality of care under the Medicare quality indicators, was often missing from the problem list within the patient's record. Although the problem list is a major document in the patient record and relatively easy to understand and complete, physicians often omitted current smoking status or did not complete the form at all (Spencer et al. 1999, 18).

The Weitzel study revealed that physicians completed 49 out of 49 items on mental status examinations when they used a checklist, whereas physicians completed only 4 out of 49 items when not using a checklist. While a checklist is an important part of documentation collection, it does not resolve the majority of clinical documentation challenges and is just one part of a CDI program strategy. In addition, there may be compliance concerns with checklist use, so the organization's compliance and legal groups need to review and approve a specific format prior to use. For example, physicians cannot use checklists to ensure they document the clinical significance of every abnormal test result in a patient's record (Weitzel and Waller 1990, 23–34).

The Devon and Novitsky research team found problems with the quality of physician operative notes. The Holli Devon study at Marquette University found the patient's health record to be an inaccurate and inadequate source of information about symptoms experienced by patients with acute myocardial infarctions. The research also found surgeons' operative notes to contain numerous deficiencies. In a teaching-hospital setting, researchers found fewer deficiencies in operative notes dictated by attending physicians than those dictated by residents, but in both cases, there was a significant failure to produce high-quality operative notes (Devon 2004, 547).

Novitsky found that 28 percent of the operative reports residents dictated contained errors. Accurate and complete operative reports are essential for medical and legal purposes. They serve as an important communication tool for all healthcare personnel involved in the care of a particular patient. These dictations delineate operative indications and justify the treatment. In addition, a full description of positive and negative findings, as well as the thought process behind them, may influence not only the quality of care for the patient, but also the outcome of a malpractice lawsuit (Novitsky et al. 2005, 627).

The EHR environment has added an extra challenge to the practice of high-quality clinical documentation. Resident physicians enter the clinical setting with a more fragmented approach to documentation. The paper record that previously read like a chronological scenario within the various sections of the health record has been replaced with templates that encourage fill-in-the-blank and drop-down data entry, and multiple views of the data that often do not give an intuitive review of the entire patient stay. Physicians rely on electronic notifications and prompts to enter key phrases, encouraging specificity that may be incorrect if the author does not use thoughtful consideration. The increase in the amount of documentation especially within the progress note section of the EHR is often a result of copying and pasting clinical data in multiple locations, making it hard to determine key information on any given date. Copying and pasting dates can result in inaccurate clinical diagnostic and treatment recordings. To mitigate some of these documentation challenges, the CDI department should diligently look for aberrant documentation patterns and provide intervention and education where needed. For example, CDI specialists must watch for overuse of key phrases that are often the topic of clarification requests in physician documentation. CDI practitioners should also observe attending physician notes and compare for consistent record keeping by the resident physicians.

⊙ Evidence-Based Documentation: The Theory of High-Quality Clinical Documentation

Because clinical documentation in patient health records is highly regulated by governmental and accreditation agencies, any theory concerning it must begin with regulatory and legal requirements. Medicare Conditions of Participation require all healthcare providers to maintain patient health records and dictates they follow these guidelines:

- The health record must contain information to justify admission and continued hospitalization, support the diagnosis, and describe the patient's progress and response to medications and services.
- All patient health record entries must be legible, complete, dated, timed, and authenticated in written or electronic form by the person responsible for providing or evaluating the service, consistent with hospital policies and procedures.
- All records must document the following, as appropriate:
    - A medical history and physical examination completed and documented no more than 30 days before or 24 hours after admission or registration, but prior to surgery or a procedure requiring anesthesia services.
    - An updated examination of the patient, including any changes in the patient's condition, when the medical history and physical examination are completed within 30 days before admission or registration.
    - An admitting diagnosis.
    - Results of all consultative patient evaluations and appropriate findings by clinical and other staff involved in the care of the patient.
    - Documentation of complications, hospital-acquired infections, and unfavorable reactions to drugs and anesthesia.
    - Properly executed informed consent forms for procedures and treatments specified by the medical staff, or by federal or state law if applicable, that require written patient consent.
    - All practitioners' orders, nursing notes, reports of treatment, medication records, radiology and laboratory reports, vital signs, and other information necessary to monitor the patient's condition.
    - A discharge summary with the hospitalization outcome, case disposition, and provisions for follow-up care.
    - A final diagnosis with completion of health records within 30 days following discharge (CMS Conditions of Participation 2014).

The Office of Inspector General (OIG) was established at the Department of Labor (DOL) by the Inspector General Act of 1978 to identify potential fraud, waste, and abuse of the Medicare Part A and B programs through improper payments and to review for quality issues related to the delivery of healthcare services in hospitals, nursing facilities, home health, and hospice services (OIG 2015). The OIG uses Medicare Administrative Contractors (MACs) to administer Medicare Parts A and B as well as to process claims for services rendered. Each year the

OIG develops a work plan that focuses on opportunities to improve the program economy, efficiency, and effectiveness. CDI programs should include pertinent OIG Work Plan topics in the CDI department goals and objectives. Examples of the work plan topics relative to CDI include

- Medical necessity of high-cost diagnostic radiology tests—Clinical documentation specialists (CDS) staff should review records for specific documentation relative to the medical necessity of high-cost tests.
- High use of physical therapists—outpatient CDI programs should focus on specific documentation substantiating the need for a high volume of physical therapy visits.
- Inpatient claims for mechanical ventilation—CDI specialists should review claims to ensure that documentation of ventilator times is clear and consistent in the health record. Inaccurate ventilator time calculation can result in overpayment or underpayment based on the 96-hour mechanical ventilation requirement for MS-DRGs 207 and 208:
  - 207 Respiratory Diagnoses with ventilator support 96+ hours
  - 208 Respiratory Diagnoses with ventilator support <96 hours
- Kwashiorkor malnutrition—CDI staff should teach providers and coders clinical indicator requirements for the coding of Kwashiorkor malnutrition. The OIG has identified this as an over-used diagnosis resulting in overpayment under the MS-DRG system (Virbitsky 2014).

Table 1.1 shows government, regulatory, and accreditation resources for health record content.

The theory of high-quality clinical documentation is a two-part, cause-and-effect theory. The first part of the theory, which identifies criteria for high quality,

Table 1.1 Resources for health record content

Resources
Medicare Conditions of Participation http://www.cms.gov/Regulations-and-Guidance/Legislation/CFCsAndCoPs/index.html
The Joint Commission http://www.jointcommission.org/
Medicare Administrative Contractor http://www.cms.gov/Medicare/Medicare-Contracting/Medicare-Administrative-Contractors/MedicareAdministrativeContractors.html
ICD-9 and ICD-10 Guidelines http://www.cms.gov/Medicare/Coding/ICD9ProviderDiagnosticCodes/index.html
OIG – 3rd Party Billing Guidance http://oig.hhs.gov/fraud/docs/complianceguidance/thirdparty.pdf

derives from legal and regulatory sources. The second part of the theory derives from the peer-reviewed research discussed earlier in this chapter. The theory of high-quality clinical documentation states that applying the seven criteria (legible, reliable, precise, complete, consistent, clear, and timely) of high-quality clinical documentation, increases clinical documentation quality and improves the accuracy of care, quality indicators, reimbursement, healthcare planning, and research (the activities that clinical documentation impacts).

Evidence-based medicine (EBM) means practicing medicine using only the best scientific data available. Just as in medical practice, physicians should only be practicing clinical documentation using the best scientific data available. *A Compelling Case for Clinical Documentation* describes in detail an interventional study performed with controls and conducted using resident physicians to test the first part of the theory of high-quality clinical documentation (Russo 2008a and 2008b).

The study found a statistically significant relationship between high-quality clinical documentation training and the improvement in physicians' clinical documentation quality (Russo and Fitzgerald 2008).

In *The Gold Standard: The Challenge of Evidence-Based Medicine and Standardization of Health Care*, the authors use the evolution of patient health records as an analogy for EBM. EBM is about creating a standard in medical care. There are four kinds of standards used in EBM:

1. Design
2. Terminology
3. Performance
4. Procedural

(Timmermans and Berg 2003)

The authors point out that like EBM, the notion of patient-centered health-record keeping, which began in the United States at the turn of the twentieth century, also encompassed all four types of standardization (Timmermans and Berg 2003). Additionally, they compare the evolution of patient record-keeping standards from the 1920s, when the American College of Surgeons was the only regulating body for health record content, to today's rigorous requirements of Medicare, The Joint Commission, and state departments of health.

Criteria for High-Quality Clinical Documentation

The seven criteria for high-quality clinical documentation require that all entries in the patient record be

1. Legible
2. Reliable
3. Precise
4. Complete

5. Consistent
6. Clear
7. Timely

(Russo and Fitzgerald 2008; Russo 2007)

The first six criteria focus on the review process and, if necessary, can be corrected after the fact; however, the last, timeliness, is one criterion that cannot be corrected after the fact since once an entry is late, it remains late. The initial definition provided for each criterion is taken from the *Oxford English Dictionary* (6th edition, 2005). Following the dictionary definition is a description of how healthcare professionals can apply the criteria to patient health record documentation. With the exception of legibility and timeliness, the dictionary entry also includes examples of documentation that *does* and *does not* meet the criteria after each definition.

Legible

Legibility means the record is clear enough for the reader to comprehend and easily decipher. The inability to read a patient record entry is usually because the physician's handwriting is indecipherable. Every regulatory body and law that addresses health record content includes discussion of legibility in clinical documentation. The most recent nod to the importance of legibility came when HIPAA gave patients the right to ask for clarification of illegible information in their records. Illegible handwriting is usually the result of a rushed or careless documentation practice. As EHR systems evolve, handwriting becomes less of an issue. However, there are other risks inherent in the rushed or careless use of an EHR that may cause a greater focus on consistency than legibility.

Reliable

Reliability means the content of the record is trustworthy, safe, and yielding the same result when repeated. Reliable criteria relate to treatment provided to the patient and whether the physician's documentation supports that treatment. For example, a physician orders a blood transfusion for a patient with an upper gastrointestinal bleed and severely low hemoglobin and hematocrit levels. The physician's diagnosis is a bleeding gastric ulcer. The diagnosis does not appear to be reliable based on the treatment the physician gave. Blood transfusion is not an accepted treatment for a bleeding gastric ulcer. If the physician documents a bleeding gastric ulcer with acute blood loss anemia (where clinically indicated), based on the treatment given, this is a reliable diagnosis.

Documentation That Does Not *Meet Reliability*

A physician admits a patient with shortness of breath and chest pain, then treats the patient with Lasix, oxygen, and Theophylline. The physician's final documented diagnosis for the patient is acute exacerbation of chronic obstructive pulmonary disease (COPD).

Documentation That Does *Meet Reliability*

The physician gave the patient Lasix to treat acute and chronic congestive heart failure (CHF). The physician amends the final progress note to reflect the final diagnosis: Acute exacerbation of chronic bronchitis and COPD; Acute and chronic CHF. In this case, the patient had bronchitis with the COPD, so the initial documentation did not meet the criteria for both reliability and precision.

Precise

Precision means the record is accurate, exact, and strictly defined. Detail, if available and clinically appropriate, is an important component of every patient's health record. The more detailed the physician's documentation, the more representative and accurate the clinical documentation in the patient's record is likely to be.

Documentation That Does Not *Meet Criteria for Precision*

A patient is admitted with chest pain, shortness of breath, fever, and cough. A chest x-ray shows aspiration pneumonia. The physician's final documented diagnosis for the patient is pneumonia.

Documentation That Does *Meet Criteria for Precision*

The physician reviews the chest x-ray and documents the patient's final diagnosis in the discharge summary as aspiration pneumonia.

Complete

Completeness means the record has the maximum content and is thorough. Complete criteria means the physician has fully addressed all concerns in the patient record. Completeness also includes the appropriate authentication by the physician or clinician, which generally includes a signature and a date. Diagnostic documentation concerns apply to anything from the patient's initial complaint (did the physician provide a working and final diagnosis?) to the ordering of tests (did the physician document the reason for the tests?) to abnormal diagnostic test results (did the physician document the clinical significance of any abnormal diagnostic test?).

Documentation That Does Not *Meet Criteria for Completeness*

A physician orders comprehensive blood chemistries. The tests show low sodium, magnesium, and potassium levels. The physician does not document diagnoses to represent any of these abnormal results, nor does he document that the results are clinically insignificant.

Documentation That Does *Meet Criteria for Completeness*

In the previous example, the physician documents the following in the patient's progress notes on the day after the test results were received:

> *Na 131 Mg 1.3 K+ 3.1; Patient dehydrated. Potassium within normal limits. Patient given CAD and hypertensive medication.*

The physician should not document a diagnosis if the clinical evidence did not support it. However, if the abnormal test results do not support a diagnosis, then the physician should document, "abnormal test results are clinically insignificant."

Consistent

Consistency means the record is not contradictory. Clinical documentation about a patient that contradicts itself from one progress note to the next or among entries from different physicians is a documentation deficiency. The overall rule is that when another physician's documentation conflicts with the attending physician's documentation, and the attending is unavailable to state otherwise, the attending physician's documentation takes precedence. However, if the attending physician has provided documentation that appears to contradict itself, he must clarify and add an addendum to the discharge summary or a final progress note.

Documentation That Does Not *Meet Criteria for Consistency*

A patient is admitted by her primary care physician with vertigo and confusion. The primary care physician documents the patient's preliminary diagnosis as transient ischemic attack (TIA) and asks for a neurology consult. The neurologist examines the patient and documents the diagnosis in his final consultation as a cerebrovascular accident (CVA). The attending physician provides no further documentation regarding the patient's diagnosis. (In this case, the attending physician and the neurologist's diagnoses are inconsistent.)

Documentation That Does *Meet Criteria for Consistency*

The attending physician is asked by the CDI specialist to re-review the neurologist's consultation. The attending physician adds a final progress note to the patient's record that states the final diagnosis is CVA.

Clear

A health record should be undoubtedly clear. Ambiguity exists when the clinical documentation does not totally describe what is wrong with the patient. This may result in physicians documenting symptoms without etiology or possible etiology. For example, if a patient presents with the symptom of chest pain and the physician provides no other insight in his documentation, the health record would be vague. If there were no clinical evidence for any diagnosis, then the appropriate documentation would be "chest pain etiology undetermined."

Documentation That Does Not *Meet Criteria for Clarity*

Patient presents with syncope. The physician orders a computed tomography (CT) scan, a magnetic resonance imaging (MRI) of the brain, an EKG, and blood tests, all of which are within normal limits. The physician's final diagnosis on discharge is syncope.

Documentation That Does *Meet Criteria for Clarity*

In the previous example, the following documentation meets criteria for clarity, assuming the appropriate clinical indicators were present:

Table 4.1 ICD-10 shift to lower MS-DRG

MS-DRG	MS-DRG Description
003	ECMO OR TRACH W MV 96+ HRS OR PDX EXC FACE, MOUTH & NECK W MAJ O.R.
177	RESPIRATORY INFECTIONS & INFLAMMATIONS W MCC
191	CHRONIC OBSTRUCTIVE PULMONARY DISEASE W CC
193	SIMPLE PNEUMONIA & PLEURISY W MCC
194	SIMPLE PNEUMONIA & PLEURISY W CC
207	RESPIRATORY SYSTEM DIAGNOSIS W VENTILATOR SUPPORT 96+ HOURS
292	HEART FAILURE & SHOCK W CC
329	MAJOR SMALL & LARGE BOWEL PROCEDURES W MCC
330	MAJOR SMALL & LARGE BOWEL PROCEDURES W CC
378	G.I. HEMORRHAGE W CC
481	HIP & FEMUR PROCEDURES EXCEPT MAJOR JOINT W CC
682	RENAL FAILURE W MCC
853	INFECTIOUS & PARASITIC DISEASES W O.R. PROCEDURE W MCC
870	SEPTICEMIA OR SEVERE SEPSIS W MV 96+ HOURS

The disadvantage is the mental challenge of coding a case in both systems at one time. When health organizations use staffing company coders to augment the process, if it is cost effective, they should have the staffing company code in ICD-9 while the facility coders use ICD-10. This results in an ICD-10-trained internal staff and decreased staffing company costs because many companies charge a higher rate for ICD-10 staff. However, the staffing company coders using ICD-9 will be unprepared for the ICD-10 implementation. This process allows for capture of both sets of codes that can be used for analysis by the facility ICD-10 implementation team.

When coders assign both ICD-9 and ICD-10 codes simultaneously, they usually begin with ICD-10 because that system involves detailed questions related to specificity. Then the encoder allows for coding in ICD-9. There may be a different set of menus for this because ICD-9 is less specific and the coding paths are different. The advantage to this method is that the coder can visualize the differences in the two systems using the same account. This enhances the training process and results in a more extensive skill set for the coder. Refer to the *Journal of AHIMA* article, "Getting the best from your ICD-10 vendor" for more information (Dimick 2011).

Table 4.2 ICD-10 Shift to Higher MS-DRG

MS-DRG	MS-DRG Description
004	TRACH W MV 96+ HRS OR PDX EXC FACE, MOUTH & NECK W/O MAJ O.R.
190	CHRONIC OBSTRUCTIVE PULMONARY DISEASE W MCC
208	RESPIRATORY SYSTEM DIAGNOSIS W VENTILATOR SUPPORT <96 HOURS
247	PERC CARDIOVASC PROC W DRUG-ELUTING STENT W/O MCC
291	HEART FAILURE & SHOCK W MCC
392	ESOPHAGITIS, GASTROENT & MISC DIGEST DISORDERS W/O MCC
460	SPINAL FUSION EXCEPT CERVICAL W/O MCC
470	MAJOR JOINT REPLACEMENT OR REATTACHMENT OF LOWER EXTREMITY W/O MCC
690	KIDNEY & URINARY TRACT INFECTIONS W/O MCC
871	SEPTICEMIA OR SEVERE SEPSIS W/O MV 96+ HOURS W MCC

The dual coding process allows for the comparison of MS-DRG assignment for the two coding systems. The IT department can provide analytic reports showing the ICD-9 and ICD-10 codes and final MS-DRG. The report should also include the reimbursement impact between the two systems. This report may then be used to perform internal or external audits of those cases with MS-DRG changes. This is a great way to provide education on coding issues and CDI challenges.

Table 4.3 provides an example of MS-DRG changes between the two systems. The principal diagnosis is alcohol withdrawal. Note that ICD-10 requires further specificity of dependence. The patient also had a melanoma of the shoulder and cellulitis of the left axilla. The surgeon performed an excision of a melanoma of the left shoulder (skin) and lymph node with biopsy and an excision of a second lesion near the site. In this case the procedure changed the MS-DRG from 988 (weight 1.7643) to 982 (weight 2.8150). Code 0HBCXZZ, excision of the melanoma skin lesion, caused the changed in the DRG.

Case Examples by Body System

The section below includes some examples of the potential shift in MS-DRG from ICD-10 codes. Healthcare organizations should use the scenarios found in these examples for coding education as well as impact projections for enhanced CDI programs. Steps to calculate the impact for these scenarios are located in the benchmarking analytics section.

Table 4.3 ICD-9 and ICD-10 Dual Coding Example

ICD-9-CM MS-DRG/Codes		ICD-10-CM/PCS MS-DRG/Codes	
MS-DRG 988 **Non-extensive** O.R. Proc Unrelated to Principal Diagnosis w CC (Wt. 1.7643)		MS-DRG 982 **Extensive** O.R. Proc Unrelated to Principal Diagnosis w CC (Wt. 2.8150)	
Alcohol withdrawal	291.81	Alcohol dependence with withdrawal, unspecified	F10.239
Malignant melanoma of skin of upper limb, including shoulder	172.6	Malignant melanoma of left upper limb, including shoulder	C43.62
Cellulitis and abscess of upper arm and forearm	682.3	Cellulitis of left axilla	L03.112
Local excision/destruction of lesion/tissue skin and subcutaneous tissue	86.3	Excision of left upper arm skin, external approach	0HBCXZZ
Biopsy of lymphatic structure	40.11	Excision of left axillary lymphatic, open approach, diagnostic	07B60ZX

Blood and Myeloproliferative Diseases

In the case example in table 4.4, a provider admits a 45-year old female with a diagnosis of anemia after lab work revealed a hemoglobin of 9.0 gm/dl and a hematocrit of 27 percent. The patient's anemia was associated with a breast carcinoma, for which she was receiving outpatient chemotherapy and radiation therapy.

Table 4.4 Case Example Blood and Myeloproliferative Diseases

Principal Diagnosis	ICD-9-CM	PDX/ MCC/ CC	DRG	Weight	ICD-10-CM	PDX/ MCC/ CC	DRG	Weight
Breast carcinoma, upper-inner quadrant	174.2		**812**	0.8162	C50.212	PDX	**597**	1.6758
Anemia, in neoplastic disease	284.89	PDX			D63.0			
Adverse effect of antineoplastic and immunosuppressive drugs, sequela	E933.1				T45.1X5S			

Case disposition: The coding guidelines related to the principal diagnoses assignments in patients with anemia in neoplastic disease will change with the ICD-10 implementation. Under ICD-9-CM guidelines, the anemia code is sequenced first:

> When admission/encounter is for management of an anemia associated with the malignancy, and the treatment is only for anemia, the appropriate anemia code (such as code 285.22, Anemia in neoplastic disease) is designated as the principal diagnosis and is followed by the appropriate code(s) for the malignancy (ICD-9-CM Official Guidelines 2011).

Under ICD-10 guidelines, the principal diagnosis is the malignancy when still present:

> When the admission/encounter is for management of an anemia associated with the malignancy, and the treatment is only for anemia, the appropriate code for the malignancy is sequenced as the principal or first-listed diagnosis followed by code D63.0 Anemia in neoplastic disease (ICD-10-CM Official Guidelines, 2011).

In this scenario, the principal diagnosis of anemia in neoplastic disease (284.89) in ICD-9-CM changes to breast carcinoma, upper inner quadrant (C50.212) in ICD-10-CM. This results in an upgraded MS-DRG change from 812 (weight 0.8162) to 597 (weight 1.6758) (Mills 2013).

Mental Disorders

In the case example in table 4.5, a 27-year-old male presents in the emergency department (ED) with a creatinine of 2.2 on admission decreasing to 1.0 after intravenous (IV) fluid treatment. The physician admitted the patient and diagnosed him with acute kidney injury. The clinical record documentation shows a history of major depressive illness, for which the patient received Cymbalta 20 mg/day twice daily during the stay.

Table 4.5 Case Example Mental Disorders

Principal Diagnosis	ICD-9-CM	MCC/CC	DRG	Weight	ICD-10-CM	MCC/CC	DRG	Weight
Acute kidney injury	584.9		**683**	**0.9512**	N17.9		**684**	0.6085
Dehydration	276.51				E86.0			
Major depressive affective disorder, single episode unspecified	296.20	CC			F32.9			

Case disposition: In the above case scenario, the major depressive episode coded in ICD-9-CM (296.20) is a complication or comorbidity (CC). In ICD-10-CM, major depressive episode requires additional specificity to be a

CC. Major depressive affective disorder, single episode (F32.9) is not a CC. This results in a downgraded MS-DRG from 683 (weight 0.9512) to 684 (weight 0.6085).

Query opportunity: The CDI or coding professional should query the physician for the specificity required in the clinical record for major depression: mild, moderate, severe, bipolar disorder, manic episode, or with psychosis. The CDI or coding professionals can also use the physician's information to catch any CCs or MCCs under ICD-10 (Coding Clinic 2002, 21 and Mills 2013).

Gastrointestinal System Disorders

In the case example in table 4.6, a 35-year-old female presents in the ED with a history of congestive heart failure (CHF). Her current symptoms are shortness of breath, pitting edema of the lower extremity, and a recent 5-pound weight gain. She also complains of bleeding from her throat. After admission as an inpatient, diagnostic tests revealed acute diastolic CHF with esophageal hemorrhage.

Table 4.6 Case Example Gastrointestinal System Disorders

Principal Diagnosis	ICD-9-CM	MCC/CC	DRG	Weight	ICD-10-CM	MCC/CC	DRG	Weight
CHF, acute diastolic	428.33		**291**	1.5097	I50.33		**293**	0.6762
Esophageal hemorrhage	530.82	MCC			K22.8			
CHF	428.0							

Case disposition: Coding of acute on chronic diastolic CHF in ICD-9-CM requires two codes (428.33 and 428.0). ICD-10-CM only requires one code (I50.33). In ICD-9-CM, the coder would assign esophageal hemorrhage as an MCC (530.82) resulting in MS-DRG 291 (weight 1.5097). In ICD-10-CM, esophageal hemorrhage NOS is not an MCC and the MS-DRG is downgraded to 293 (weight 0.6762).

Respiratory System Diseases

In the case example in table 4.7, a 67-year-old male arrives in the ED with a history of chronic obstructive asthma and chronic obstructive pulmonary disorder (COPD). His symptoms include productive cough, shortness of breath, chest tightness, and wheezing. His pulse oxygen saturation (SpO_2) was 83 percent and his $PaCO_2$ 48 mmHg. The provider diagnosed and admitted him with an acute exacerbation of both.

Table 4.7 Case Example Respiratory System Diseases

Principal Diagnosis	ICD-9-CM	MCC/CC	DRG	Weight	ICD-10-CM	MCC/CC	DRG	Weight
Chronic obstructive asthma, acute exacerbation	493.22		**191**	0.937	J44.1		**192**	0.719
COPD, acute exacerbation	491.21	CC						

Case disposition: ICD-9-CM requires two codes for acute exacerbation of COPD with exacerbation of chronic obstructive asthma (493.22 and 491.21) and both are CCs. The resulting MS-DRG for ICD-9-CM is 191 (weight 0.937). ICD-10 only requires one code (J44.1), and if there are no other MCCs or CCs coded on the account, the resulting MS-DRG is downgraded to 192 (weight 0.719).

Infectious Disease

In the case example in table 4.8, a 45-year-old male arrives in the ED with a history of human immunodeficiency virus (HIV) disease. His white blood cell (WBC) count was 16,000, temperature 101.5 F, pulse rate 94, respiratory rate 26, and his blood sugar was 140 mg/dl. His mental status is altered from his normal state. Family members suggest, "He is just not himself today." The provider diagnosed and admitted the patient with HIV disease and influenza-related sepsis.

Table 4.8 Case Example Infectious Disease

Principal Diagnosis	ICD-9-CM	MCC/CC	DRG	Weight	ICD-10-CM	MCC/CC	DRG	Weight
HIV	042		**974**	2.6849	B20		**976**	0.8774
Influenza	038.41	CC			J11.1			
Sepsis	995.91	MCC			A41.3			

Case disposition: Sepsis requires two codes in ICD-9-CM (038.41 CC and 995.91 MCC). In ICD-10-CM, sepsis code A41.3 is not an MCC. This results in a MS-DRG downgrade from 974 (weight 2.6849) to 976 (weight 0.8774).

Cardiovascular System Diseases

In the case example in table 4.9, a 72-year-old female arrives in the ED with a history of systolic and diastolic CHF with a recent weight gain of 6 pounds, shortness of breath, syncope, and nocturnal cough. Diagnostics revealed an ejection fraction of 38 percent, an x-ray positive for cardiomegaly, a pulse rate of 121, a blood pressure of 190/132, and a BNP of 600 pg/mL. The provider diagnosed and admitted her with acute on chronic systolic and diastolic CHF and malignant hypertension. The provider documented the malignant hypertension as unrelated.

Table 4.9 Case Example Cardiovascular System Diseases

Principal Diagnosis	ICD-9-CM	MCC/CC	DRG	Weight	ICD-10-CM	MCC/CC	DRG	Weight
Acute systolic and diastolic CHF	428.41		**292**	0.9824	I50.41		**293**	0.6762
Malignant hypertension	401.0	CC			I10			
CHF	428.0							

Case disposition: Acute systolic and diastolic CHF requires two codes in ICD-9-CM (428.41 and 428.0). The secondary diagnosis of unrelated malignant hypertension is coded 401.0 and is a CC. In ICD-10-CM, acute systolic and diastolic congestive heart failure requires only one code (I50.41). The unrelated hypertension is I10 but is not a CC. This results in a downgraded MS-DRG from 292 (weight 0.9824) to 293 (weight 0.6762).

Determining Impact Using Benchmarking Analytics

Effective analytics use enhances CDI programs. No program can reach maximum efficiency without identifying trends. Healthcare professionals use trends to

- Establish high reimbursement risk or high volume focus MS-DRGs
- Determine the root cause of high risk diagnoses and procedures
- Develop interdepartmental and facility-wide corrective action plans
- Create and implement effective stakeholder education programs (which include the physician, CDIP, and coder)

Healthcare organizations can use the previous case scenarios as a starting point to estimate the impact of ICD-10-CM/PCS on their facility. Following the steps below can help estimate this impact for the above case scenarios:

1. Identify the annual case volume and weight for the following MS-DRGs *where the only MCCs or CCs listed are secondary diagnoses in each corresponding case scenario table above.* The only exception is MS-DRG 812 where the PDX changes the MS-DRG and not the presence of an MCC or CC.
   a. 812 RED BLOOD CELL DISORDERS without MCC (All cases are counted)
   b. 683 RENAL FAILURE with CC
   c. 291 HEART FAILURE AND SHOCK with MCC
   d. 191 CHRONIC OBSTRUCTIVE PULMONARY DISEASE with CC
   e. 974 HIV W MAJOR RELATED CONDITION with MCC
   f. 292 HEART FAILURE AND SHOCK with CC

2. Determine the IPPS hospital-specific base rate
3. Create an Excel spreadsheet using table 4.8 format
4. Compare the payments to determine the potential loss for each MS-DRG

Table 4.10 presents a report view of the estimated impact for these high risk-focused MS-DRGs under ICD-10. The table includes the annual volume for each high risk MS-DRG in the first column. Next are the MS-DRGs with corresponding descriptions, followed by the weight and estimated payment under the ICD-9 grouper. The estimated payment calculation is

Volume × Weight × Hospital-Specific Base Rate = Estimated Payment

The more detailed calculation for actual payment includes the wage index, indirect medical education costs, disproportionate share payments, and cost outlier adjustments. Specific details for calculating MS-DRG payments are located at http://www.tricare.mil/drgrates/. The finance department can provide the hospital specific base rate. Most base rates are within the range of $5,000 to $8,000. Table 4.10 uses $5,000 in the calculation.

Facilities should compare the ICD-9-CM versus ICD-10-CM/PCS code sets for dual-coded accounts reimbursed under MS-DRGs to determine which MCCs and CCs ICD-10-CM/PCS includes, and which principal diagnoses changed with the implementation. The information technology (IT) department should provide the analytic reports needed for this project.

Table 4.11 provides a sample report format. This format can be used by the CDI manager to develop a facility-specific impact report if one is not available.

Table 4.10 High Risk MS-DRG Impact: ICD-10-CM

Vol	MS- DRG ICD-9-CM Grouper		Wt.	Est. Payment	MS- DRG ICD-10-CM/PCS Grouper		Wt.	Est. Payment
265	812	RED BLOOD CELL DISORDERS W/O MCC	0.8162	$1,081,465	597	MALIGNANT BREAST DISORDERS W MCC	1.6758	$2,220,435
456	683	RENAL FAILURE W CC	0.9512	$2,168,736	684	RENAL FAILURE W/O CC/ MCC	0.6085	$1,387,380
193	291	HEART FAILURE & SHOCK W MCC	1.5097	$1,456,861	293	HEART FAILURE & SHOCK W/O CC/MCC	0.6762	$652,533
325	191	CHRONIC OBSTRUCTIVE PULMONARY DISEASE W CC	0.937	$1,522,625	192	CHRONIC OBSTRUCTIVE PULMONARY DISEASE W/O CC/MCC	0.719	$1,168,375
75	974	HIV W MAJOR RELATED CONDITION W MCC	2.6849	$1,006,838	976	HIV W MAJOR RELATED CONDITION W/O CC/ MCC	0.8774	$329,025
245	292	HEART FAILURE & SHOCK W CC	0.9824	$1,203,440	293	HEART FAILURE & SHOCK W/O CC/MCC	0.6762	$828,345
Total				$8,439,964				$6,586,093
Variance								$1,853,871

Table 4.11 Congestive Heart Failure ICD-9-CM to ICD-10-CM Impact Report

Account #	ICD-9 MS-DRG	Payment	ICD-9 Codes	ICD-10 MS-DRG	Payment	ICD-10 Codes	Payment Variance	CDIP/ Coder Comment
10000	292	$4,969	428.41	293	$3,362	I50.41	**$1,608**	Coding guideline
			401.0			I10		
			428.0					

The following is a list of steps for estimating the facility-specific impact for the case scenarios presented in this chapter. This exercise helps determine whether the effect of ICD-10 implementation will be positive or negative. The steps include

1. Begin dual coding all or focused DRG cases
2. Discuss analytic report layout with the IT department
3. Run the *High Risk MS-DRG Impact: ICD-10-CM* report to identify those cases with varying MS-DRGs
4. Analyze each case to determine the root cause of DRG change
5. Document the reason for change in the comment field (for example, a coding guideline, an MCC or CC change, or a principal diagnosis change)
6. Correlate the findings by MS-DRG and develop work plan for correction of root cause through education of stakeholders (physicians, CDIP, coders)

Conclusion

The projected reimbursement impact for ICD-10 implementation is negative 1.4 percent according to a study performed by a team at 3M Health Information Systems in 2013 (Mills 2013). Facilities will benefit from the analysis of hospital-specific case scenarios proven to create an MS-DRG change. The change in MS-DRG is based on varying guidelines for principal diagnosis and secondary diagnosis MCC and CC assignment within the two coding systems. Trend analytics based on dual coding activities are useful for establishing focused MS-DRGs education for physicians, CDIPs, and coders.

Chapter Quiz

1. All of the following are deficiencies in ICD-9-CM related to new advances in medicine, except:
   A. Measurement of healthcare services
   B. Quality measurement
   C. Use of clinical indicators
   D. Tracking of public health issues

2. All of the following are key deficiencies related to reimbursement posed by ICD-9-CM, except:
   A. Exactness
   B. Coding conventions
   C. Quality
   D. Flexibility

3. What is suggested as a requirement for reflection of current medical practices and supports worldwide epidemiology?
   A. Advanced quality measures
   B. Enhanced healthcare services
   C. Increased tracking of health issues
   D. New coding system

4. Which item below is not an improvement found in ICD-10-CM?
   A. Influenza
   B. Obstetrics
   C. Diabetes
   D. Laterality

5. A 3M study suggested that the reimbursement impact on the implementation of ICD-10-CM/PCS would be what?
   A. Agonizing
   B. Minimal
   C. Extensive
   D. Extraordinary

6. What is the estimated negative impact of the top 25 MS-DRGs mentioned in the text?
   A. 0.05 percent
   B. 0.85 percent
   C. 1.4 percent
   D. 2.6 percent

7. What is the first step required to determine the facility specific impact of ICD-10 implementation?
   A. Create analytic report formats
   B. Determine root cause of MS-DRG change
   C. Contact the IT department to determine which analytic reports are currently available
   D. Begin dual coding

8. What is the principal tool used by CDI programs to enhance efficiency?
   A. Quality measures
   B. Analytics
   C. Risk mitigation
   D. Health issues tracking

9. All of the items below are reasons that trends are measured except:
   A. Developing corrective action plan
   B. Implementing stakeholder education programs
   C. Department operational budgets
   D. Establishing high risk/volume focus

10. All of these items below are steps for estimating the impact on reimbursement by ICD-10-CM/PCS on your facility, except:
   A. Determine the IPPS hospital-specific base rate
   B. Identify annual case volume and weight for MS-DRGs
   C. Compare payments to determine potential loss for each MS-DRG
   D. Compile a Word document summarizing all analytics

REFERENCES

CMS. 2014. ICD-10 Overview. Retrieved from https://www.cms.gov.

Coding Clinic, Third Quarter. 2002. Effective with discharges Acute Renal Failure Due to Dehydration.

Dimick, C. 2011. Getting the best from your ICD-10 vendor. AHIMA Library. Retrieved from: http://library.ahima.org/xpedio/groups/public/documents/ahima/bok1_049130.hcsp?dDocName=bok1_049130.

Mills, R., R. Butler, R. Averill., E. McCullough, M. Bao. 2013. Estimating the impact of the transition to ICD-10 on Medicare inpatient hospital payments. Retrieved from: http://library.ahima.org.

Chapter 5

Assessing Cli[...] Documentation

The Importance of a Clinical Documentation Assessment

An assessment is a snapshot in time that gives the clinical documentation improvement (CDI) review team or CDI specialists a starting point for their activities. Unless the review team is familiar with the organization's documentation and the data it produces, it cannot determine whether its efforts to improve clinical documentation have been successful. Reviewing actual documentation and data prior to investing in a CDI program prevents the CDI review team from acting on assumptions.

For example, the management team may believe there is a quality problem with clinical documentation based on discussions, a change in case mix, and a few examples of documentation problems identified in patient records during the coding process. In this case, the organization should perform an objective analysis of both data and documentation for two reasons. First, an analysis determines whether the perceived problem exists. Second, the analysis, if performed consistently with the recommendations in this chapter, provides a valid baseline for measuring the impact of any CDI efforts.

If the organization already has a CDI program in place, it can use the information in this chapter to validate its current baseline. The organization can also use the information to determine whether current analyses include all of the necessary components. If not, then the organization can use this chapter to include some new baseline analytics in the process. Finally, if there is a program in place that only focuses on inpatient documentation, the organization can use this information to analyze outpatient or long-term care data and create a baseline for those care areas. In every case, it is important to include analyses of both data and documentation for any assessment.

Data Review

Every healthcare organization produces significant amounts of data on an ongoing basis. As noted in the introduction to this book, organizations use this data for everything from reimbursement and quality indicators to research and planning. "When the information is used for decision making, it leads to knowledge creation for common understanding. Repeatable use of knowledge leads to development of best practices which, applied over time to achieve organizational goals, leads to behavior change" (AHIMA 2014a). Using data for decision-making is even more important when the decisions involve a new or established CDI program.

What Data Matters?

There are two types of data to consider in the CDI process. The first is the data the organization itself produces. The second is the data that others produce about the organization. An organization produces data from coding, data collected for quality indicators, other specialized data collected for the organization's mortality and morbidity review (MMR), or other internal clinical committees or groups.

An organization collects a significant amount of data it must prioritize to focus its efforts and obtain maximum benefit from this data review. There are certain general guidelines included in this chapter, but data varies for each organization based on individual needs. One of the first questions to ask is at what level of aggregation should the organization look. Many organizations want to begin at a high level and drill down to the details if it discovers a problem or unexpected finding in the high-level data. For coded data, one of the highest levels of aggregation is by diagnosis-related group (DRG). The organization may also want to consider reviewing data by severity level or by the presence or absence of complication and comorbidity (CC) codes. One of the most detailed levels of data is found at the diagnosis or procedure code level. Table 5.1 shows hospital severity levels from the All Patient Refined (APR) grouper broken out by service type. This shows another way to drill into high-level data. The review begins with data by severity. Within each severity level, the report specifies the type of service. This type of data review can help determine whether there may be specific problems in certain clinical departments.

Table 5.1 Hospital severity levels from the APR grouper based on service type

Service	Minor (Level 1)	Moderate (Level 2)	Major (Level 3)	Extreme (Level 4)
Internal Medicine	40%	32%	25%	3%
Cardiology	35%	35%	28%	2%
Neurology	30%	40%	27%	3%
General Surgery	28%	42%	25%	5%
Orthopedic Surgery	45%	40%	14%	1%

In table 5.1, the orthopedic service shows 45 percent of patients with severity level 1 and only 14 percent of patients with severity level 3. These two numbers show that orthopedic patients have lower severity levels than patients in all other services. This is a reason to expect orthopedic patients to be less severely ill than those in all other services are. If not, this data finding is a red flag that orthopedic services may have a more significant problem with documentation practices than other services.

Data that others produce about the organization has an impact on patient perception, accreditation status, and reimbursement. These data types include Medicare quality indicators, Joint Commission's Quality Check, private quality organizations like Healthgrades, and state-specific quality programs such as the Medisgroup data abstracting used by states like Colorado and Pennsylvania (PHCCCC 2006). An example of the Healthgrades search screen to review physician and hospital profiles appears in figure 5.1.

Hospitals with one star are providing care below the quality expected, those with three stars are providing care at the level of quality expected, and those with five stars are providing better quality care than expected for the diagnosis or procedure analyzed. If an organization has a one- or three-star rating that it believes should be a five-star rating, documentation may be the reason. Furthermore, analysis at this level allows comparison of ratings by service type as Healthgrades provides ratings by diagnosis and procedure. Additional information on quality indicators may be found on http://www.healthgrades.com./

Using Criteria to Screen the Data

Everything is relative, and the data needs a valid comparison. Three sources of comparative data include

- Normative data from a broad representative population
- Regulatory guidance such as the Centers for Medicare and Medicaid Services (CMS 2014a; CMS 2014b; CMS 2014c)
- The organization's own benchmarks or trends over time

National normative data can be used by the CDI department for benchmarking peer hospital case mix indices and other metrics, but it is much more relevant to use data from hospitals that are similar in size, teaching status, and geographic status. Some organizations have their own information staffs that can obtain detailed levels of data. In addition, the data can be purchased for reasonable rates from organizations like the American Hospital Directory (AHD) (http://www.ahd.com/). Other sources of data may be found in the regulatory guidance provided by the Office of the Inspector General (OIG), Medicare, Quality Improvement Organizations (QIOs), and other governmental agencies.

For example, Hospital Compare, found at www.medicare.gov/hospitalcompare/compare.htm, publishes CC rates or certain DRG pair proportions that raise a red flag for the review team. Finally, the organization can use its own benchmarks to screen data (so long as this is consistent with legal and regulatory requirements). Ideally, an organization will develop its own set of criteria based on the three sources.

Figure 5.1 Example of hospital quality ratings by Healthgrades

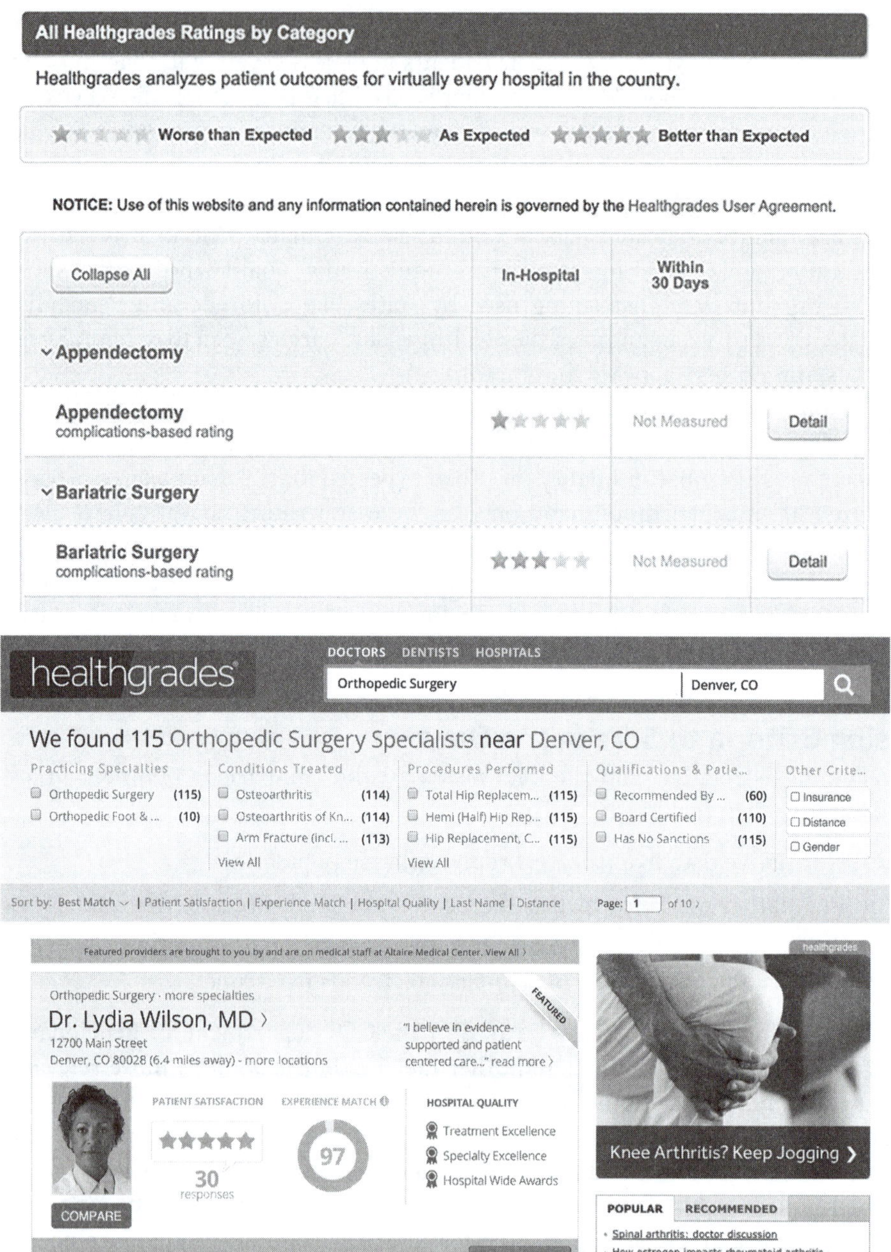

Used with permission from Healthgrades. Healthgrades, headquartered in Denver, Colorado, is the leading online resource for comprehensive information about physicians and hospitals. Today, more than one million people a day use the Healthgrades websites to search, compare, and connect with hospitals and physicians based on the most important measures when selecting a healthcare provider: experience, hospital quality and patient satisfaction. For more information about Healthgrades, visit http://www.healthgrades.com.

Deciding What Data to Review

Once the CDI review team decides which criteria to use, it needs to determine what data to review. Ultimately, there are two things that drive the team reviews: the criteria used to screen the data for decision making and the purpose of the review.

For example, what is the team trying to get out of the data review? For high-quality clinical documentation, one of the criteria is completeness. One way to apply the criteria to aggregate level data is to identify patient records with vague principal diagnoses.

While these may be valid from a high-level data perspective, a vague or symptomatic principal diagnosis can be a red flag. Table 5.2 illustrates this type of data. Medicare was separated out from other payers since the age difference may impact the data. The table represents discharges for a 300-bed hospital over the course of a year. The hospital in this case was concerned about the high numbers of chest pain and vertigo cases. At a minimum, this type of data analysis can provide the organization with enough information to know it should further explore the issue of clinical documentation quality.

Table 5.2 Discharges for a 300-bed hospital during a 12-month period

	Number Medicare Inpatients	Average Length of Stay	Average Charges	Average Cost	Medicare CMI	CMI Adjusted Avg. Cost
Cardiology	1,162	4.0	$50,340	$5,588	1.0594	$5,275
Cardiovascular Surgery	1,012	4.6	$214,020	$20,299	3.7449	$5,420
Gynecology	12	3.3	$96,608	$9,907	1.1377	$8,708
Medicine	1,671	6.3	$66,588	$8,235	1.2344	$6,671
Neurology	326	4.3	$61,362	$6,991	1.0965	$6,376
Neurosurgery	13	6.3	$135,412	$15,470	2.8146	$5,496
Obstetrics	12	2.3	$19,774	$3,931	0.6711	$5,857
Oncology	48	5.2	$81,634	$8,650	1.4007	$6,176
Orthopedic Surgery	155	7.0	$147,823	$15,769	2.2627	$6,969
Orthopedics	113	4.3	$46,564	$5,355	0.9452	$5,665
Psychiatry	25	4.2	$52,480	$5,554	0.9275	$5,988
Pulmonology	598	5.3	$66,025	$7,680	1.2796	$6,002
Surgery	464	9.2	$227,228	$32,532	3.9227	$8,293
Surgery for Malignancy	45	5.1	$170,671	$18,185	1.8789	$9,679
Urology	395	5.1	$71,986	$8,729	1.1713	$7,453
Vascular Surgery	172	4.2	$120,784	$12,879	2.2572	$5,706
TOTAL	6,224	5.41	$103,593	$11,764	1.8588	$6,329

www.ahd.com. Used with permission.

Recommended Data to Review

This section presents a list of recommended data to review. It is important, however, to ensure the data review is reflective of the organization. This list is intended as a general guide only. Each organization should create a data review that accomplishes the organization's specific objectives.

Discharges by Service and by Major Diagnostic Category

It is important that the CDI review team understands what are the most common services occasioning the patient's admission to the hospital. It is particularly important to review the data by service if CDI uses an indicator other than major diagnostic category (MDC). For example, the cases can be grouped by admission diagnosis code range. Then, the CDI review team can compare discharges by admitting service with discharges by MDC.

Lack of agreement between the two may point to a problem with clinical documentation. For example, when cardiologists are admitting a significant number of patients with chest pain to the hospital, discharges by MDC may show a lower number of cardiac admissions than discharges by service. This difference represents a potential problem with precision in documenting a principal diagnosis.

Discharges by DRG

Most organizations review data by DRG on a regular basis as part of their case mix analysis. For clinical documentation purposes, organizations should review actual DRG data against its expectations. For example, an organization may believe there have been few, if any, inpatient admissions for chest pain since it opened the chest pain clinic. If an analysis of DRG level data reveals several cases in the chest pain DRG, this is a red flag for documentation.

Case Mix Index

Most organizations review case mix index (CMI) over time, both overall and by specialty. For clinical documentation analysis purposes, an unexpected change in CMI signals a possible problem with clinical documentation. For example, if the CMI for orthopedic surgery has dropped for the past six months with no change in admitting physicians or types of surgery performed, it is probable that the orthopedic surgeons are not completely documenting all diagnoses in their patients' records.

Table 5.3 is an example of data about the organization that is available from the American Hospital Directory (AHD 2014). This data derives from MedPAR data, so it is usually more than a year old. While it is a starting point for analysis, ultimately more current data provided by the organization's IT or finance staff is desirable.

Complication and Major Complication Rates

Changes in rates, or rates that are inconsistent with an organization's expectations or normative data, may indicate a problem with clinical documentation quality. Table 5.4 is an example of a report that shows overall CC capture rate by all medicine, all surgical specialties together, and by each specialty. The comparison with peer norms for Medicare cases is helpful in determining whether rates appear to be lower or higher than an organization's norms. Any inconsistency provides support for further clinical documentation review and analysis.

Table 5.3 Examples of data that can be obtained from the American Hospital Directory

	Number Medicare Inpatients	Average Length of Stay	Average Charges	Average Cost	Medicare CMI	CMI Adjusted Avg. Cost
Cardiology	1,162	4.0	$50,340	$5,588	1.0594	$5,275
Cardiovascular Surgery	1,012	4.6	$214,020	$20,299	3.7449	$5,420
Gynecology	12	3.3	$96,608	$9,907	1.1377	$8,708
Medicine	1,671	6.3	$66,588	$8,235	1.2344	$6,671
Neurology	326	4.3	$61,362	$6,991	1.0965	$6,376
Neurosurgery	13	6.3	$135,412	$15,470	2.8146	$5,496
Obstetrics	12	2.3	$19,774	$3,931	0.6711	$5,857
Oncology	48	5.2	$81,634	$8,650	1.4007	$6,176
Orthopedic Surgery	155	7.0	$147,823	$15,769	2.2627	$6,969
Orthopedics	113	4.3	$46,564	$5,355	0.9452	$5,665
Psychiatry	25	4.2	$52,480	$5,554	0.9275	$5,988
Pulmonology	598	5.3	$66,025	$7,680	1.2796	$6,002
Surgery	464	9.2	$227,228	$32,532	3.9227	$8,293
Surgery for Malignancy	45	5.1	$170,671	$18,185	1.8789	$9,679
Urology	395	5.1	$71,986	$8,729	1.1713	$7,453
Vascular Surgery	172	4.2	$120,784	$12,879	2.2572	$5,706
TOTAL	6,224	5.41	$103,593	$11,764	1.8588	$6,329

www.ahd.com. Used with permission.

Severity Levels (MS-DRGs and APR-DRGs)

If the CDI review team has access to the MS-DRG and the all patients refined (APR) DRG grouper, it is helpful to look at the organization's severity levels for both groupers. While MS-DRGs are used for Medicare reimbursement, the APR-DRG grouper is used for quality indicators such as Healthgrades' analysis and by many states for Medicaid reimbursement. Changes in rates or inconsistency with expectations or normative data may indicate a problem with clinical documentation quality.

Medicare Quality Indicators

Since Medicare quality indicators are important for both reimbursement (pay for performance) and accreditation (Joint Commission uses many of the same measures), it is essential to be familiar with the organization's outcomes data. These measures act as tools to assess healthcare, process, outcome, patient perception,

Table 5.4 Complication and comorbidity (CC) capture rates-combined and by specialty

Medical Service	Hospital Statistics				Comparative Statistics			
	Cases	CMI	CC/ MCC Rate	MCC Rate	Cases	CMI	CC/ MCC Rate	MCC Rate
Burns					1,600	2.7716	73.4%	0.0%
Cardiology	1,421	1.0045	57.3%	31.1%	1,834,648	1.0167	63.8%	36.3%
Cardiovascular Surgery	1,243	3.2674	30.9%	24.0%	610,319	3.3600	37.2%	27.8%
Gynecology					46,738	0.9469	28.8%	42.2%
Medicine	1,436	1.0791	62.8%	34.1%	2,678,606	1.1374	57.0%	36.8%
Neurology	299	1.0748	59.0%	23.0%	643,559	1.0991	53.9%	27.2%
Neurosurgery					55,145	3.1580	65.2%	33.4%
Obstetrics					3,072	0.7099	64.0%	0.0%
Oncology	33	1.3910	87.9%	42.4%	147,532	1.5550	86.8%	38.5%
Orthopedic Surgery	168	2.2923	51.2%	22.6%	948,657	2.1970	30.5%	12.4%
Orthopedics	96	0.8576	27.1%	21.9%	231,042	0.9247	29.3%	21.3%
Psychiatry	12	0.9377	41.7%	41.7%	563,709	0.8260	13.2%	13.2%
Pulmonology	569	1.2359	71.4%	30.0%	1,461,294	1.3117	71.5%	35.8%
Surgery	440	3.3857	81.1%	43.3%	629,125	3.5514	75.7%	39.8%
Surgery for Malignancy	38	1.2592	18.4%	0.0%	53,196	1.5992	45.2%	20.4%
Urology	484	1.2889	67.6%	43.2%	694,502	1.1467	59.7%	37.2%
Vascular Surgery	234	2.1787	59.8%	34.0%	204,650	2.0186	55.5%	26.8%
TOTALS	6,473	1.7394	56.2%	31.4%	10,807,394	1.5113	56.6%	32.4%

www.ahd.com. Used with permission.

organization structure, and systems that provide high-quality patient care (CMS, 2014a; CMS, 2014b; CMS, 2014c). CMS contracted with Florida Medical Quality Assurance Inc.(FMQAI) to develop the Medication Measures Special Innovation Project (CMS 2014b). The key objectives for this project are to

- "Maintain previously developed medication measures and develop new medication measures with the potential for National Quality Forum (NQF) endorsement;
- Adapt/specify existing NQF-endorsed medication measures and develop new measures for implementation in CMS reporting programs, such as:
  - The Hospital Inpatient Quality Reporting (IQR) Program,

- The Hospital Outpatient Quality Reporting (OQR) Program,
  - The Physician Quality Reporting System (PQRS), and
  - Others as directed by CMS, such as long-term care settings and ambulatory care settings;
- Continue to develop new medication measures that address the detection and prevention of adverse medication-related patient safety events that can be used in future Quality Improvement Organization (QIO) Statements of Work and in CMS provider reporting programs; and
- Identify and specify up to five new adverse event measures (non-medication-related) that could be used in future QIO programs and CMS provider reporting programs in the hospital setting (inpatient and/or emergency department)" (CMS 2014b).

FMQAI developed the set of CMS-recommended core measures in the inpatient setting based on several factors:

- "Conditions that contribute to the morbidity and mortality of the most Medicare and Medicaid beneficiaries
- Conditions that represent national public health priorities
- Conditions that are common to health disparities
- Conditions that disproportionately drive healthcare costs and could improve with better quality measurement
- Measures that would enable CMS, States, and the provider community to measure quality of care in new dimensions, with a stronger focus on parsimonious measurement
- Measures that include patient and/or caregiver engagement" (CMS 2014b).

The quality, CDI, and HIM departments monitor the recommended core measures for the adult population in table 5.5. The CDI practitioner can assist where there is a trend of deficient clinical documentation and intervene during the patient stay. An example of this would be patients who do not have a recorded

Table 5.5 Recommended Core Measures

Adult
1. "Controlling High Blood Pressure 2. Use of High-Risk Medications in the Elderly 3. Preventive Care and Screening: Tobacco Use: Screening and Cessation Intervention 4. Use of Imaging Studies for Low Back Pain 5. Preventive Care and Screening: Screening for Clinical Depression and Follow-Up Plan 6. Documentation of Current Medications in the Medical Record 7. Preventive Care and Screening: Body Mass Index (BMI) Screening and Follow-Up 8. Closing the referral loop: receipt of specialist report 9. Functional status assessment for complex chronic conditions" (CMS, 2014).

CMS 2014

calculated body mass index (BMI) within the past six months with a follow-up plan documented during the current reporting period.

Secondary Diagnoses

The number of secondary diagnoses for inpatient cases provides some insight into the level of detail in documentation available to the coding staff for code assignment. If a CDI or coding professional uses this measure for CDI, the review team needs to ensure its members are familiar with the coding guidelines at the hospital and understand any possible limitations. The team may also want to delete one-day stays from the data since they can skew overall averages. Table 5.6 uses severity levels to stratify numbers of secondary diagnoses. This table reveals that the number of secondary diagnoses for this hospital in all cases is less than that of peer hospitals. It points in particular to a possible significant problem with surgery cases since the peer norm figure is 6.6 secondary diagnoses on average, while the hospital has only 4.2 secondary diagnoses for surgery cases. Services and physicians can stratify secondary diagnoses for more detail.

Analytic Report Examples

In addition to the reports discussed above, CDI program monitoring requires additional detail level analytics. Each facility should assess the capabilities of existing software for use in the CDI program. CDI-specific software programs are available through consulting and software firms that specialize in this product line. CDI tracking tools provide a place for entering concurrent case review information. In addition, the software allows for entry of information on the query and the response by the provider. Chapter 16 describes additional information on this tool. The output of the data entered into the tracking tool is often reported in a CDI activities scorecard. Table 5.7 provides an example of a CDI program scorecard. This report provides summary information on the following:

- Total cases available for review (initial or follow-up)
- Number of cases reviewed by the CDIP and coding staff
- Submitted queries
- Provider response rates
- Provider agreement rates
- Top service lines
- Top query topics

The exact format of the report varies with the software vendor.

The second type of report necessary for monitoring and tracking the CDI program is an internal and peer benchmarking report. The CDI software vendor or internal health information system vendors generate internal benchmarking reports.

Table 5.6 Comparison of secondary diagnoses

Number of secondary diagnoses for:	Number	Peer Norms
All inpatient cases	5.3	6.8
Medicine cases	5.6	7.2
Surgical cases	4.2	6.6
Severity Level 1 cases	2.6	2.8
Severity Level 2 cases	5.3	5.5
Severity Level 3 cases	8.6	9.0
Severity Level 4 cases	11.8	12.0

Table 5.7 CDI program scorecard

Summary Report				Allen&Shariff HEALTHCARE CONSULTING	
Time Period: 5/1/14 - 5/31/14		**CDIP**		**Coder**	
CDIP FTEs: 3		**Total**	**Target**	**Total**	**Target**
Total Cases		637		652	
Initial Case Review (ICR)		601	605		
ICR %		94%	95%		
ICR per Day		29	30		
Follow-up Case Review (FCR)		1202	1242		
FCR %		63%	65%		
FR per Day		57	59		
Query (Total)		144	145	65	0
Query (Rate)		24%	25%	10%	15%
Provider Response Rate		90%	95%	90%	95%
Provider Agreement Rate		80%	85%	80%	85%
Top Service Lines Queried		**Top 5 Queries**			
Cardiology	12	Acute Renal Failure		26	
General Surgery	7	Acute Respiratory Failure		17	
Hospitalists	82	Congestive Heart Failure		32	
Internal Medicine	14	Encephalopathy		15	
Orthpedic Surgery	15	Excisional Debridement		27	
Other	14	Other		27	

Used with permission from Allen & Shariff Healthcare, LLC

Capture Rate

Capture rate is one of the key indicators used to monitor a successful CDI program. Capture rate is the percentage of cases where an MCC or CC is present within those MS-DRGs that include them. Table 5.8 shows an executive level detailed report on medical and surgical service capture rates. The report provides a trend for the baseline period, current period, last three months, current month, and the 80th percentile. The 80th percentile of hospitals within peer groups by bed size can be used by the CDI team as a target for CMI and capture rates. The baseline period is typically the most recent 12-month period prior to the program start, and no less than a minimum of six months. The 80th percentile is a peer group comparison using Medicare Provider and Analysis Review (MEDPAR) data. Peer group comparisons commonly include similar hospitals according to size groups or specialty areas such as academic medical centers. The report includes graphical depictions of the medical and surgical capture rates for ease of discussion during executive presentations.

CDI Multispecialty Impact

The CDI Impact by Specialty report provides a monthly trend comparison of each MDC or service line. The report is useful for drilling down and determining the services with potential coding or clinical documentation issues. For example, the report in table 5.9 shows the nervous system MDC (neurology or neurosurgery) with a total number of cases at 57 for month one and 42 for month two. The percent total relative weight is 10.07 percent in month one and 7.84 percent in month two meaning the percentage of patients and severity decreased in month two.

This decrease may be due to a surgeon on vacation or seasonal changes in patient population. The calculated decrease in actual reimbursement for the service was $182,911. The CMI decreased 0.02 during the period. This report may also be used to compare each quarter rather than each month. When large shifts are identified, the next step is to drill down to the MS-DRG level and determine root causes of the service line fluctuation.

CDI Specialty MS-DRG Impact

The next step in assessing changes in the specialty area is to drill down to the MS-DRG level to determine the impact trend and success of the program. This report provides each MS-DRG for a specified service line. In addition, the volume, relative weight, payment variance, and CMI can be compared over two periods (monthly or quarterly). A review of the volume change within a specific MS-DRG might indicate the reason for the CMI change during the period. A review of each MS-DRG within a designated pair or triplet may explain the reason for the CMI change, for example, a lower CC capture rate.

After identifying the high volume MS-DRGs with lower CMI variance, an audit of these focused MS-DRGs may reveal the reason for the change, such as a new physician, coder, or CDIP. The information gleaned from the audit can be used during training sessions. In table 5.10, MS-DRG triplet Acute Myocardial Infarction shows the volume change between month one and month two as well as a shift from lower weighted MS-DRGs (without MCC/CC and with CC). The higher weighed MS-DRG 280

Table 5.8 Capture Rates-Medical and Surgical

CaptureRates — Allen&Shariff HEALTHCARE CONSULTING

		Baseline		Current Period		Last 3 Months		Current Month		80th Percentile
		Jan 2012-Jun 2012		*Jul 2012-Oct 2012*		*Aug 2012-Oct 2012*		*Oct 2012*		
		Vol	%	Vol	%	Vol	%	Vol	%	%
	Medical Capture Rates:									
Subgroup	**MCC Pairs** MCC vs.Without MCC	901	26.0%	648	29.9%	492	30.5%	163	27.6%	**27.7%**
Subgroup	**CC/MCC Pairs** CC/MCC vs. Without CC/MCC	11	63.6%	9	55.6%	9	55.6%	7	57.1%	**57.9%**
Subgroup	**Triplets** CC+MCC vs. Without CC/MCC	1275	79.9%	790	78.9%	581	79.7%	213	86.9%	**71.7%**
	MCC vs. CC	1019	48.6%	623	48.2%	463	47.1%	185	50.8%	**42.9%**
	Surgical Capture Rates:									
Subgroup	**MCC Pairs** MCC vs.Without MCC	519	17.7%	348	19.5%	254	21.3%	93	19.4%	**17.9%**
Subgroup	**CC/MCC Pairs** CC/MCC vs. Without CC/MCC	121	38.8%	92	41.3%	68	39.7%	30	33.3%	**40.5%**
Subgroup	**Triplets** CC+MCC vs. Without CC/MCC	1177	70.1%	792	70.7%	570	71.2%	218	69.7%	**70.1%**
	MCC vs. CC	825	45.2%	560	47.7%	406	46.8%	152	50.0%	**45.9%**

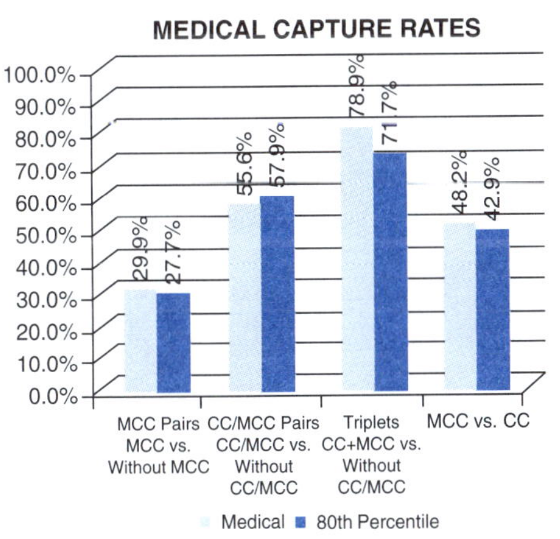

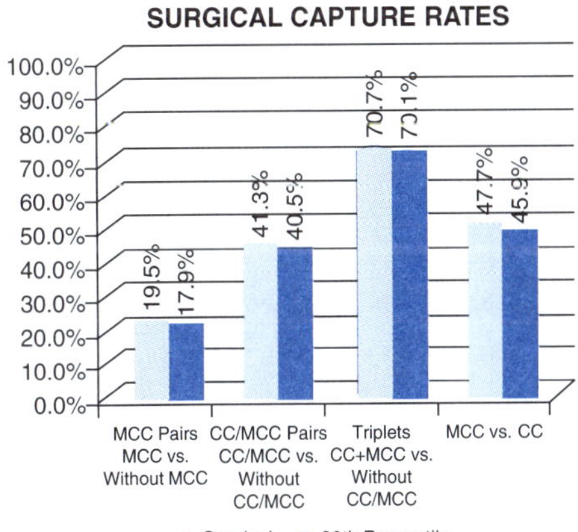

Used with permission from Allen & Shariff Healthcare, LLC

Table 5.9 CDI Multi Specialty Impact

CDI MULTI SPECIALTY IMPACT — Allen&Shariff HEALTHCARE CONSULTING

Bed Size	>499
Facility	**Sample Large Hospital**
Hospital Specific Rate	**$8,000**
MedPAR Fiscal Yr	**2012**

CMI Change	**0.059**
Actual Month Gain/Loss	**$(125,663)**
Estimated Gain/Loss for CDI Improvements Based on Month 1 Volume in Month 2	**$320,111**

MDC	MDC Description	Month 1 MDC		Month 2 MDC		Actual Payment		Volume-based CMI		
		MDC Vol	% Total Rel Wt	MDC Vol	% Total Rel Wt	Vol Var	Payment Variance	Month 1 CMI	Month 2 CMI	CMI Var
01	Nervous system	57	10.07%	42	7.84%	-15	$(182,911)	1.31	1.29	-0.02
02	Eye	2	0.35%	1	0.19%	-1	$(9,232)	1.05	0.00	-1.05
03	Ear, Nose, Mouth & Throat	9	1.59%	8	1.49%	-1	$(23,123)	1.00	0.82	-0.18
04	Respiratory System	34	6.01%	34	6.34%	0	$70,145	1.04	1.81	0.77
05	Circulatory System	184	32.51%	174	32.46%	-10	$(167,122)	2.31	2.33	0.02
06	Digestive System	68	12.01%	45	8.40%	-23	$(150,471)	1.15	1.34	0.19
07	Hepatobiliary System & Pancreas	10	1.77%	24	4.48%	14	$221,479	1.27	1.60	0.34
08	Musculoskeletal System & Connective Tissue	44	7.77%	47	8.77%	3	$(57,290)	2.34	2.08	-0.26
09	Skin, Subcutaneous Tissue & Breast	23	4.06%	13	2.43%	-10	$(82,655)	1.19	1.35	0.16
10	Endocrine, Nutritional & Metabolic	31	5.48%	30	5.60%	-1	$(70,058)	1.26	1.05	-0.21
11	Kidney & Urinary Tract	51	9.01%	53	9.89%	2	$27,350	1.27	1.34	0.07
12	Male Reproductive System	2	0.35%	6	1.12%	4	$55,392	1.15	1.39	0.24
13	Female Reproductive System	5	0.88%	7	1.31%	2	$20,966	1.04	1.07	0.04
16	Blood & Blood Forming Organs & Immunological Disorders	5	0.88%	10	1.87%	5	$58,152	1.01	1.15	0.14
17	Myeloproliferative Diseases & Disorders, Poorly Differentiated Neoplasms	11	1.94%	8	1.49%	-3	$(52,802)	1.58	1.44	-0.14
18	Infectious & Parasitic Diseases (Systemic or Unspecified Sites)	15	2.65%	22	4.10%	7	$199,563	1.73	2.15	0.42
21	Injuries, Poisonings & Toxic Effects of Drugs	9	1.59%	8	1.49%	-1	$4,745	1.57	1.92	0.35
22	Burns	0	0.00%	0	0.00%	0	$-	0.00	0.00	0.00
23	Factors Influencing Health Status & Other Contacts w/ Health Services	4	0.71%	2	0.37%	-2	$(13,977)	0.69	0.64	-0.05
24	Multiple Significant Trama	0	0.00%	0	0.00%	0	$-	0.00	0.00	0.00
25	Human Immunodeficiency Virus Infections	0	0.00%	1	0.19%	1	$22,173	0.00	2.51	2.51
ALL		2	0.35%	1	0.19%	-1	$4,012	1.98	3.19	1.22
Total		**566**		**536**		**-30**	**$(125,663)**			
				CMI Comparison				**1.710**	**1.769**	**0.059**

Used with permission from Allen & Shariff Healthcare, LLC

Table 5.10 CMI by Specialty MS-DRG Impact

CMI IMPACT BY SPECIALTY REPORT — Allen&Shariff HEALTHCARE CONSULTING

Bed Size	>499
Facility	Sample Large Hospital
Hospital Specific Rate	$5,000
MedPAR Fiscal Yr	2012

Actual Month Gain/Loss $67,671

MS-DRG	MDC Circulatory System MS-DRGs	Weight	Month 1 MDC		Month 2 MDC		Actual Payment	
			MDC Vol	% Total Rel Wt	MDC Vol	% Total Rel Wt	Vol Var	Payment Variance
280	ACUTE MYOCARDIAL INFARCTION, DISCHARGED ALIVE W MCC	1.7431	26	9.29%	28	9.79%	2	$17,431
281	ACUTE MYOCARDIAL INFARCTION, DISCHARGED ALIVE W CC	1.0568	1	0.36%	1	0.35%	0	$-
282	ACUTE MYOCARDIAL INFARCTION, DISCHARGED ALIVE W/O CC/MCC	0.7551	5	1.79%	4	1.40%	-1	$(3,776)
283	ACUTE MYOCARDIAL INFARCTION, EXPIRED W MCC	1.6885	17	6.07%	17	5.94%	0	$-
284	ACUTE MYOCARDIAL INFARCTION, EXPIRED W CC	0.7614	90	32.14%	87	30.42%	-3	$(11,421)
285	ACUTE MYOCARDIAL INFARCTION, EXPIRED W/O CC/MCC	0.5227	34	12.14%	25	8.74%	-9	$(23,522)
286	CIRCULATORY DISORDERS EXCEPT AMI, W CARD CATH W MCC	2.1058	5	1.79%	12	4.20%	7	$73,703
287	CIRCULATORY DISORDERS EXCEPT AMI, W CARD CATH W/O MCC	1.0866	22	7.86%	28	9.79%	6	$32,598
288	ACUTE & SUBACUTE ENDOCARDITIS W MCC	2.7956	12	4.29%	8	2.80%	-4	$(55,912)
289	ACUTE & SUBACUTE ENDOCARDITIS W CC	1.7891	16	5.71%	15	5.24%	-1	$(8,946)
290	ACUTE & SUBACUTE ENDOCARDITIS W/O CC/MCC	1.2359	25	8.93%	26	9.09%	1	$6,180
291	HEART FAILURE & SHOCK W MCC	1.5031	1	0.36%	5	1.75%	4	$30,062
292	HEART FAILURE & SHOCK W CC	0.9938	2	0.71%	4	1.40%	2	$9,938
293	HEART FAILURE & SHOCK W/O CC/MCC	0.6723	3	1.07%	5	1.75%	2	$6,723
294	DEEP VEIN THROMBOPHLEBITIS W CC/MCC	0.9439	6	2.14%	3	1.05%	-3	$(14,159)
295	DEEP VEIN THROMBOPHLEBITIS W/O CC/MCC	0.6287	7	2.50%	11	3.85%	4	$12,574
296	CARDIAC ARREST, UNEXPLAINED W MCC	1.3013	5	1.79%	4	1.40%	-1	$(6,507)
297	CARDIAC ARREST, UNEXPLAINED W CC	0.6063	0	0.00%	0	0.00%	0	$-
298	CARDIAC ARREST, UNEXPLAINED W/O CC/MCC	0.426	2	0.71%	1	0.35%	-1	$(2,130)
299	PERIPHERAL VASCULAR DISORDERS W MCC	1.3647	0	0.00%	0	0.00%	0	$-
300	PERIPHERAL VASCULAR DISORDERS W CC	0.9666	0	0.00%	1	0.35%	1	$4,833
301	PERIPHERAL VASCULAR DISORDERS W/O CC/MCC	0.6681	1	0.36%	1	0.35%	0	$-
Total			**280**		**286**		**6**	**$67,671**
					CMI Comparison			

Used with permission from Allen & Shariff Healthcare, LLC

increased by two with a total reimbursement gain of $17,431. This could be due to a recent education program for the cardiologist on clinical documentation requirements for common MCC/CCs found in cardiology patients.

CDI Specialty MS-DRG Benchmark

Peer benchmarking reports are useful at the start of a new CDI program to determine the potential opportunity for improving reimbursement. The reports may also be used to monitor focused MS-DRGs needing improvement to identify possible quality issues related to inaccurate coding. This report provides a look at the designated service line MS-DRGs and MS-DRG utilization compared to peer facilities. Table 5.11 provides information for the cardiology service, including the MS-DRG 280-282 triplet group, Acute Myocardial Infection. For MS-DRG 280, the peer utilization 50.5 percent compared to the facility utilization 60.80 percent indicates a higher than average usage of this higher weighted MS-DRG. This may indicate a coding compliance issue. Those MS-DRGs that are above the peer utilization should be audited for accurate coding or an overutilization of specific MCC diagnoses by the provider. In both cases, additional education is needed for remediation. The report indicates an underutilization of MS-DRG 289 acute and subacute endocarditis with CC. Peer utilization is 19.9 percent compared to the facility at 11.6 percent. This MS-DRG should also be audited for missing CCs.

CDI Dashboard

The example reports offer a starting point for facilities to craft their own scorecards and dashboards. The exact content of these dashboards should be related to the areas of focus found through study of CDI data to be most important to clinical documentation improvement within the specific facility. The following list provides a broad range of options for the monthly CDI dashboard data elements. The CDI task force can use these elements design a set of internal reports that will assist in tracking specific metrics for the dynamic CDI process. Where specific metrics are no longer needed, other areas of focus should be added as opportunities for clinical documentation are identified. Some indicators allow for the establishment of facility specific thresholds. These can be trended over time to show program impact and department-specific improvements. Reporting these impact trends offers a way to show appreciation for departments with significant improvements:

- "Total discharges available to review/Actual CDI reviews percentage
  - By financial class, DRG payer vs. no DRG payer
- Physician clarification impact percentage
  - The number of clarifications placed by a CDI that had an impact on the DRG
- Severity clarification percentage
  - The number of clarifications that resulted in a severity change
- Physician response to CDI specialist
  - The number of times a physician responds to a CDI question
- Physician response turnaround time, e.g., is there a bill-hold issue
- Physician agreement with CDI specialist

    - For non-agreements, try to understand from the physician why there was a non-agreement, e.g., did not understand the query, did not have enough clinical information to make a judgment, etc. This collaboration fosters better queries and better understanding on both sides
    - For agreements, trend if impact was for principal diagnosis, major complication/co-morbid and complication/co-morbid conditions (MCC/CC), procedure, present on admission/hospital-acquired condition (POA/HAC), etc.
- CDI specialist/coder DRG match
    - Use as learning opportunities for both CDI and coding
- Baseline medical/surgical case mix index (CMI)—set at time of initial program assessment
- Trending actual CMI to goal CMI
    - Can break the trend into medical and surgical CMI
- Physician specialty/service line CMI
- Actual CMI—medical and surgical—based on population CDI program reviews, e.g., Medicare only or all inpatient discharges, etc.
    - May want to exclude OB, newborn, psych, rehab, etc.
    - Most healthcare facilities review CMI over time, both overall and by specialty. There is quite a bit of controversy over using CMI as your only metric to measure CDI program success, as there are many variables that are included in CMI.
    - It is important to have a clear understanding of the implications of changes in CMI and how a CDI program may impact it. Some examples of other metrics that could affect the CMI include but are not limited to:
        - Census
        - Surgeries being performed as outpatient rather than inpatient
        - Loss of a physician group or surgical group
        - Addition/deletion of services such as CT surgery, neurosurgery, or adding a specific service line
- DRG Proportions
    - Low/high DRGs
    - Opportunities for DRG movement, e.g., from DRG 193-195, Simple Pneumonia, to DRG 177-179, Respiratory Infections & Inflammations.
- Medical/surgical MCC/CC capture rates
- Threshold metrics and benchmarks
    - >80 percent total discharges reviewed
    - 15–20 percent physician clarification impact
    - >50 percent severity clarifications
    - >80 percent physician response to clinician
    - >80 percent physician agreement with clinician
    - >75 percent CDS/Coder DRG match
    - CMI to be determined by each facility
    - 80 percent MCC/CC capture rate (AHIMA CDI Toolkit 2014).

Table 5.11 CDI Specialty MS-DRG Impact Projection

CDI SPECIALTY MS-DRG IMPACT PROJECTION — Allen&Shariff HEALTHCARE CONSULTING

Bed Size	>499
Facility	Sample Large Hospital
Hospital Specific Rate	$5,000
MedPAR Fiscal Yr	2012

MS-DRG	Cardiology DRG Description	DRG WGT	Geometric Mean LOS	Peer Utilization	Facility Utilization	Utilization Variance	Reimbursement Impact	Pair/Triplet Impact
280	ACUTE MYOCARDIAL INFARCTION, DISCHARGED ALIVE W MCC	1.7431	4.7	50.5%	60.8%	(10.3%)	$(48,204)	
281	ACUTE MYOCARDIAL INFARCTION, DISCHARGED ALIVE W CC	1.0568	3.1	26.2%	28.8%	(2.6%)	$(10,526)	
282	ACUTE MYOCARDIAL INFARCTION, DISCHARGED ALIVE W/O CC/MCC	0.7551	2.1	15.5%	5.9%	9.6%	$28,957	$(28,125.00)
283	ACUTE MYOCARDIAL INFARCTION, EXPIRED W MCC	1.6885	3.0	78.9%	92.7%	(13.8%)	$(9,860)	
284	ACUTE MYOCARDIAL INFARCTION, EXPIRED W CC	0.7614	1.8	11.8%	3.3%	8.5%	$3,230	
285	ACUTE MYOCARDIAL INFARCTION, EXPIRED W/O CC/MCC	0.5227	1.4	5.0%	1.5%	3.5%	$1,097	$(3,184.00)
286	CIRCULATORY DISORDERS EXCEPT AMI, W CARD CATH W MCC	2.1058	4.9	21.5%	39.1%	(17.6%)	$(154,700)	
287	CIRCULATORY DISORDERS EXCEPT AMI, W CARD CATH W/O MCC	1.0866	2.4	73.9%	55.8%	18.1%	$87,925	$(86,742.00)
288	ACUTE & SUBACUTE ENDOCARDITIS W MCC	2.7956	7.8	72.8%	75.3%	(2.5%)	$(1,775)	
289	ACUTE & SUBACUTE ENDOCARDITIS W CC	1.7891	5.7	19.9%	11.6%	8.3%	$10,109	
290	ACUTE & SUBACUTE ENDOCARDITIS W/O CC/MCC	1.2359	3.9	3.4%	11.8%	(8.4%)	$(6,025)	$1,814.00
291	HEART FAILURE & SHOCK W MCC	1.5031	4.6	43.3%	39.4%	3.9%	$34,940	
292	HEART FAILURE & SHOCK W CC	0.9938	3.7	33.2%	42.2%	(9.0%)	$(120,321)	
293	HEART FAILURE & SHOCK W/O CC/MCC	0.6723	2.6	18.8%	10.8%	8.0%	$69,222	$(17,663.00)
294	DEEP VEIN THROMBOPHLEBITIS W CC/MCC	0.9439	4.0	71.9%	14.2%	57.7%	$18,700	
295	DEEP VEIN THROMBOPHLEBITIS W/O CC/MCC	0.6287	3.1	25.0%	1.5%	23.5%	$8,075	$1,155.00
296	CARDIAC ARREST, UNEXPLAINED W MCC	1.3013	1.9	70.1%	96.0%	(25.9%)	$(2,465)	
297	CARDIAC ARREST, UNEXPLAINED W CC	0.6063	1.2	15.6%	0.0%	15.6%	$887	
298	CARDIAC ARREST, UNEXPLAINED W/O CC/MCC	0.426	1.0	8.5%	0.0%	8.5%	$332	$(258.00)
299	PERIPHERAL VASCULAR DISORDERS W MCC	1.3647	4.4	26.4%	20.3%	6.1%	$30,509	
300	PERIPHERAL VASCULAR DISORDERS W CC	0.9666	3.6	40.8%	55.8%	(15.0%)	$(39,034)	
	Note: Based on National Average MedPar data							

Used with permission from Allen & Shariff Healthcare, LLC

Data Considerations for Reviewing Outpatient Clinical Documentation

Most clinical documentation assessments seem to focus, at least initially, on inpatient documentation. However, outpatient stays now drive an increasing percentage of healthcare systems' revenue. Therefore, every organization should include outpatient clinical documentation in its CDI initiatives.

Data review opportunities for outpatient analyses are more abundant than for inpatient analyses. This is partly because the CDI team cannot reduce outpatient cases to 500 or so categories like the DRG system used for inpatient cases. While there are some aggregations via the ambulatory payment classifications (APCs), one outpatient can be assigned more than one APC by the APC grouper. Furthermore, not all outpatient cases have APCs. Therefore, in some instances, the analysis remains at the code level for some outpatients.

Organizations can create their own reporting system for outpatient analysis. AHD provides a web-based resource to generate reports such as those shown in tables 5.12 and 5.13 (AHD 2014). These include

- Top 20 medical diagnoses
- Top 20 APCs
- Number of cases
- Financial information

In table 5.12, one of the top five diagnoses is 285.9, Anemia NOS. This may raise a red flag for the level of precision in documentation. While only actual record review confirms whether a problem exists, this type of data review can justify investing in a record review. In table 5.13, the most expensive procedure is for a diagnostic cardiac catheterization (APC 0080). The charge alone for these cases may justify a review to ensure the documentation was accurate.

Documentation Review

Documentation review allows CDI professionals to determine if clinical documentation that does not meet the criteria for high quality is causing problems seen in the data. Because they are reviewing only a sampling, they may need some additional verification. However, by using the suggestions that follow, the review should produce a result that is highly representative of the clinical documentation for the organization's overall patient base.

Concurrent vs. Retrospective Review

There are two ways to review clinical documentation in patient records: concurrently or retrospectively. Reviewing records concurrently requires the reviewer to be on the unit where the patient is receiving treatment. The concurrent review takes place after the provider has recorded documentation, but before the provider discharges the patient. While technically, this is not a concurrent review of the documentation, it is a review concurrent with the patient's stay.

Table 5.12 Statistics for the top 20 medical diagnoses

ICD-9 Code	ICD-9 Description	Total Payment	Number Patient Claims	Average Charge	Average Cost	Average Payment	Total Outlier Amount	National Average Charge
V580	RADIOTHERAPY ENCOUNTER	$4,122,061	1,308	$11,520	$3,461	$3,151	$18,919	$6,773
V581	CHEMOTHERAPY ENCOUNTER	$1,743,963	1,755	$6,184	$1,598	$993	$123,099	$7,359
28522	ANEMIA NEO DIS	$953,915	1,691	$3,635	$1,015	$564	$190,180	$3,159
41401	CAD	$446,410	213	$8,027	$1,840	$2,095	$790	$6,309
2859	ANEMIA NOS	$359,570	785	$2,398	$795	$458	$58,740	$1,564
1985	SEC MALIG BONE	$323,846	371	$4,052	$974	$872	$13,387	$3,114
185	MALIGN PROSTATE	$260,317	384	$2,952	$800	$677	$3,408	$3,477
2880	AGRANULOCYTOSIS	$251,534	376	$3,258	$879	$668	$31,064	$1,883
78659	CHEST PAIN NEC	$235,678	221	$4,077	$961	$1,066	$869	$2,882
V7612	SCREEN MAMMO	$228,930	3,843	$175	$33	$59	$0	$207
V6709	F/U SURGERY NEC	$226,928	707	$1,170	$342	$320	$851	$1,028
72402	SPINAL STENOSIS-	$211,599	748	$1,126	$315	$282	$900	$1,395
V7283	OTH PREOP EXAM	$197,265	1,974	$567	$136	$99	$4,234	$575
78057	OTH SLEEP APNEA	$186,736	313	$2,288	$2,749	$596	$0	$1,960
2113	BEN NEO BOWEL	$180,566	369	$1,902	$527	$489	$5,859	$1,935
78650	CHEST PAIN NOS	$179,248	390	$2,380	$552	$459	$1,492	$2,014
5920	CALC OF KIDNEY	$174,352	104	$6,674	$1,732	$1,676	$1,692	$2,613
79439	ABN CARDIO STUD	$155,047	78	$7,568	$1,719	$1,987	$73	$5,820
V5332	Fit DFIBRILLATOR	$152,409	22	$34,412	$7,838	$6,927	$1,113	$16,407
20280	OTH LYMP UNSP	$139,535	112	$4,673	$1,224	$1,245	$7,146	$3,353
	All Other	$10,569,388	31,392	—	—	—	—	—
	TOTAL FOR ALL CLAIMS	$21,338,924	47,240	—	—	—	—	—

www.ahd.com. Used with permission.

In a retrospective review, the reviewer assesses the documentation after discharge and usually after the coding professional codes the record. The retrospective review takes place prior to billing or after, depending on the organization's common policies and procedures. The advantage to reviewing records after coding, but prior to billing, is that if there are changes made that affect the coding, the reviewer can make them before submitting the bill. The disadvantage to reviewing records prior to billing is that it significantly limits the population from which the sample is drawn, thereby possibly making the findings less reliable.

Table 5.14 lists the advantages and disadvantages of both the concurrent and the retrospective approaches to record review. Another option to consider is performing a review that includes both a retrospective and a concurrent review.

Table 5.13 Top 20 ambulatory payment classifications (APCs)

APC Number	APC Description	Total Payment	Number Patient Claims	Units of Service	Average Charge	Average Cost	Average Payment	National Average Charge
0300	Level I Rad Tx	$2,051,416	1,159	12,314	$541	$164	$166	$430
0080	Diag Card Cath	$959,830	501	501	$3,027	$738	$1,915	$3,688
0733	Non esrd epoetin alpha	$760,787	2,243	83,833	$95	$22	$9	$40
0304	Level I Rad TX	$618,749	3,296	7,200	$313	$95	$85	$317
0143	Lower GI Endo	$610,824	1,477	1,478	$1,275	$360	$413	$1,088
0612	High Lev ED Vis	$486,810	2,089	2,097	$634	$248	$232	$563
0303	TX Device Construction	$444,627	1,031	2,903	$524	$159	$153	$551
0260	Level I Xray	$425,613	8,816	10,192	$204	$39	$41	$171
0849	Rituximab, 100	$374,195	192	1,454	$1,954	$457	$257	$1,166
0206	Lev II Nerve Inj	$349,685	1,360	1,360	$630	$225	$257	$651
0714	New Tech Lev IX	$349,071	246	246	$4,016	$766	$1,418	$3,605
0332	CAT	$332,109	1,795	1,796	$1,042	$193	$184	$1,033
0280	Level III Angio	$318,244	429	451	$1,945	$494	$705	$1,623
0710	New Tech Lev V	$285,849	171	710	$2,726	$846	$402	$1,121
0823	Docetaxel,20 mg	$259,003	225	1,278	$1,249	$292	$202	$869
0267	Level III Dx Ultrasound	$254,713	1,921	1,926	$473	$185	$132	$561
0117	Chemo by Infus	$243,120	1,163	1,252	$602	$182	$194	$349
0905	Immune globulin	$234,727	265	8,281	$334	$78	$28	$172
0305	Level II TX Rad	$227,139	1,068	1,159	$770	$233	$195	$763
0291	Level II DX Nuc Med	$224,181	1,058	1,060	$820	$152	$211	$803
	TOT FOR TOP 20	$9,810,692	30,505	141,491	—	—	—	—
	SERV MIX IND =	2.575						

www.ahd.com. Used with permission.

Collecting a Sample for Retrospective Review

Some of the initial issues to consider for sampling include identifying the population, determining the size of the sample, and selecting the methodology for the review. For example, some organizations may exclude normal newborn cases or certain one-day-stay cases from their documentation review. When an organization excludes any segment of the population, someone should document the exclusion as well as the rationale for eliminating these cases. Recording this information allows replication of the study for use in future comparisons.

Once the organization has clarified the population, it must determine the sample size. A documentation review needs to be representative, but not necessarily scientific. The review team should consider the size of the sample population and specific areas of focus previously identified. "Directors and managers should obtain

Table 5.14 Advantages and disadvantages of concurrent and retrospective reviews

Review Type	Advantages	Disadvantages
Concurrent	• Real time intervention with physicians to make changes identified during the audit • Greater reliability of the recommended query • Ability to mimic the activity of a clinical documentation program and provide subjective information about how successful the actual process could be	• Review time and cost can be increased significantly because the reviewers must locate cases unit by unit • Sample selection is not random, so the findings will not be generalizable to the entire patient population
Retrospective	• Review time and cost is less than concurrent review since records can be identified and pulled prior to starting the work • Random sample selection is possible, making the results of the review generalizable across the entire patient population	• The ability to determine a concurrent query retrospectively may be difficult in some cases and may result in under or over estimation of the impact • The ability to act on any findings that may impact reimbursement may be limited due to payer time constraints

a representative sample of 2 percent of the required productivity standards per patient type coded by the coder for the time frame selected for the review. If the audit has a broad focus (for example, beyond individual coder rates), a larger, more statistically valid sample size is recommended" (Brownfield, 2009). Should a statistically valid sample be necessary, Section 8.4: Use of Statistical Sample for Overpayment Estimation in the Medicare Program Integrity Manual, chapter 8 is a good resource for determining the sampling methodology. Some organizations may engage statisticians and apply other methodologies for sample selection. The most important consideration is that, over time, the organization uses the same methodology for all sample selections. This allows the results to be comparable. If the organization modifies the methodology even slightly, results will not be comparable from study to study.

After determining the number of cases in the sample, the review team must determine the methodology to select the records. Random sampling is optimal since it is generally representative of the overall patient population (Medicare Program Integrity Manual, Section 8.4 2011), and a representative sample is most likely to yield study findings that a CDI review team could identify as opportunities for improvement. Some organizations stratify by payer or even service. Ultimately, if the sample size is large enough, it includes cases that are representative of the entire patient population.

Collecting a Sample for Concurrent Review

Unless the organization is large, with several hundred discharges per day, it is impossible to obtain a random sample selection for an efficient concurrent review.

One way to approach the concurrent review process is to replicate the activities of a CDI program. Essentially, reviewers conduct their assessment of the records in the same manner that clinical documentation specialists would. While an organization cannot generalize the results of such a review over the entire patient population, it can report on the findings as representative of a two-week period of CDI review. If a team approaches a review in this manner, a retrospective review of at least 100 records provides a good sample size.

There is a way to conduct a concurrent review using a random-type sampling methodology (Babbie 1999). It is not as reliable as the sample selection methodology for retrospective review, but it provides more representative results than the scenario previously described. First, the reviewers must prepare to spread out the review over a four- to eight-week period so that sampling is not biased by the short timeframe. Smaller hospitals should use the eight-week period, while larger hospitals can use the four-week period. Each day, using the census listing, reviewers select a random number of patients for review. If the reviewer already reviewed a patient, he or she would throw out the record and add a replacement record. By using random number generators found on the Internet, this sample selection will be is as objective as possible.

Reviewing the Documentation

When reviewing records for clinical documentation, it is most important to focus the review solely on the documentation. In a retrospective review, the reviewer may have a tendency to allow the coding assigned to the records influence him or her. Thus, reviewing the records without referencing the coding provides the most reliable results.

Individuals with clinical expertise as well as training in clinical documentation review should perform the review. In organizations that do not have clinical documentation experts available internally, a team consisting of a nurse reviewer and a coding professional can provide the appropriate skill set. The team, however, must be trained in the principles of high-quality clinical documentation as well as the organization's specific objectives for the review. Trusted external consultants offering subject matter expertise in CDI can provide the necessary resource if they are not available within the facility.

The objectives become very important during the analysis phase. In this phase, the review team should identify not only opportunities for querying physicians, but also what the impact would be if the response were positive. For example, in some cases, a query response may change the coding, the DRG assignment, or both. In other cases, the query response may change reporting for quality indicators. In some cases, the response may affect severity leveling, while in others it may influence more than one performance outcome.

The most reliable and consistent methodology for reviewing clinical documentation is to use the criteria for high-quality clinical documentation to identify wherever documentation is deficient (Russo 2008). This methodology also ensures the review is compliant. When a query is recommended by the CDI specialist or coder, especially in a retrospective review, it is best to have the agreement of at least two reviewers before including it in a final report.

Reporting and Acting on Findings

The primary purpose of the report of findings from the clinical documentation review is to determine whether the review identified one or more problems with the quality of clinical documentation. If the answer is yes, then the review team should include additional detail to the report that specifies the number and type of problems found. It is important to state the findings in an objective, factual format. Then, the organization can use the report to draw logical conclusions based on the data. Some examples of how to report the findings are discussed with the CDI team and coders. The report should include detailed data specific to the needs and goals of the organization.

Table 5.15 shows the differences in severity levels if the documentation in the reviewed records was complete on the units or at the time of coding. In the best-case scenario, if documentation was completed concurrently by the CDI specialist or concurrent coder, the percentage of level 3 cases would increase from 22 percent to 32 percent. This finding alone supports the recommendation to implement a complete CDI program.

Table 5.16 is an example of a CMI analysis performed on the records in the review. The table lists the current CMI along with projected CMI. Projected CMI is CMI with improved clinical documentation. The actual CMI opportunity can be calculated by the CDI manager by adding up all of the relative weight differences

Table 5.15 Differences in severity levels depending on documentation

Severity Level	Current Documentation	Complete Documentation at Coding	Complete Concurrent Documentation
Minor (Level 1)	20%	17%	15%
Moderate (Level 2)	57%	54%	51%
Major (Level 3)	22%	28%	32%
Extreme (Level 4)	1%	1%	2%

Table 5.16 Case mix index (CMI) comparison analysis

Medicare Payers only:			
	Current	**Projected**	**Opportunity**
Medical CMI:	1.0635	1.1107	+.0472
Surgical CMI:	2.4615	2.4781	+.0166
All Other Payers:			
	Current	**Projected**	**Opportunity**
Medical CMI:	0.8033	0.8424	+.0391
Surgical CMI:	1.8921	1.9249	+.0328

from the review and dividing that number by the total number of discharges for the payer for a year.

In table 5.15, the overall Medicare impact is .0472 for medical and .0166 for surgical. The economic value of that opportunity is determined by multiplying the improved opportunity for medical (.0472) or surgical (.0166) by the hospital's blended rate.

The conclusion to the clinical documentation review process is a decision to move forward (or not) with a CDI program. The more careful thought and preparation that goes into the assessment process, the more reliable and sustainable the CDI program that emanates from it is likely to be.

Conclusion

A clinical documentation assessment is an important prerequisite to implementing a CDI program. First, a review team should review the organization's data for inconsistencies and patterns that do not meet target norms. Second, using results of the data review, the reviewer should assess clinical documentation in patient records. The review team should carefully select the sample and the methodology for review and use the same methods for each review so they can compare results over time. Finally, the team should gather results, analyze findings, make recommendations, and prepare and deliver the report to the appropriate managers in the organization.

Chapter Quiz

1. What should the facilities interested in investing in a CDI program perform on data and documentation?
   A. Quality analysis
   B. Objective analysis
   C. Internal audit analysis
   D. Revenue cycle analysis

2. When analyzing coding data, what system has one of the highest levels of aggregation?
   A. POA
   B. APC
   C. CMI
   D. DRG

3. Which reimbursement method allows for multiple assignments for each encounter and allows for the analysis of clinical documentation to remain on the coding level?
   A. POA indicators
   B. APC
   C. CPT-4
   D. MS-DRG

4. During the review of clinical documentation, on what is it imperative to focus the review?
   A. Current provider documentation
   B. Vital sign flowsheets
   C. Problem lists
   D. POA indicators

5. Review of inconsistencies or patterns that do not meet DRG target norms, allows this data to be used for what purpose?
   A. Quality improvement process
   B. Internal physician audits
   C. Revenue cycle analysis
   D. Clinical documentation assessment

6. What are the two types of data the review team should consider in the CDI analysis process?
   A. Patient severity; length of stay data
   B. Number of errors in consultation reports; delinquency rates by providers
   C. Data produced by the organization; data produced by others about the organization
   D. Number of CCs and MCCs; CMI discrepancies

7. Most organizations review data on a regular basis by ______, as part of _______ analysis.
   A. Service type; regulatory
   B. Diagnostic-Related Group; case mix
   C. Auditing; case mix index
   D. Specialty; revenue cycle

8. Changes in these two rates may suggest problems with clinical documentation?
   A. Major complication or comorbidity and complication or comorbidity
   B. DRG; case mix
   C. Primary and secondary diagnostics
   D. Level of severity; Medicare quality indicators

9. Which type of review takes place while the patient is still in the hospital and when the patient leaves the hospital?
   A. Initial; subsequent
   B. Primary; secondary
   C. Pre-billing; post-billing
   D. Concurrent; retrospective

10. The ____________ is one of the key indicators used to monitor a successful CDI program.
    A. APC
    B. CDI review
    C. Capture rate
    D. Retrospective review

REFERENCES

AHIMA. 2014a. The role of analyzing healthcare data: Health data analysts aggregate, evaluate, and validate information for key healthcare stakeholders. *Journal of AHIMA* 85(5):54-55.

AHIMA. 2014b. Clinical documentation improvement toolkit. Retrieved from: http://library.ahima.org/xpedio/groups/secure/documents/ahima/bok1_050585.pdf.

American Hospital Directory. AHD. 2008. http://www.ahd.com/.

Babbie, E. 1999. *The Basics of Social Research.* Albany, NY: Wadsworth Publishing Company.

Brownfield, D.M. and C. Didier. Making the most of external coding audits: From preparation to recommendations. *Journal of AHIMA* 80(7): 34–38.

Centers for Medicare and Medicaid Services. 2014a. Quality Measures. Retrieved from: http://www.cms.gov/Medicare/Quality-Initiatives-Patient-Assessment-Instruments/QualityMeasures/index.html.

Centers for Medicare and Medicaid Services. 2014b. *Recommended Core Measures.* Retrieved from: http://www.cms.gov/Medicare/Quality-Initiatives-Patient-Assessment-Instruments/QualityMeasures/index.html.

Centers for Medicare and Medicaid Services. 2014c. *Proposed Clinical Quality Measures for 2014.* Retrieved from: http://www.cms.gov/Medicare/Quality-Initiatives-Patient-Assessment-Instruments/QualityMeasures/ProposedClinicalQualityMeasuresfor2014.html.

Healthgrades. 2015. http://www.healthgrades.com.

IPRO. 2005a. Coding for quality: Documentation tips for the top seven DRGs revised 2005, Hospital Payment Monitoring Program. http://providers.ipro.org/index/hpmp

IPRO. 2005b. Coding for Quality: Documentation tips for the top ten denied DRGs, Hospital payment monitoring program. http://providers.ipro.org/index/hpmp

Medicare Program Integrity Manual, Chapter 8, Section 8.4. 2011. Centers for Medicare and Medicaid Services. Retrieved from: http://www.cms.gov/Regulations-and-Guidance/Guidance/Manuals/Downloads/pim83c08.pdf.

Pennsylvania Health Care Cost Containment Council (PHCCCC). 2006. Cardiac Surgery in Pennsylvania 2005–2006. http://www.phc4.org/reports/cabg/06/docs/cabg2006keyfindings.pdf.

Russo, R. 2008. *A Compelling Case for Clinical Documentation.* Bethlehem, PA: DJ Iber Publishing.

Chapter

6 Moving Forward with a CDI Program

Making the decision to move forward with a clinical documentation improvement (CDI) program is an essential choice for every organization. The decision should be based on an objective assessment of the organization's current clinical documentation practices. Using this information, the organization should create a vision statement for its CDI program, and include the goals for the CDI staff (Russo 2008). In addition, the organization must be prepared to support the program with appropriate resources and staffing. This chapter addresses the crafting of a vision statement for CDI and how to gain organizational support for the program.

Key Decision Makers

Before proceeding with the creation of a vision statement for clinical documentation and the CDI program, it is necessary to have the right individuals in place to participate in the decision-making process. The CDI leadership should strive to make a good decision that organization will embrace. Leaving out a key player during the visioning process means potential failure, or at the very least, a significant setback for the program.

Because CDI is an interdisciplinary process, it is essential to include leaders in each of the functional areas that affect the CDI process. While each organization varies, suggested participants include

- Chief medical officer (CMO)
- Chief financial officer (CFO)
- Chief information officer (CIO) (or appropriate representative from information technology [IT])

- Chief compliance officer
- Chief nursing officer (depending on the organization)
- Other key physicians, especially from areas that show high opportunity
- Director of health information management (HIM)
- Vice president of outpatient services (if outpatient services are in the scope of the client's need)
- Director of case management
- Director of quality
- Emergency department director

Creating a Vision for Clinical Documentation and the Clinical Documentation Improvement Program

When developing a new CDI program or improving an existing one within the organization, CDI leadership needs to ask the following question before spending any (or any more) of the organization's resources on this effort. Why do we want to improve clinical documentation? In essence, ask, "What does our organization hope to achieve by implementing a new or upgrading the current CDI program?"

In developing a CDI vision statement, the organization should begin with its own values, vision, and mission statements. The CDI vision statement should flow naturally from these broader statements reflecting the organizational values and overall direction. The CDI vision statement does two things. First, it provides a purpose for the program. Second, it provides a way to get the attention of the physicians and other clinicians whose documentation the effort is attempting to improve.

Research shows that unless the vision is specific to the program and the organization, it is unlikely to succeed and be sustainable (Porras and Collins 1996; Collins 2001). Some of the reasons for implementing a CDI program include the following:

- The healthcare team caring for the patient has an interest in the highest quality clinical documentation. Without complete and accurate documentation, the best treatment is not possible. The healthcare team provides one of the strongest arguments for having a CDI program: high-quality care for patients.
- Organizations that measure quality use the hospital's publicly available data to create quality scorecards for the hospital. These scorecards rate the hospital by type of diagnoses providers treat and surgical procedures they perform (http://www.healthgrades.com/), how the hospital treated certain diagnoses (Medicare quality indicators [http://www.cms.hhs.gov/] and the Leapfrog Group [http://www.leapfroggroup.org/]), and how frequently providers performed certain surgeries (https://www.vimo.com/) among others. The clinical documentation in patient records drives the organization's *perceived quality*, which is the public's perception of its quality of care based on these reports.

- Patients have a greater interest in obtaining, maintaining, and understanding their patient records. The patient owns the information in the record, and under the Health Insurance Portability and Accountability Act (HIPAA), the patient has the right to ask someone in the organization to explain the content, correct it, or even rewrite the information if it is illegible (HIPAA 1996). The motivation for high-quality clinical documentation in this instance is patient satisfaction. Patients' requests to review their records have increased in recent years. Well-kept, easy-to-read, complete health records will likely begin to play a more prominent role in patient satisfaction (Gunter 2002).
- An organization's healthcare planning relies largely on the data it gathers (Johnson 2001). An organization uses details about the types of patients it is treating, how it is treating them, as well as clinical details about symptoms and diagnoses. All this information is generated from the clinical documentation in health records, translated into coded data by HIM professionals. The organization needs accurate and complete information to make good decisions (Russo 2008).
- The same clinical documentation is used by attorneys in medical malpractice or other legal claims against the hospital, by payers as the basis for payment by health plans, and for research and reporting to government and regulatory agencies. These examples are more operational in nature than the first four uses mentioned.

Healthcare organizations should consider all of these issues when creating a CDI vision statement. Ultimately, a CDI vision statement should embrace the issues that CDI leadership believes are most significant to the organization and be a natural extension of the organization's overall mission statement.

Initial Structure: Program Committees

This section presents time-tested CDI structures proven effective in implementing or redesigning the program. The initial structure for a CDI program, in most organizations, should be two guided committees. These committees consist of one that operates at the strategic level of the organization and another that operates at the day-to-day, or operational, level of the organization. Over time, these committees may change into a formalized department with an executive team member who is responsible for clinical documentation and CDI practices. Most organizations should begin with the committee structure and determine, over time, what long-term structure will work best in their environment to support and maintain high-quality clinical documentation.

Governance or Oversight Committee

Support from the top is essential to the success of a CDI program. Therefore, the governance or oversight committee should be composed of members of executive management, the physician advisor or leader for clinical documentation and CDI, and the manager of the CDI program. In general, the oversight committee should include the chief executive officer (CEO), the chief financial officer (CFO), the chief marketing officer (CMO), the chief compliance officer, the chief information officer (CIO), a physician, a CDI leader, and a CDI program manager. Committee composition may vary by the size and complexity of the organization. For example in a very large organization, the vice president of operations or the chief operating officer (COO) may sit on the committee in lieu of the CEO, and a vice president of reimbursement may sit on the committee in lieu of the CFO.

The amount of time the committee needs to spend in meetings gradually decreases after program implementation. In the beginning, it may be best to have a joint meeting for all members of both the oversight and the day-to-day committees. At this meeting, members review specific responsibilities of each group. The chair of the oversight committee manages this meeting with the chair of the operations committee. During this joint committee meeting, each group agrees to its responsibilities and communicates its expectations about what it needs from the other group. During the initial implementation phase, the oversight committee may meet every other week. Then, during the remainder of the first year, the oversight committee should meet monthly.

During year two, when additions and adjustments are being made to the program by the CDI governance and management, the oversight committee may choose to meet every quarter. Finally, as clinical documentation and CDI become an operationalized function within the organization, the oversight committee will likely stop meeting. A standing executive-level committee, often a quality initiative, or other strategic committee usually replaces them. However, the responsibilities of the oversight committee do not stop. Even after year two, the committee should conduct an annual program review to identify strengths and weaknesses of the program or to implement new processes.

During its time of operation, the oversight committee has five key responsibilities. First, the group must obtain and maintain support from the medical staff. This is the most essential role the oversight committee plays. Initially, the committee must determine the strategy for obtaining physician support and, through its own actions, demonstrate the importance of the CDI initiative. In addition to obtaining support, the oversight committee should also determine the chain of command it will use to manage physicians who are either unresponsive or uncooperative with the CDI program staff. The oversight committee is responsible for obtaining initial program funding through the organization's budget and maintaining that funding for some period, usually up to two years. After that time, the organization has likely operationalized the function and included it as a budget line item. The oversight committee should also identify the key metrics it will use to measure program success. This committee reviews those metrics regularly and provides feedback to the operations group on how they perceive the program is moving. Five key responsibilities of the oversight committee are to

- Obtain and maintain medical staff support
- Create a chain of command to manage uncooperative physicians
- Support the program financially

- Determine key metrics to be reviewed at the strategic level
- Provide feedback to the CDI operational group

Operational Committee or CDI Task Force

The operational committee or CDI task force comprises the individuals who are responsible for the day-to-day management of and support for the CDI program. The members of this committee are likely to include the CDI program manager, the physician leader for CDI, the health information manager, the coding manager, the quality indicators manager, a data analyst, a financial analyst, or the case mix manager. Depending on the structure of the program, the director of case management may also participate on this committee. The quality indicators manager is the individual in the organization who supervises the abstraction of data for quality indicator purposes. Because of the overlap in responsibilities, someone from this function should be involved in CDI so they can identify and implement any synergies that allow the organization to operate more efficiently. A data analyst (or similar individual) should be involved to allow easily accessible data. CDI specialists may or may not be involved with the committee. Generally, for organizations with a large number of CDI specialists (five or more), they will not be included in the operations meetings. However, for organizations with only a few CDI specialists, they may be included in the meetings. In smaller organizations, the CDI specialists are likely to play a role in program management and may multitask within the program. In this case, it makes sense to include all members in the operations committee. For larger organizations, including all CDI specialists would be inefficient for program operations. Because of the operational nature of the CDI program, this group should not include a member of the compliance team. The day-to-day operational involvement of a compliance team member conflicts with the CDI specialist's responsibilities for reviewing and auditing organizational activities

The operations committee should meet weekly during the first few months of the program. There are a number of activities the committee needs to coordinate, and these weekly meetings help facilitate them. After the first few months, the operations committee meets monthly for the first two years of program operation. In the second year, the members of the committee change. For example, the data analyst and financial analyst may no longer be needed on the committee.

There are seven primary responsibilities of the operations committee. They include the initial responsibilities of hiring and training program staff as well as training physicians and other clinicians in high-quality clinical documentation practices. As the committee hires and trains CDI program staff members, the staff members assume more and more of the operational responsibilities. Moreover, the operational committee plays a support and review function. On an ongoing basis, the operations committee is responsible for ensuring the query process along with any other activities necessary to obtain high-quality clinical documentation. Other responsibilities of the operations committee include reviewing CDI program data, supervising the design of auditing clinical documentation and CDI functions, supervising the design of follow-up training for physicians, and reporting key metrics to the oversight committee. The seven primary responsibilities of the operations committee are to

- Hire and train staff
- Oversee the training of physicians and other clinicians
- Implement and oversee activities for obtaining high-quality clinical documentation through day-to-day activities such as location of record review activities and one-on-one training with the positions
- Review program data for tracking and measuring
- Supervise the design of auditing clinical documentation and CDI functions
- Supervise the design of follow-up training for physicians
- Report on key metrics to the oversight committee

There is one caveat for small and focused organizations. In organizations with fewer than 50 beds, the committee structure can be greatly streamlined by the CDI governance team, and individuals may take on the roles of multiple members of a committee. The committee structures recommended above assume that an organization is operating with at least 150 beds. Organizations with fewer than 150 inpatient beds should use the suggested committee structure to determine which activities it needs to perform and assign individuals to those roles. The activities the organization needs to complete remain the same regardless of the size of the organization. Each organization just needs to determine how it can best accomplish those activities.

Figure 6.1 demonstrates a typical committee structure for a clinical documentation program.

Figure 6.1 Clinical documentation committee structure

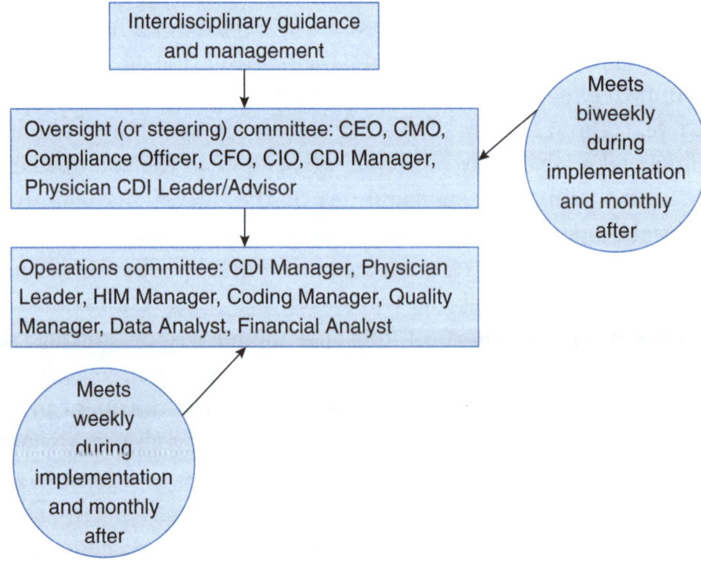

⊙ Communicating to the Organization

As with any new function, it is necessary for an organization to start a strategic communications process about clinical documentation and the CDI program to ensure the success and sustainability of the program. This is really part of the oversight committee's responsibility for obtaining support from the medical staff for the CDI program. The operations committee is involved in disseminating the message, but the initial communication must come from the top of the organization. The message about clinical documentation and the CDI program coming from the CEO and other executives in the organization emphasizes to the physicians the importance of both the program and the physicians' participation in the program.

The Communication Process

Communication about the CDI process should begin in advance of any program training or operationalizing. Letting the physicians know about the program prepares them for the coming activities and, if done appropriately, helps obtain the physicians' support for the program.

The organization should consider three key concepts in communication:

- ***WHO*** *communicates it*—From whom will communications come?
- ***HOW*** *will it be communicated*—What media will the CDI program use?
- ***WHAT*** *is communicated*—What information will the CDI staff communicate?

The initial communication regarding the program should come from the top of the organization, for example, from the CEO. Subsequent communications can come from the CMO or the physician leader for CDI. The media selected for communication may vary since physicians in each organization may value one type of communication over another. The primary means of communication include in-person meetings and electronic communications such as email. The best way to communicate is through multiple media. For example, an in-person meeting with the CEO and members of the medical staff, in which the CEO discusses the program and then follows up with an e-mail or hard copy letter (depending on the organization), is likely to send the most powerful message (Patterson et al. 2002).

Once someone from the CDI program staff communicates the message about the program to physicians and all managers in the organization, additional follow-up communications are necessary. These communications should come from a physician. The importance of physician involvement is discussed later in this section. These communications should begin to introduce the physicians to more details about the CDI program and the CDI program staff. Physicians should share details about the staff's qualifications, the training programs, and the query process in these communications. If the physician uses e-mail, he or she should dedicate each e-mail to one aspect of the program since other physicians are not likely to read the contents of a lengthy e-mail.

Some organizations have successfully used marketing communications in addition to personal communications to announce the CDI program. For example, organizations have used posters in the physicians' lounge, announcements, and brief articles in the medical staff newsletter. These tactics are helpful in some organizations, but the organization should only use them after sending a formal communication from the CEO and CMO to the medical staff. Members of the medical staff should not find out about a CDI program by reading a brochure or poster in the lounge. Figure 6.2 shows a sample letter to the medical staff from the CEO describing the CDI program.

Once the program staff determines who will communicate the information and how, it is essential to determine the exact message. The beginning of this chapter addressed the importance of creating a program vision that is linked directly to the organization's vision and mission statements. The concepts of quality of care, perceived quality, and patient satisfaction are key reasons for program implementation. These reasons are important to physicians and should be included in the message. *While accurate reimbursement is usually a key goal of a CDI program, it should not be the only goal, and the program staff should not lead the medical staff to think of it as the primary reason for the program.*

Physicians should understand how the goals of the CDI program align with their goals. If an organization has identified quality and patient satisfaction goals as the vision for CDI, these goals will probably strike a chord with the physicians. It is important to include this information in the initial message to them. In addition, the communication should include the benefits the physicians experience when they improve their clinical documentation in the hospital. Next, the message should communicate what the hospital's expectations are regarding physician involvement in the CDI process. The communication should explain the physicians' responsibilities realistically, with a focus on using a limited amount of their time. Finally, the message should share with the physicians any benefits they can expect from the hospital. This may include a meal during the training program and CME credits. The sample letter in figure 6.2 summarizes the information the message to the physicians should include.

Physician Support

Physician support is the key to the success and sustainability of the CDI program. The organization should identify initial physician supporters prior to the formal communications about the program. In addition to the CMO or vice president of medical affairs, the program should have a physician advisor or CDI leader by the time the organization makes the announcement. The communication can include the physician leader's name so other physicians can contact the leader with questions about the program. In addition, the organization should create a strategy that brings other physician leaders into the fold to support CDI as early as possible. Which physicians participate varies by organization.

The chiefs of service may be a good group to involve. If the organization employs physicians (hospitalists, physician group practices, or others), they should all learn about the program prior to the initial communication to the medical staff. These individuals can help clarify questions other physicians may have. They can also demonstrate support for the process.

Other physicians that an organization may want to inform early in the process include the *informal* medical staff leaders. These are physicians who everyone

Figure 6.2 Sample letter from the CEO to the medical staff

Date

James Smith, MD
214 Elm Street
Providence, RI 10034

Re: Clinical Documentation Program

I hope you were able to attend the medical staff meeting last week where I described the hospital's clinical documentation program, which will begin in March. I wanted to provide you with some additional detail about the program. As well as the benefits to our organization overall, the program will provide you with some documentation training opportunities that you can use in your private practice as well as with patients in the hospital.

Research has shown that physician clinical documentation in patient records is directly linked to quality indicators, quality of care, and the efficiency of healthcare operations. In addition, patients are twice as likely to request and read copies of their health records today than they were 10 years ago. And, under HIPAA patients have the right to request modifications to their health information. Based upon this research and our desire to maintain high quality care and high levels of patient satisfaction, we are implementing a clinical documentation program. This program teaches the criteria for high-quality clinical documentation and program staff use the criteria to review patient records for opportunities for improvement.

I am asking for your support of this clinical documentation initiative. Your responsibilities to the program include attendance at an initial documentation training program and continued attendance at follow-up training two to three times per year. In return, the hospital will provide you with lunch or dinner and CMEs for every hour of training you attend. In addition, you may be asked to clarify documentation in your patient records by one of the clinical documentation specialists, who will be located on the nursing units. If asked, you will need to clarify your documentation in the patient's record.

If you have any questions about the program or would like additional information on the research conducted to justify implementing the program, I would be happy to share that with you. You can also find additional information about the program, including program staff names and contact information, in the physicians' lounge and in the current medical staff newsletter.

Thank you for your time and involvement in this process. I appreciate the work you do with our healthcare system and the contributions that your practice of medicine makes to our community.

Sincerely,

CEO

cc:

CFO, CMO, CIO, Compliance Officer (Oversight Committee Members)

respects but do not hold specific formal positions within the organization. Every organization has a few of these leaders. It may be wise for the CMO or the CEO to meet with these physicians individually prior to the initial announcement. An informal lunch to discuss CDI along with other key initiatives of the organization can solidify support from these informal leaders. The more physician support the organization obtains for the CDI program in its early stages, the higher the likelihood of success and sustainability.

Customizing the CDI Program

Each facility has a unique set of goals and objectives for the CDI program. The members of the CDI taskforce should develop these objectives using a collaborative effort. This collaboration can bridge the gap between professionals such as "physicians, case management, coding professions, quality management, and financial services" (AHIMA 2014).

Possible goals and objectives for the program include

- Obtaining clinical documentation that captures the patient severity of illness and risk of mortality
- Identifying and clarifying missing, conflicting, or nonspecific physician documentation related to diagnoses and procedures
- Supporting accurate diagnostic and procedural coding and MS-DRG assignment, leading to appropriate reimbursement
- Promoting health record completion during the patient's course of care, which promotes patient safety
- Improving communication between physicians and other members of the healthcare team
- Providing awareness and education
- Improving documentation to reflect quality and outcome scores
- Improving coders' clinical knowledge (AHIMA 2014)

The CDI task force should add more goals and objectives based on the answers to the questions below. By reviewing the effectiveness of the current program and its success over time, the CDI task force can determine the best program type for the facility. The task force should understand which payers reimburse under a DRG-based system so the task force can include these payers in the CDI process. Once the task force identifies the payers, it needs to determine the annual patient volume for each payer to establish staffing levels. The task force should consider the collaborative efforts of the coding department related to the query process and how effective these efforts are in supporting the existing program. Some of the questions to consider include

- Is this a new or existing CDI program?
- How long has the program been in existence?
- Is the program effective?

- Has a new DRG system been implemented? If so, what type of DRG and which payer implemented the new system?
- Which payers reimburse based on DRGs and what type?
- What is the annual inpatient volume for these payers?
- Is adequate CDI staff available to cover the review of all DRG-based payers?
- Does the inpatient coding staff submit queries? If so, who tracks them?

Once the task force identifies the goals and objectives, it should select the approach best suited for the facility's needs. There are several types of customized approaches for the program, including

1. Implementing a new CDI program
2. Refreshing an existing CDI program
3. Staffing an existing CDI program
4. Comprehensively managing an existing CDI program

New CDI Program

Facilities should consider a new program if they have not implemented one in the past or if a past program is no longer functioning. There are key elements of a new program required for successful implementation and sustainability. A new program typically consists of five elements: governance, staffing, training, communication, and analytics. Each of the given have corresponding tasks listed below:

- Governance
    - Establishing a governance committee
    - Establishing a CDI task force
    - Monitoring the program
        - Analyzing monitoring reports
        - Auditing to determine root causes of identified issues
        - Developing a monthly action plan
        - Presenting to a governance committee quarterly (monthly during program start up)
- Staffing
    - Determining necessary staffing levels
    - Hiring CDI staff
- Training
    - Training medical staff
    - Training CDI and coding staff
        - Classroom
        - One-on-one
- Communication
    - Communicating at a high level with medical and ancillary department staff
    - Communicating and celebrating program success to stakeholders (medical staff, CDI professionals [CDIP], and coders)

- Analytics
  - Establishing standard analytic monitoring reports
  - Establishing target CMI benchmarks
  - Benchmarking against peer hospitals to determine possible reimbursement impact and quality issues
  - Determining which payers to include and annual inpatient volume
  - Analyzing data to determine the volume of patients under DRG payers

Refreshed CDI Program

The refreshed CDI program is a good option for facilities that already have a CDI program in place, but not operating at its maximum potential. This may be due to factors such as staff attrition, new staff requiring training, new medical staff requiring training, medical staff cooperation issues, new DRG-based payer, facility or physician-related quality score issues, and mortality indicator issues. When any of these circumstances occur, the organization may not need to implement all the steps for a new CDI program. Table 6.1 outlines factors requiring a refreshed program along with the required tasks for implementation.

Staffing Existing CDI Program

Staff attrition or a new DRG-based payer can result in staffing gaps that are difficult for organizations to fill. Organizations may have trouble finding an effective program without outside assistance. Consulting firms and staffing vendors offer contract CDIP staff that can fill positions or assist with hiring necessary staff.

Table 6.1 Factors/Tasks to Refreshing a CDI Program

FACTOR	RECOMMENDATION
Newly hired CDIP	Classroom or one-on-one training
New medical staff or medical staff cooperation issues	CDI presentations at department meetings, one-on-one with monitoring, one-on-one follow-up
New DRG based payer	Analytics to determine volume, focused DRGs and impact potential, physician education, CDIP and coder classroom and one-to-one training, revision of standard analytic reports to governance, monitor progress and feedback loop to education
Quality or mortality score issues	Analytics to determine root cause, case audit to determine whether coding or clinical documentation issue, education for physicians, CDIP and coders, monitoring for improvement and feedback loop to education

These companies provide complete staffing project management, including hiring, training, and transitioning vendor staff to facility employees. Using a staffing company is the quickest way to staff a program. As the organization hires and trains employees, it can replace the vendor staff. If the budget does not allow for this option, organizations can hire and train employees over a period of three to four months.

Comprehensive Management of Existing CDI Program

When the facility does not have a CDI manager with the experience and skills necessary to oversee a program, the organization can bring in a consultant manager to establish or maintain the program. The consultant assists with hiring an experienced manager and provides training once the manager arrives. This management option works for large programs that require extensive oversight beyond the capability of current management due to time requirements or lack of appropriate experience and skill sets. The program includes a contract manager who steps in to establish or refresh an existing program. A facility manager may be present as a trainee in the process. The contract manager completes all the necessary steps as specified above. In addition, the manager brings contract staff as necessary to fill open positions until the facility hires and trains staff. This option also works when CDIP staff is new and requires classroom and one-on-one training. The one-on-one training is most effective when there is a three to one student ratio. Large facilities may need more than one trainer. The contract manager establishes a standard set of analytics to track the success of the program and is accountable to the governance committee and department director.

Conclusion

It is essential for every organization to develop a vision statement for its CDI program. This statement guides the organization and its physicians towards the ultimate key outcomes of CDI: high-quality care, high-perceived quality, improved patient satisfaction, and accurate reimbursement. It is important to involve the correct stakeholders when creating the vision. It is also important to involve physicians in the vision process as well as in the initial communication to medical staff.

The CEO should take the lead in communicating with the medical staff about the CDI program. However, the organization should inform physician leaders and physician employees about the program first so they are available to respond to questions and concerns that members of the medical staff may have about the CDI program. These activities are likely to improve the success and sustainability of the program. The type of CDI program best suited for the organization is an important consideration.

Chapter Quiz

1. What is one important reason for having a CDI vision statement?
   A. It is usually part of the administrative operating policy.
   B. It provides a purpose for the program.
   C. It provides justification for the investment in CDI.
   D. The Joint Commission requires it for certification.

2. Prior to creating a vision statement for clinical documentation and CDI, what is the first necessary step?
   A. Hold an HIM interdepartmental meeting for suggestions
   B. Invite discussion by essential leaders in areas that might impact CDI process
   C. Let the leading physicians and hospital directors design a rough draft
   D. Browse the Internet for peer recommendations and suggestions

3. Which committee should be comprised of executive management, a physician advisor, a leader for clinical documentation and CDI, and the manager of a CDI program?
   A. Operational
   B. Executive leadership
   C. Clinical documentation improvement
   D. Oversight

4. What committee is comprised of individuals responsible for day-to-day management and support for the CDI program?
   A. Executive leadership
   B. Oversight
   C. Clinical documentation improvement
   D. Operational

5. What is the most essential role the oversight committee plays?
   A. Supervise the design of follow-up training for physicians
   B. Obtain and maintain support from the medical staff
   C. Oversee training of physicians and other clinicians
   D. Obtain contract resources to support day-to-day needs

6. Which hospital leader should provide the initial announcement for the CDI program the organization installs?
   A. Director of HIM
   B. Chief information officer
   C. Chief medical officer
   D. Chief executive officer

7. When refreshing an existing CDI program, what is one of the recommendations when quality or mortality scores decline?
   A. Case audit to determine if it is a coding or clinical documentation issue
   B. Analytics to determine focused DRG's impact
   C. Request operational oversight committee re-evaluate data
   D. Review major complications or comorbidities compared to peer data

8. What is one of the key concepts in communication regarding CDI the organization should consider?
   A. High-quality graphics
   B. The cost of the communication
   C. What media the organization will use to communicate it
   D. Use of word of mouth

9. What is the key to success and sustainability of the CDI program?
   A. Physician support
   B. Quality vision statement
   C. Executive communication
   D. Clinical documentation improvement

10. The operational committee is responsible for which process on an ongoing basis?
   A. Communicating with medical staff
   B. Querying for high-quality clinical documentation
   C. Revising the vision statement
   D. Analyzing metrics for program success

REFERENCES

45 CFR 160.101, 164.102(a), and 164.500(e). HIPAA Privacy Rule. 1996. http://www.access.gpo.gov/nara/cfr/waisidx_07/45cfr160_07.html.

AHIMA. 2014. Clinical Documentation Toolkit. Retrieved from: http://library.ahima.org/xpedio/groups/secure/documents/ahima/bok1_050585.pdf.

Collins, J. 2001. *Good to Great: Why Some Companies Make the Leap… And Others Don't.* New York: Harper Collins Publishers.

Gunter, K. 2002. The HIPAA privacy rule: Practical advice for academic and research institutions. *Healthcare Financial Management* 56(2):50–56.

Johnson, D.E. 2001. HIPAA is a new weapon and career opportunity. *Heath Care Strategic Management* 19(2):2–3.

Patterson, K., J. Grenny, R. McMillan, and A. Switzler. 2002. *Crucial Conversations: Tools for Talking When Stakes are High.* New York: McGraw Hill.

Porras, G., and J. Collins. 1996. *Built to Last: Successful Habits of Visionary Companies.* New York: Harper Collins Publishers.

Russo, R. 2008. *A Compelling Case for Clinical Documentation: Use Clinical Documentation to Achieve Strategic Alignment with Your Medical Staff,* volume 1. Bethlehem, PA: DJ Iber Publishing.

Part II

Implementing a Clinical Documentation Program

Chapter

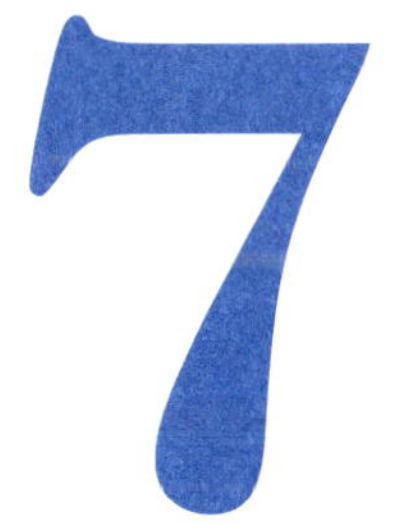

Staffing the Program

The clinical documentation improvement (CDI) program needs structure to ensure continued success and sustainability. When considering the structure to support the program, an organization must address clinical documentation at four levels: reporting, management, staffing, and physician leadership. The organization should apply general guidelines for staffing and management within the context of its dynamics. Every organization is unique in its culture and dynamics. Ultimate success in clinical documentation depends on tailoring the program's structure to fit the organization.

Program Reporting

Before making any structural determinations, an organization should decide to which C-suite executive the CDI program will ultimately report. Because the program involves clinical documentation and relies upon physicians for success, the chief medical officer (CMO) or vice president of the medical staff is the optimal reporting structure. In organizations with a new or less than optimal medical staff management function, it may be necessary to design a different short-term strategy. Implementing a new function requires strong leadership. Organizations can use the recommendations presented in this chapter to develop the best long-term strategy for CDI program management and support, but in the short term, the CDI program staff may need to report to another administrative function that ultimately reports to the chief executive officer (CEO) or chief operating officer (COO), with a dotted-line reporting relationship to the CMO.

⊙ Physician Leaders

Physician leadership is essential to a successful and sustainable CDI program (Marco and Buchman 2003; Keogh and Martin 2004). Ideally, a program should incorporate four levels of physician leadership: two official levels and two unofficial levels. The two official levels of leadership include the physician at the executive level and the physician designated as the CDI program advisor or leader. In addition, the organization should develop physician CDI leaders within the medical staff and within the medical staff leadership group.

First, the physician executive in charge of the CDI program should preferably be the CMO or the vice president of medical affairs. This executive must be involved in designing and communicating the clinical documentation program from the start. The physician executive should also be involved in identifying other physicians who support and manage the program and who encourage the entire medical staff.

Second, the CDI program must have a physician officially designated as the physician leader for CDI, also known as the physician advisor or champion. Ideally, this physician should be a full-time employee of the hospital. However, for smaller organizations, the physician may be a part-time employee. Organizations without appropriate resources to support the program with physician management can contract with an external organization with expertise in clinical documentation. This strategy should be temporary until the organization secures its own physician leader for the program.

The physician leader for CDI should have experience and expertise consistent with the responsibilities demanded by the CDI program, as listed in table 7.1. The physician leader must be involved in all formal training provided to physicians. The physician leader also serves in a support role to the CDI program specialists. The leader should be available to answer questions the program staff has and assist in particularly challenging reviews. When the CDI specialist encounters a problematic physician, the physician leader is responsible for obtaining cooperation from the physician. The physician leader for CDI serves on the oversight and operations committees. Finally, the physician leader oversees the clinical documentation audits and makes judgment calls when there are particularly challenging documentation problems. Ideally, the physician CDI program leader should report directly to the CMO. Depending on the organization size and if the physician leader is a full-time employee, the physician may manage the entire CDI function, or the program

Table 7.1 Responsibilities of the physician leader for CDI

Responsibilities of the Physician Leader for CDI
• Conducts initial and follow-up clinical documentation training with program staff • Manages physician responsiveness to queries and cooperation with program staff • Supports CDI specialists • Assists in CDI reviews that are particularly challenging • Manages clinical documentation audits • Serves on the oversight and operations CDI committees

staff may report directly to the CMO or other executive level manager. Table 7.1 presents the general responsibilities of the physician leader for CDI.

The physician leader for CDI should have certain experience and qualifications. "In general, the physician advisor will act as a liaison between CDI specialists, [health information management (HIM)] coders, and providers to facilitate complete and accurate documentation to support the diagnosis, treatment, medical necessity, and severity of illness, which in turn substantiate accurate code assignment and correct DRG assignment" (AHIMA 2014). Ideally, the physician leader should be well versed in the principles of high-quality clinical documentation, but the right individual can learn this skill. CDI specialists usually accomplish this by educating healthcare providers to

- Correlate between clinical language and coding guidelines
- Reflect the true picture of a patient's severity of illness
- Capture services, treatment, and utilization for the organizations
- Translate classification codes to individual physician profiles
- Ensure documentation supports code assignments
- Interpret coded data in quality measures and reporting
- Understand payment methodologies (AHIMA 2014)

CDI specialists can also accomplish this by collaborating with HIM coding to

- Review health record documentation on a concurrent and retrospective basis
- Discuss clinical issues identified in record review activities such as specificity of congestive heart failure (CHF)
- Discuss clinical criteria for disease processes, such as sepsis or respiratory failure
- Assist in developing appropriate and compliant provider queries
- Review hospital-acquired conditions (HACs) and treatment complications (AHIMA 2014)

When the physician leader for CDI does not have existing expertise in CDI, the organization can bring in an external physician to teach and temporarily supplement the responsibilities of the physician leader (Russo 2008).

Table 7.2 contains the qualifications of a physician leader for CDI. The table includes two columns, one for the ideal qualifications and one for minimum qualifications. Because it is so difficult to find physicians trained in the CDI process, organizations can use the minimum qualifications to identify a physician who they can then train further on CDI processes.

In addition to the official physician program support, it is also important to ensure the structure allows the development of unofficial physician supporters for the CDI program. This activity should be a designated responsibility of both the CMO (regardless of the reporting relationship) and the physician leader for CDI. The organization should charge these leaders with obtaining support for CDI from service chiefs, any physicians employed by the healthcare organization, and the

Table 7.2 Qualifications of a physician leader for CDI

Skill	Ideal	Minimum
Formal education	Currently licensed MD or DO; board certified in specialty of physicians in the training group	Currently licensed MD or DO
Training received in clinical documentation	40 hours or more; certification	At least 40 hours
Experience in clinical documentation	5 years of practice; currently treating patients	3 years of practice and currently treating patients on at least a part- time basis
Experience providing classroom instruction	40 hours or more of classroom instruction	At least 40 hours of classroom instruction
Experience providing practical instruction	100 hours or more of on-unit or in-office instruction including observation and feedback	At least 40 hours of on-unit or in-office instruction including observation and feedback
Communication	Ability to negotiate with peers	Ability to negotiate with peers

unofficial physician leaders who are on the medical staff. The CMO is likely to have more success with obtaining support from physicians in most of these situations, but the physician leader for CDI should be involved in the relationship development activities as well.

The advent of the electronic health record (EHR) came with improvements as well as challenges related to clinical documentation. Overall, the EHR has increased the amount of documentation based largely on the ease of entry. Physicians can now enter clinical information in templates by selecting key words or phrases from a drop down menu or by adding free text. Templates are an excellent tool for the physician leader or advisor to use for CDI. As the program staff identifies CDI issues, the physician advisor should consider if the use of a template can correct the problem. For example, where further specificity is missing from a diagnosis of CHF, the CHF template provides automated drop down options for acute versus chronic and diastolic versus systolic. If a template provides the solution, the physician advisor and CDI team leader should meet with the physician department chair and the IT department to develop a solution. One change of this nature can eliminate the need for hundreds of queries.

Beyond the template, the health information system scans the clinical record and identifies key terminology for answering questions related to specificity. Figure 7.1, CHF CDI EHR Work Flow, provides a technology-based solution to gather specificity for CHF in the clinical record. In figure 7.1, the physician documents heart failure in the EHR. The system pop-up appears whether the documentation reflects CHF or heart failure. This process also includes a reminder to the physician to consider ordering an echocardiogram if the patient has not had

Figure 7.1 CHF CDI EHR workflow

Attending physician enters heart failure in patient record
1) CHF
2) Congestive heart failure
3) Heart failure
Echocardiogram within last 6 mo?
NO
System Pop-up "Is there an Echocardiogram order?
YES
System Pop-up Showing results of echo or cardiac cath report
Physician orders echocardiogram results recorded in system
Echo results indicate CHF?
NO
Ejection fraction in cardiac cath report or clinical record <= 35%?
YES
Should ejection fraction be recorded as a final diagnosis?
NO
END
YES
Pop-up physician query "For diagnosis of heart failure, do the following apply? Acute, acute on chronic, diastolic, systolic?"
YES
Physician response to query
NO
YES
Pop-up box selection:
• Acute
• Chronic
• Acute on Chronic
• Diastolic
• Systolic
HIM coder assigns CC/MCC
HIM coder assigns Unspecified CHF no CC/MCC assignment

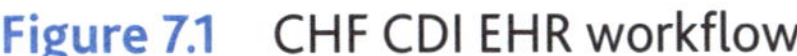

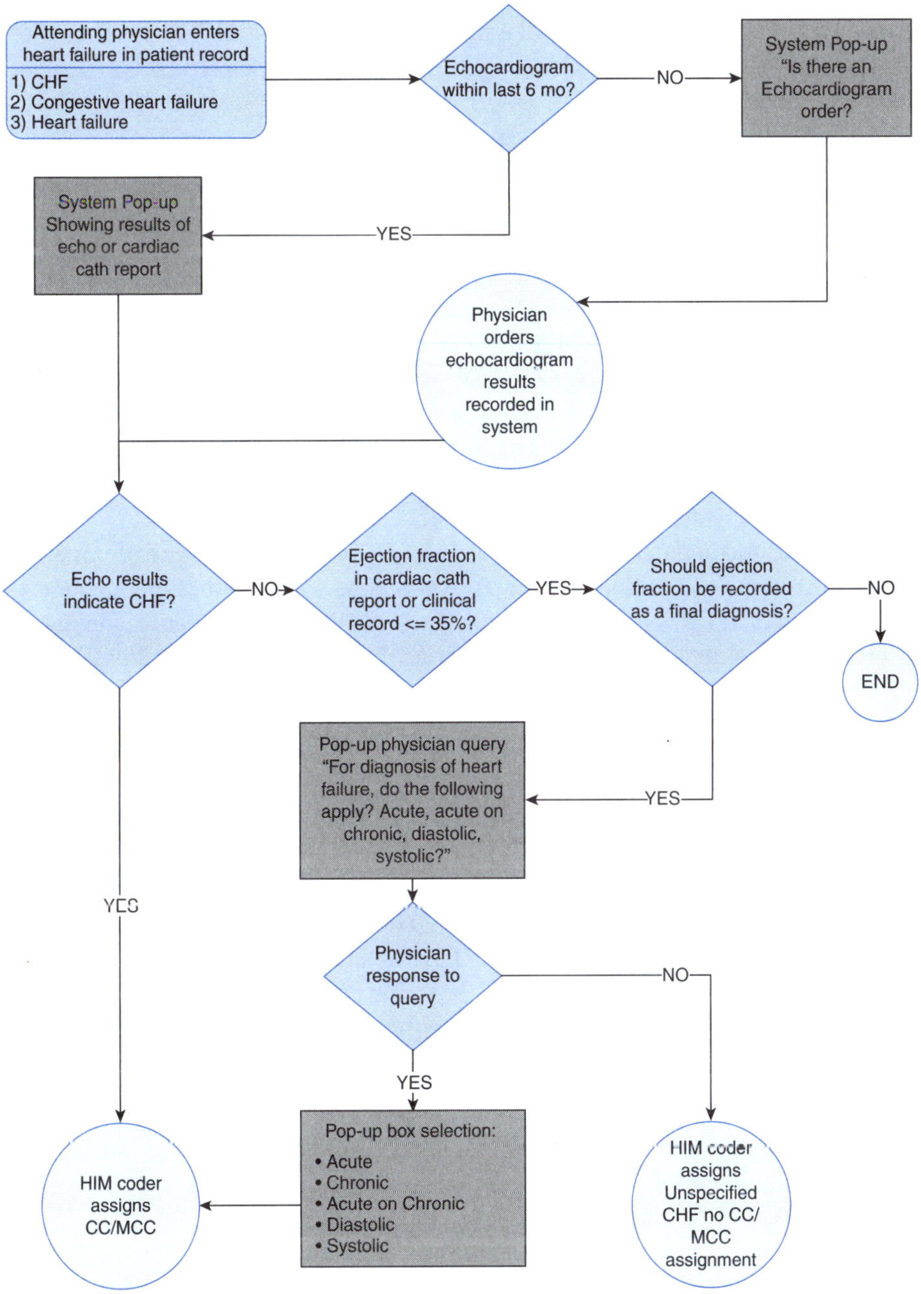

one in six months. If the provider performed the procedures, he or she provides the results of the echocardiogram for the physician. The physician is asked by the system to view the ejection fraction and to consider any value below 35 percent when documenting the final diagnosis. A system pop-up box appears showing the physician the key phrases: acute, chronic, acute on chronic, diastolic, and systolic. The use of templates and pop-up alerts can greatly improve the clinical specificity needed for accurate International Classification of Diseases (ICD) code assignment. For more information using technology for CDI, refer to chapter 16.

Program Management

The structure of the program depends on the size of the organization as well as how many functions the organization initially staffs for CDI. Reporting relationships vary throughout the industry. The CDI manager may report to the HIM, quality, or case management director. If the CDI manager is at the director level, the reporting relationship may be with the CMO, CFO, or revenue-cycle vice president. However, except in large organizations or organizations with long-term CDI in all areas, this structure is unlikely to be effective or efficient for the organization. It is probable the CDI program manager will initially report to a director for another function. Therefore, the CDI program structure should address both program management and the day-to-day department reporting structure.

If clinical documentation will not be an independent department initially in the organization, where does it belong? Common, workable options include the departments of HIM, case management, and quality management. The specific criteria for choosing a department that houses the CDI function should include the following:

- The efficiency and effectiveness of the department—The best choice is a department that has met or exceeded its key metrics consistently for at least the last three years. It is difficult for an efficiently run department to take on new responsibilities and nearly impossible for an inefficient department to do so.
- A visionary department director—CDI is a dynamic concept for most organizations. The manager of the CDI function must be capable of creative, out-of-the-box thinking for the program to be successful. A well-oiled department with a manager who has been responsible for the same three functions for the past 10 years is not the best choice for housing the CDI function.

Every organization is different in terms of strengths and weaknesses. Organizations that apply these criteria when choosing the function location have an increased chance of success (Grol et al. 2002).

Most organizations require a separate CDI management position. This individual is responsible for managing the clinical documentation staff, all training, and the query process, collecting program data, and reporting key metrics, as well as representing the CDI program as a committee member. In some organizations, the CDI program manager may also be responsible for reviewing records, being visible on the unit, and querying physicians when appropriate. The CDI program manager interacts regularly with the physician leader for CDI.

The CDI program manager should have some clinical or HIM background, record review experience, and extensive experience in training, especially with physicians. In addition, the manager should have experience with healthcare coding and reimbursement systems. The manager must also be able to communicate effectively with physicians, motivate staff, and be comfortable with ambiguity and change. When the CDI program is new or the organization is refreshing an existing program, the program needs to morph into a functional operations unit so the CDI manager can look ahead. Figure 7.2 shows a sample position description for a CDI program manager. This organization combined the CDI manager position duties with some reimbursement-related activities to make the position into a full-time position. Depending on the organization's needs, the specifics of the duties for the CDI manager may vary.

Figure 7.2 Clinical documentation improvement manager position description

Job Description: Clinical Documentation Improvement Manager

General description:
The manager of documentation improvement and reimbursement is responsible for ensuring that clinical documentation within the health system is consistent with the services and care provided to patients. The manager acts as a coordinator of physician clinical documentation, coding, and reimbursement processes in working towards high-quality clinical documentation and meeting key metrics for all services provided in the system.

Experience:

The successful candidate should:

1. Have a minimum of five years work experience in coding and health information management with progressive management responsibilities
2. Be familiar with all government healthcare reimbursement systems
3. Have experience working collaboratively with diverse groups in a healthcare environment
4. Be successful in interacting effectively with physicians
5. Possess excellent speaking, writing, and teaching skills
6. Have the ability to analyze large amounts of data to identify trends

Education:

1. Bachelor's degree in health information management, nursing, or equivalent
2. Current certification in a health information management or coding discipline recommended
3. If not a clinician, must have completed clinical coursework with the ability to understand disease processes

Specific responsibilities:

Interdisciplinary:

The manager of documentation improvement and reimbursement will function primarily as an interdisciplinary functional manager who focuses on ensuring physician documentation meets criteria for high quality clinical documentation. To that end, the manager will have access to physicians and clinical staff to participate in and assist in ensuring the ongoing documentation improvement effort is successful.

The manager:

1. Coordinates the activities of the documentation improvement committee
2. Ensures that the documentation improvement committee is continuously used primarily as a vehicle to promote documentation improvement for accurate reimbursement on an ongoing basis
3. Oversees the documentation improvement efforts of clinical documentation specialists and other program staff as necessary
4. Provides ongoing education to medical staff on documentation concerns
5. Works with finance department on continuous case mix modeling and assessment
6. Participates in the rejections and claims review process with patient accounting to ensure both compliance and accurate reimbursement
7. Tracks trends in documentation concerns and implements corrective action
8. Directs coding activities to ensure accurate, consistent, and compliant coding for all services
9. Creates and updates documentation tools on an ongoing basis
10. Uses the claims denials, auditing, and testing processes to design and conduct follow-up CDI education with physicians

Inpatient services:

1. Tracks case mix through both retrospective and concurrent means
2. Provides feedback to clinical documentation improvement specialists, case managers, coders, physicians, and other clinicians involved in the documentation improvement effort
3. Recommends and implements corrective actions when deficiencies are identified

Outpatient services:

1. Designs a case mix tracking system for APCs
2. Implements a documentation improvement program for outpatient services

3. Recommends and implements corrective actions when deficiencies are identified

Physician services:

1. Designs a documentation proficiency tracking system for system-based pro-fee billing and coding
2. Implements a documentation improvement program for pro-fee billing and coding
3. Recommends and implements corrective actions when deficiencies are identified

Benchmarks:

1. Measures the effectiveness of documentation tools
2. Trends and quantifies the effectiveness of coding
3. Evaluates the success of concurrent documentation improvement on an ongoing basis

Program Staff

The CDI program staff members, or CDI specialists, are responsible for the day-to-day activities of the program. Initially, the activities consist of training and record review. Once initial training for all physicians and clinicians finishes, the program staff focuses on record review, querying, and ongoing physician education. They may also be involved in conducting follow-up education with physicians. In addition, as clinical documentation activities expand into various patient care areas, the CDI specialists may have the opportunity to take on additional responsibilities.

The CDI specialists should have a clinical or health information background with record review experience. They should be able to effectively communicate with physicians and skillfully review clinical documentation to determine where it fails to meet the criteria for high quality. Experience with computer programs, data entry, and data analysis is very important. They should be effective trainers. In addition, current or prior experience in the healthcare organization is helpful. Prior experience with clinical documentation training and record review using the criteria for high-quality clinical documentation is ideal. It is likely that many organizations will need to provide initial training to new clinical documentation improvement practitioners (CDIPs), so experience and qualifications will be the determining factors in deciding whom to hire. The organization should manage the employment interview as an investigative process. The interviewer(s) should have experience in CDI management as well as a list of relevant questions. Figure 7.3 is a list of questions interviewers can use when interviewing candidates for a CDI specialist position (AHIMA Toolkit 2014).

Figure 7.3 Questions for prospective CDI specialist

SAMPLE INTERVIEW QUESTIONS FOR A CDI SPECIALIST

Knowledge and Skills Questions:
Financial: Describe your understanding of a case mix index (CMI), diagnosis-related groups (DRGs), major complications and comorbidities (MCCs), and complications and comorbidities (CCs).
How is CDI important to the organization's revenue cycle?
Clinical: Where would you expect to find clinical documentation in a health record?
How much clinical training or experience do you have?
The CDI specialist position requires clinical knowledge. What references would you need as a part of this position and why?
Coding: What is a principal diagnosis?
What is a secondary diagnosis?
How often are ICD codes updated?
Interpersonal: Explain a situation in which you have had to compromise and why?
How would you interact with a negative person?
Communication: Give me an example of how you have communicated a difficult decision.
What is your preferred mode of communication, verbal or written, and why?
Leadership: Tell me about a leadership position you have been in, professionally or personally.
Are you a member of a professional association? Why and for how long?
Team Player: Tell me about the best team you have been a part of professionally or personally.
Explain what a high-functioning team is.
When working on a team, what role do you usually take and why?
Organization: How do you organized yourself each day?
How do you achieve a work-life balance?

Behavior Questions:
Positive: Tell me about a time in your life that you have been disappointed and why.
How do you handle a challenge? Give me an example.
How do you find ways to make sure your job is more rewarding?
Outgoing: What motivates you and why?
Tell me about a time you had to use your verbal communication skills in order to convey an important point.
Give me an example of when you have had to "read" or "gauge" another person during an interaction.
Energetic: Tell me about your favorite activities.
Share an example of how you motivate others.
Give me an example of when you did more than what an employer expected of you.
Independent: Tell me about a time when you were responsible for a project.
Give me an example of a goal that you reached and explain how you achieved it.
Responsible: Who is your role model and why?
Tell me about a time when you worked effectively under pressure.
How do you handle a variety of different functions in your job?
Flexible: Tell me about a time when you have had to make a last-minute schedule change.
Tell me about a time when you had to develop an innovative approach to completing a task or assignment.
How do you minimize stress in your life?

(Source: AHIMA CDI Toolkit 2014)

Health Information and Coding Interface

The goal of every CDI program is to obtain high-quality documentation on a patient's record while the patient is still in house. A program staff member can obtain some degree of concurrent documentation quality through training. The member must achieve the rest of the documentation goal by using a record review and query process. An effective program should be able to capture 70 to 75 percent of query responses concurrently. Someone needs to obtain the remainder retrospectively. The most efficient way to capture retrospective queries is through the coding process (Russo 2001). Therefore, it is essential to have the coding staff interface with the CDI program staff. The coding staff should understand when there are outstanding concurrent queries upon discharge of the patient. The coding professional should generate a retrospective query to the physician so long as the justification for the query still exists when the patient is discharged. Depending on the program structure, the CDI staff may or may not be directly reporting to the HIM department. Wherever the program reports, the CDI program manager should ensure there is a daily interface between the CDI specialists and the coding staff.

Figure 7.4 illustrates a CDI program structure that shows interface and integration with both the departments of case management and HIM. In this example, the CDI function does not report to either function directly, and uses physician liaisons to assist with continuing program interfaces.

Figure 7.4 Sample clinical documentation improvement organization chart

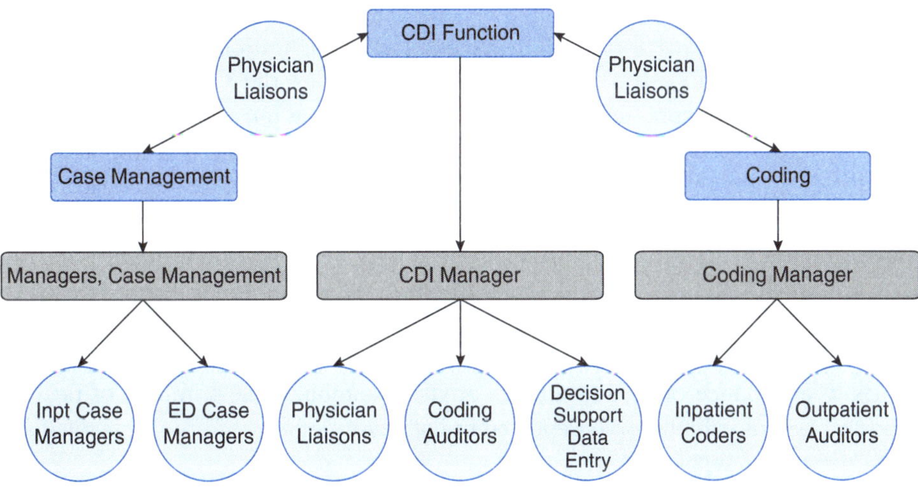

CDI Implementation Workplans

The primary stakeholder of the CDI program (for example, the manager, consultant, or physician leader) should prepare a project work plan to keep the program on track. The work plan should include the tasks required for both implementation and on-going monitoring, the responsible party, due date, completion date, the status of the task, and a comment field. The CDI task force that oversees the operations of the project should discuss the workplan and determine steps, time frame, and responsibilities of each task. Workplan vary with the goals and objectives of the program.

New CDI Program

Table 7.3 provides the steps for implementing a new CDI program. The plan includes the required key work steps. As the organization establishes more detailed work steps, they should add them to the plan. For example, detailed work steps for task number 1 might include

- Identifying software available to create analytic reports. These reports may be identified by internal information technology [IT], finance, or an external consulting firm.
  - Schedule a meeting with the consulting firm or the finance and IT departments, and the team leader
  - View a demonstration of the software
  - Discuss the demonstration and make a decision on the source of reports
  - Obtain consulting firm proposals
  - Contract with consulting firm
  - Obtain benchmarking reports
- Reviewing benchmarking reports and establishing target CMI (overall, medical, and surgical)
- Establishing a list of high-volume high-risk focused MS-DRGS for an audit

Table 7.3 represents a new CDI program implementation workplan example using a Microsoft Excel spreadsheet. Step 1 includes the CDI assessment the organization should conduct prior to the program. The purpose of this task is to identify the CDI program's potential impact. Peer benchmarking is important for this step. The industry standard is the 80th percentile CMI benchmark for the facility peer group (3M 2012). Refer to table 7.4 for an example of a peer facility CMI comparison report. After reviewing the peer benchmark and identifying the potential impact, the next step is to set the target CMI for the program. Based on the example in table 7.4, the peer benchmark CMI for the bed size 400 to 599 is 1.8945 for both medical and surgical services. The average peer CMI is 1.7788. This results in a variance of 0.0803 and a potential reimbursement impact of positive $1,932,671. This calculation is repeated in the example report for both medical and surgical services separately.

After establishing the CMI targets, the next step (task number 2) is the audit process. The organization should select a sample of 50 to 100 high-volume cases with CC and without MCC and CC for review. The review should include an evaluation of accurate coding and opportunity for query based on clinical indicators. The organization should identify and extrapolate the potential reimbursement impact of the change in MS-DRG for the sample cases over the total annual number of cases with CC and without MCC and CC. This number is also an indicator of the

Table 7.3 New CDI program implementation workplan

New CDI Implementation Workplan						
Task #	**Task**	**Responsible Party**	**Due Date**	**Completion Date**	**Status**	**Comments**
Phase 1						
1	Conduct CDI assessment with analytics to include target CMI, focused MS-DRGs, and reimbursement impact	Finance Director or Consultant	Mar 2014	Mar 2014	Complete	
2	Conduct coding/clinical documentation audit of 50-100 records on focused MS-DRG to validate findings	Consultant	Mar 2014	Mar 2014	Complete	
3	Establish CDI Governance Committee (CEO, CMO, CFO, CDI Physician Advisor, Medical Staff Department Chiefs, HIM Director, Nursing Director, Finance Director, Care Management Director, CDI Manager/Director (Team Lead))	CMO,CFO and or CDI Team Leader	Apr 2014	Apr 2014	Complete	
4	Establish CDI Task Force (CDI Physician Advisor, HIM Director, Nursing Director, Finance Director, Care Management Director, CDI Manager/ Director (Team Lead))	Team Leader	Apr 2014	Apr 2014	Complete	
5	Determine DRG based payers and patient volumes that will be included in concurrent review	Finance Director or Consultant	Apr 2014	Apr 2014	Complete	
6	Determine staffing levels required for program (one CDIP per 2500 annual discharges)	Team Leader	Apr 2014	Apr 2014	Complete	
7	Determine outside consulting support if needed, establish budget and start date	Team Leader	May 2014	May 2014	Complete	
8	Interview and hire CDIP staff	Team Leader	May 2014		In Progress	
9	Develop or purchase classroom program content (include key body systems: neurology, respiratory, circulatory, GI, hepatobiliary, musculoskeletal, integumentary, endocrine, renal, blood diseases, and infectious disease)	Team Leader or Consultant	Jun 2014		Pending	
10	Determine staff requiring training (CDIP, coders, and physicians)	CMO, Team Leader	Jun 2014		Pending	
11	Identify method of capturing concurrent review information (recommend tracking software)	Team Leader or Consultant	Jun 2014		Pending	

(Continued)

Table 7.3 New CDI program implementation workplan *(Continued)*

New CDI Implementation Workplan						
Task #	**Task**	**Responsible Party**	**Due Date**	**Completion Date**	**Status**	**Comments**
12	Plan and conduct two-week classroom training (Include body system chapter discussions, corresponding case discussions of audits conducted in step two, and method of capturing review data (software or worksheet))	Team Leader	Jun 2014		Pending	
13	Determine number of concurrent review trainers needed for six weeks one-on-one (recommend three trainers to one staff trainee)	Team Leader and consultant	Jun 2014		Pending	
14	Develop plan for one-on-one including target number of reviews per day and nursing unit assignments	Team Leader	Jun 2014		Pending	
15	Conduct concurrent review training	Team Leader and consultant	Jul 2014			
16	Organize meeting with Chief Medical Officer (CMO) to plan physician training program	Physician Advisor and Team Leader	Jun 2014		Pending	
17	Schedule, communicate, and present medical staff CDI education	Physician Advisor and Team Leader	Jun 2014		Pending	
Phase II - On-going Monitoring						
18	Determine source of tracking reports to monitor program (recommend software)	Team Leader	Jun 2014		Pending	
19	Schedule Governance (quarterly) and Task Force meetings (monthly)	Team Leader	Jun 2014		Pending	
20	Review monthly monitoring reports	Governance Committee, Task Force, Team Leader	Sept 2014		Pending	
21	Conduct quarterly audits of cases concurrently and post-coding to determine coding issues and missed queries (recommend external audit resource)	Consultant	Oct 2014		Pending	
22	Develop remediation plan including stakeholder (physician, CDIP, coder) education	Consultant	Oct 2014		Pending	

Table 7.4 Peer Facility CMI Comparison

Bed Size	400-599
Facility	Sample Medical Center
Hospital Specific Rate	$5,000.00
Program Begin Period	May-15
MedPAR Fiscal Yr	2012

MS-DRG Payers	ALL MS-DRGs		MEDICAL MS-DRGs		SURGICAL MS-DRGs	
Annual Volume	**National Data (MedPAR 2012)**	**Facility Data**	**National Data (MedPAR 2012)**	**Facility Data**	**National Data (MedPAR 2012)**	**Facility Data**
Medicare Cases	6,987,648	4,812	4,288,069	3 655	2,699,579	1,157
National Average/Facility CMI Baseline	1.7788	1.8142	1.5659	1.6425	2.6715	2.5991
National CMI Benchmark (80th %)	1 8945		1.6971		2.7607	
CMI Variance		0.0803		0.0546		0.1616
Reimbursement Impact		**$1,932,671**		**$997,815**		**$934,856**
Capture Rates						
MCC	26.20%	24.88%	29.87%	26.59%	22.53%	21.70%
CC	24.18%	21.94%	25.15%	23.42%	23.21%	19.33%
WO	49.62%	46.13%	44.98%	41.23%	54.25%	51.06%
National MCC	33.92%		36.77%		31.06%	
National CC	30.18%		28.64%		31.71%	

potential impact of the program and a validation for the peer comparison report. Organizations should use cases within the audit with coding or missing queries as sample cases during classroom training.

The third task provides for the establishment of an oversight or governance committee. It is essential that the key stakeholders are involved and visible in the program. Members of the governance committee should include the CEO, the CMO, the chief financial officer (CFO), the CDI physician advisor, the medical staff department chiefs, the HIM director, the nursing director, the finance director, the care management director, and the CDI manager or director (team lead).

The fourth task includes creating a CDI task force as the working committee that oversees the day-to-day project and the completion of most tasks. The committee should include the same participants as the governance committee.

Task numbers 5 through 7 involve identifying the target patient population. The organization should review all DRG payers concurrently through the CDI program. Each DRG system has unique coding and clinical documentation challenges. The CDI program should address each for accurate reimbursement and reflection of patient severity and quality levels. Industry surveys show that 30 percent of the hospitals surveyed report full-time equivalent (FTE) to annual patient discharges at 2,000 or higher (ACDIS 2010). That many discharges per FTE is a challenging yet achievable target to use for estimating staffing levels. Consider outside consulting support for the classroom and one-on-one training. These activities are time consuming and may not be possible for facility managers with other daily operational duties. It is also important to have subject matter experts who have implemented successful programs in the past. Check references for consultants and ask if the programs implemented were sustainable over time. In addition, consulting firms offer software for monitoring the program, daily input, case review data, and tracking concurrent review activities including queries and responses.

The eighth task includes interviewing and hiring staff, which is a critical success factor for the CDI program. Refer to the program staff section above for recommendations on staff selection.

Tasks 9 through 17 involve training key stakeholders (physicians, CDIPs, and coders). CDIPs and coders often participate in a two-week formal classroom program. The classroom training includes discussions on these major disease classifications (MDCs): neurology, respiratory, circulatory, gastrointestinal, hepatobiliary, musculoskeletal, integumentary, endocrine, renal, blood diseases, and infectious disease. The group should discuss actual cases identified during the audit in task number 2. During the discussion, each trainee should be allowed to present a case discussion. The leaders can successfully deliver one-on-one training by using one trainer for every three to four trainees. The trainer will first show the student how to review a case, and then ask the student to review and present findings. The one-on-one training should last a minimum of six weeks. The physician advisor, chiefs of the medical service, and the CDI team leader should hold a meeting to discuss physician training. The leaders need to consider carefully the type of communication they provide to the medical staff regarding the CDI program and training. Use the approach "less is better" with the physician sessions. Short presentations of 10 to 15 minutes that focus on one or two concepts with one or two examples are most successful.

Tasks 18 through 22 relate to phase II of the program, which includes tracking the program's success. This is done via monitoring reports created internally with the IT and finance departments' support or by purchasing software designed for this purpose. The CDI task force should review reports monthly. The task force should conduct a quarterly presentation for the CDI governance committee. Keeping the senior executives involved ensures that the program be visible to the entire facility. The task force should share program success not only with the governance group but also with the stakeholders (physicians, CDIPs, and coders).

Refresh CDI Program

It is not difficult to find a CDI program that is no longer effective. This can occur for various reasons such as staff attrition, lack of senior executive support, lack of high-level program visibility within the organization, budget constraints, or medical staff complacency. The tasks required to refresh the program vary with the facility's current situation. The original governance committee should discuss the current program's successes and failures in detail and create a new set of goals and objectives. Next, the task force can begin developing a refresh CDI workplan. The task force should carefully consider the current staffing levels, existing medical staff support and compliance, tracking and concurrent review software effectiveness, and workflow of the CDI process related to concurrent review and coding. The task force should identify any or all of these factors prior to developing the workplan. Table 7.5 provides a sample refresh CDI workplan.

Conclusion

Every clinical documentation program must have structure and support to ensure its success and sustainability. Program management should include both a physician leader and a CDI manager. Program staffing should be composed, at least initially, of CDI specialists charged with concurrent querying and training, who interface regularly with coding professionals on the retrospective query process. In the ideal structure, the CDI program reports directly to the CMO. In organizations where this direct reporting relationship is not possible, it is still important to ensure the program reports up through the CMO or that there is a dotted-line reporting relationship between the CDI function and the CMO.

Table 7.5 Refresh CDI Implementation Workplan

Task #	Task	Responsible Party	Due Date	Completion Date	Status	Comments
Phase 1						
1	Conduct CDI assessment with analytics to include target CMI, focused MS-DRGs, and reimbursement impact	Finance Director or Consultant	Mar 2014	Mar 2014	Complete	
2	Conduct coding/clinical documentation audit of 50-100 records on focused MS-DRG to validate findings	Consultant	Mar 2014	Mar 2014	Complete	
3	Reconvene CDI Governance Committee (CEO, CMO, CFO, CDI Physician Advisor, Medical Staff Department Chiefs, HIM Director, Nursing Director, Finance Director, Care Management Director, CDI Manager/Director (Team Lead))	CMO, CFO, and/or CDI Team Leader	Apr 2014	Apr 2014	Complete	
4	Reconvene CDI Task Force (CDI Physician Advisor, HIM Director, Nursing Director, Finance Director, Care Management Director, CDI Manager/Director (Team Lead))	Team Leader	Apr 2014	Apr 2014	Complete	
5	Determine any changes in DRG-based payers and patient volumes that will be included in concurrent review	Finance Director or Consultant	Apr 2014	Apr 2014	Complete	
6	Determine staffing levels required for program including changes in DRG-based payers (one CDIP per 2500 annual discharges)	Team Leader	Apr 2014	Apr 2014	Complete	
7	Determine outside consulting support if needed for additional staffing or classroom refresher	Team Leader	May 2014	May 2014	Complete	
8	Interview and hire CDIP staff (as needed)	Team Leader	May 2014		In Progress	
9	Develop or purchase classroom refresher course for high-volume, high-risk DRGs based on analytics and DRGs below or well above national benchmarks	Team Leader or Consultant	Jun 2014		Pending	

10	Determine staff requiring training (CDIP, coders, and physicians)	CMO, Team Leader	Jun 2014		Pending	
11	Plan and conduct one-week classroom training for existing CDIPs and coders. A full two-week course should be provided for new CDIPs.	Team Leader	Jun 2014		Pending	
12	Conduct one-on-one training for CDIPs (six weeks for new CDIPS, two-weeks for existing staff)	Team Leader and consultant	Jun 2014		Pending	
13	Develop plan for one-on-one including target number of reviews per day and nursing unit assignments	Team Leader	Jun 2014		Pending	
14	Meet with Physician Advisor to plan required training, communicate educational session schedule, present to physicians	Physician Advisor and Team Leader	Jun 2014		Pending	
15	Identify physicians requiring additional one-on-one and conduct meetings	Physician Advisor and Team Leader	Jun 2014		Pending	
Phase II - On-going Monitoring						
16	Reestablish tracking reports to monitor program	Team Leader	Jun 2014		Pending	
17	Reconvene governance (quarterly) and task force meetings (monthly)	Team Leader	Jun 2014		Pending	
18	Review monthly monitoring reports	Governance Committee, Task Force, Team Leader	Sept 2014		Pending	
19	Conduct quarterly audits of cases concurrently and post-coding to determine coding issues and missed queries (recommend external audit resource)	Consultant	Oct 2014		Pending	
20	Develop remediation plan including stakeholder (physician, CDIP, coder) education	Consultant	Oct 2014		Pending	

Chapter Quiz

1. Which executive must be involved in designing communication of the clinical documentation program from the start?
   A. Revenue cycle leader
   B. Health information director
   C. Clinical documentation consultant
   D. Physician executive

2. What must happen in order to obtain ultimate success with regard to clinical documentation?
   A. Give proper attention to the mission statement
   B. Align physician leaders with executive management structure
   C. Adopt a program structure that fits the organization
   D. Dotted-line organization between physician leaders and CDI leaders

3. The advent of the EHR has increased the amount of documentation largely due to:
   A. CDI
   B. Joint Commission requirements
   C. Ease of entry
   D. Reporting

4. What is the minimum recommended length of training in clinical documentation for the CDI physician leader?
   A. 3 to 6 months
   B. 1 to 3 months
   C. 100 hours
   D. 40 hours

5. When the CDI program encounters a problematic physician, who should control and resolve the situation?
   A. Physician leader for CDI
   B. VP of revenue cycle
   C. Medical staff leader
   D. Informal peer CDI leader

6. Who must be a creative and out-of-the box thinker in order for the CDI program to be a success?
   A. Director of HIM department
   B. Director of CDI department
   C. Director of physician leadership
   D. Director of executive management

7. The CDI specialist is required to handle which day-to-day activities?
   A. Track program costs and savings
   B. Direct the flow of the CDI program as it evolves
   C. Resolve any problems with problematic physicians
   D. Training staff and physicians and health record review

8. Who should be an effective physician communicator, and excellent at reading clinical documentation and data to uncover low-quality clinical documentation?
   A. Clinical documentation director
   B. Physician leader
   C. Clinical documentation improvement practitioner
   D. Physician executive

9. A goal of every CDI program is to obtain high-quality clinical documentation _________.
   A. Before the CDI team finishes installing the CDI program
   B. Prior to the patient being discharged from the hospital
   C. Before recovery audit contractors discover inaccuracies and deficiencies
   D. Before the revenue cycle auditors discover deficiencies

10. An effective CDI program should be able to capture 70 to 75 percent of the query responses _______.
   A. Concurrently
   B. Retrospectively
   C. Consecutively
   D. Simultaneously

REFERENCES

ACDIS. 2010. 2010 CDI Program Benchmarking Survey, pp. 32–44.

AHIMA. 2014. Clinical Documentation Toolkit. Retrieved from: http://library.ahima.org/xpedio/groups/secure/documents/ahima/bok1_050585.pdf.

3M Health Information systems. 2012. A case study in coding compliance: Achieving accuracy and consistency, pp 1–8.

Grol, R., R. Baker, and F. Moss. 2002. Quality improvement research: Understanding the science of change in health care. *Quality and Safety in Health Care* 11(2):110–111.

Keogh, T. and W. Martin. 2004. Managing unmanageable physicians: Leadership, stewardship and disruptive behavior. *Physician Executive* 30(5):18–22.

Marco, A.P., and D. Buchman. 2003. Influencing physician performance. *Quality Management in Health Care* 12(1):4–42.

Russo, R. 2008. *A Compelling Case for Clinical Documentation: Use Clinical Documentation to Achieve Strategic Alignment with Your Medical Staff*, volume 1. Bethlehem, PA: DJ Iber Publishing.

Russo, R. 2001. The application of knowledge management principles to compliant coding activities. *Topics in Health Information Management* 21(3):18–22.

Chapter 8 Physician Training

Introduction

Physician training in high-quality clinical documentation programs is the keystone of every clinical documentation improvement (CDI) program. Unfortunately, physicians do not receive clinical documentation training during medical school or in most residency programs. Therefore, the members of the typical medical staff have had little to no exposure to a formal clinical documentation training program (Cascio et al. 2005). Ideally, every healthcare system or organization involved in training physicians on clinical documentation practices should be using the same program content and methodology for training.

This chapter proposes the use of a scientifically validated method for clinical documentation training known as the CAMP Method (coaching, asking, mastering, and peer learning). The method draws upon the adult-learning theory of self-efficacy and uses the components of coaching, asking, mastering, and peer learning to teach physicians the principles of high-quality clinical documentation. This method is statistically proven using the CAMP Method to produce higher quality and sustainable clinical documentation in physician trainees. Moreover, the CAMP Method is proven to produce significantly better documentation results than the traditional training provided in most physician CDI training programs. The typical program involves a team consisting of a physician trainer and a clinical documentation expert who lecture physicians for about 45 minutes, using PowerPoint slides and handouts. However, experience with CDI training reveals that many organizations provide even less than the typical 45 minutes of training.

There are three challenges for healthcare organizations in moving forward with a comprehensive physician-training program for clinical documentation.

- First, the organization must obtain the support of the executive team for such an initiative. The importance of support from the senior management team (and how to obtain it) is addressed in chapter 6 of this book.
- Second, the organization must identify the appropriate resources for training. Resources include qualified trainers, training materials, and a budget to pay for the training.
- Third, physicians must attend the training (Parochka and Paprockas 2001). Physician support for the program, including attendance at training sessions, should be the initial responsibility of the executive management team. Ultimately, the physicians must perceive some intrinsic or personal value in the training.

The CAMP Method attempts to demonstrate value for the physicians by using research based on the scientific method to support it. Physicians are trained as scientists and typically only accept proof of effectiveness of treatment (or in this case, training) when it has been scientifically proven. They may be more likely to accept rigorously tested training such as the CAMP Method. In addition, using the case study method for training and the actual practice of clinical documentation skills during training is an essential part of an effective training program. The CAMP Method uses two 2-hour programs (four total hours) to train physicians in the core components of high-quality clinical documentation. Each organization needs to assess the value of comprehensive CDI training, like that proposed in the CAMP Method, and determine the best approach for training its medical staff.

Program Instructor

Research has shown that professionals learn best from a peer whom they trust and respect (Bandura 2000). Moreover, learning from a peer, coupled with coaching, asking, and mastering (as described in this chapter), results in more sustainable training. For optimal training outcomes, it is essential that a physician peer perform the CDI training. It is also important that the trainees perceive the physician trainers as credible communicators of the training topic. In the case of CDI training, there are few physician experts available to act in that role. Therefore, the best instruction for a physician CDI training program involves a training team. The team should comprise a physician instructor and a clinical documentation expert. These two individuals, delivering the information together, will likely contribute to an optimal training outcome (Bandura 1986; Lenz and Shortridge-Baggett 2002). A team of a physician instructor and a clinical documentation expert at The Hospital of the University of Pennsylvania originally conducted the training program for the CAMP Method study with resident physicians.

Chapter 7 describes in detail the inclusion of a physician leader for CDI on the team. This physician leader can also serve in the training role. If an organization does not have a physician leader on its CDI team initially, it can hire a physician consultant to function in this role in the short term. The key to having an effective training team is including both a clinical documentation expert to train on content as well as a physician peer who can share experiences with peers. The physician trainer is also valuable for managing the physician trainees and assuring them that they are capable of practicing high-quality clinical documentation. In addition, it does not involve a significantly greater amount of time than their current practices take.

The non-physician trainer should be an individual who is well versed in clinical documentation principles, quality indicators, and coding and reimbursement methodologies. This individual is likely to be a health information management (HIM) professional or a nurse with the appropriate training in coding and reimbursement. The non-physician trainer must be comfortable training both small and large groups of physicians and work well with the physician trainer. It is important for the team members to plan their roles in the training process. Table 8.1 contains the ideal and minimum qualifications for a non-physician trainer. Table 7.2 in chapter 7 shows the ideal and minimum qualifications for the physician leader or trainer.

Program Attendees

The question of which physicians should attend CDI training must be addressed early in the process. Ideally, all physicians should be responsible for completing basic clinical documentation training. In reality, this may be limited by training capabilities of the organization and the willingness of physicians to participate. The best approach is to prioritize and organize the CDI physician trainees. The exact methodology for prioritizing varies by organization. Important issues for an

Table 8.1 Qualifications for nonphysician clinical documentation trainer

Skill	Nonphysician Trainer Ideal	Nonphysician Trainer Minimum
Formal education	Bachelor's degree or above in a clinical area; current licensure or accreditation; academic training in pathophysiology and health information	Bachelor's degree or equivalent with licensure or accreditation in a clinical or healthcare area
Training received in clinical documentation	80 hours or more and certification, if possible	At least 80 hours
Experience in clinical documentation	Experience documenting in patient records; at least five years reviewing documentation in patient records and treating patients	At least five years reviewing documentation in patient records
Experience providing classroom instruction	40 hours or more of instruction	At least 40 hours of instruction
Experience providing practical instruction	160 hours of on-unit or in-office observation and feedback	At least 100 hours of on-unit or in-office observation and feedback

organization to consider in identifying the physicians to train include the value to the organization and the likelihood of cooperation from the physicians. Using these criteria, the organization should give top priority to the physicians who admit the largest numbers of patients and historically have been supportive of organizational initiatives. This may be the organization's hospitalist group or internal medicine physicians. An example of a training plan for a teaching hospital that employs hospitalists follows.

Physicians from the hospitalist group are often the top priority for CDI training in many organizations. Hospitalists often take on the role of the patient's primary care physician when a patient is hospitalized. Hospitalists should therefore have a predominant role in CDI training. The physician must carefully balance training with clinical responsibilities because hospitalists carry a very high patient load. Hospitalists, if employed by the organization, can bring value not only in improved inpatient documentation, but also in professional-fee documentation (Rifkin et al. 2007).

Residents are often the first-line documenters for inpatient cases. Although they should not be the sole documenters, residents play an important role in any CDI initiative. Programs are most successful if the initial training is provided annually to first-year residents. The organization should clearly define the residents' continuing documentation responsibilities and involve them in years two, three, and four. However, as long as the comprehensive CDI training is provided to each first-year class, by the fourth year of operations, any teaching hospital that adopts this process will have a full complement of residents armed with high-quality clinical documentation skills.

As with hospitalists, residents carry a heavy workload, and current Department of Health and Human Services (HHS) requirements limit the number of hours residents can spend in the hospital in a patient-care role. The CDI trainer needs to plan carefully with the director of resident education. A benefit of CDI training for the residents is that they can use the training to meet one of the Accreditation Council of Graduate Medical Education (ACGME) competency requirements, which requires hospitals to train residents to be familiar with healthcare systems (Barden et al. 2003; Phillbert et al. 2002). Clinical documentation, quality indicators, the Health Insurance Portability and Accountability Act (HIPAA) and patient rights, and reimbursement systems, all of which trainers cover during the basic CDI program, fulfill this requirement.

Hospital-employed physicians should be a high priority on the CDI training list. If an organization owns any physician practices or employs other physicians within the system, those physicians should be expected to attend CDI training early in the process. Because physician employees of a health system generate documentation related to both hospital care and office-based care, they can begin applying the concepts of high-quality clinical documentation they learn in the initial training in their office practices. These office practices may also be a good place for eventual expansion of the CDI program beyond the acute care setting (Robinson 1998).

Every hospital has a small group of physicians, usually about 10 to 15 percent of the attending staff, who are responsible for the majority of hospital admissions. CDI trainers should identify and target these individuals for early training. While some view training as a benefit, in that it increases a physician's skill set, the hospital's executive team should make it clear to the physicians that CDI training is a responsibility. This is the message that, in particular, the high-admitting physicians need to hear. Hopefully, because high-admitting physicians have a significant impact on an organization's economic state, the executive team and other managers have positive relationships with them. This makes good business sense, and the CDI program staff can use it to obtain support from the high-admitting physicians for both attendance at training sessions and overall support for the program.

Members of the medical staff generally divide into two groups: those that support new hospital initiatives and those that do not support new hospital initiatives. It is likely that the organization can also identify physicians on either end of this spectrum. Some physicians will be strong supporters of any hospital initiative and will step up to the plate to help in any way they can. These physicians should begin training as early as possible since they are likely to advocate the value of the training and the program to their peers. This information communication can strengthen program support.

Other physicians will be strong opponents of any hospital initiatives. Unfortunately, the negative attitude of these physicians can begin to influence other members of the medical staff. It is important to identify physicians in both of these groups and create a strategy for CDI training. The CDI trainers may need to rely on communications from the CEO and other executive team members to convince the naysayers. The naysayers will be the most difficult group to convert, but the earlier the trainers begin working with them, the greater the positive impact will be for the organization.

Table 8.2 illustrates a sample training schedule for a teaching hospital that employs hospitalists and primary care physicians. Trainers need to consider both the physician's time and willingness to participate, as well as training resources, when designing the training plan, which should also include a plan for makeup sessions for physicians who cannot attend the initial training.

⊙ Methodology

Because the CAMP Method is proven through the experimental method to produce a statistically significant positive difference in clinical documentation quality and sustainability over either traditional training or no training, it is the method that this book proposes (Russo and Fitzgerald 2008). The CAMP acronym stands for the four components used in teaching: coaching, asking, mastering, and peer learning. These components are derived from the theory of self-efficacy, a proven adult-learning model (Bandura 2000; Bandura 1986; Lenz and Shortridge-Baggett 2002) and are briefly described as follows:

Coaching involves reinforcing and encouraging participants about their abilities to perform the function. Here, the physician trainer shares experiences about clinical documentation with the trainees. Coaching should be interactive, and the physician should ask for feedback from the trainees. The physician trainer

Table 8.2 Sample 2-year clinical documentation training plan for physicians

Physician	Month																							
Group	1	2	3	4	5	6	7	8	9	10	11	12	13	14	15	16	17	18	19	20	21	22	23	24
Hospitalists																								
Medicine																								
Medicine specialties																								
General surgeons																								
Surgery specialties																								
OB/GYN Newborn																								
ED Physicians																								
Radiologists																								
Anesthesiologists																								
Residents																								
Fellows																								
Employed primary care physicians																								
Employed specialists and surgeons																								
Session 1 makeup for medicine specialties																								
Session 2 makeup for medicine specialties																								
Session 1 makeup for surgical specialties																								
Session 2 makeup for surgical specialties																								

should be able to manage responses from the trainees so that other physician trainees can benefit from this interactive experience. Essentially, the feedback loop here becomes another form of peer learning.

Asking involves soliciting feedback from the physician participants in a specific manner and at a specific time. At a minimum, the trainers should ask the physicians at the beginning of the program about their concerns regarding the training. This activity helps to eliminate any misconceptions. It also reduces or extinguishes underlying negativity some physicians may have harbored during the training process. The physician trainer and the non-physician trainer must be prepared for physician responses and be able to manage these responses to ensure the program proceeds as planned.

Mastering involves practical application of the principles demonstrated and discussed during the training program. Here, physician trainees have an opportunity to practice high-quality clinical documentation. The trainers provide the physicians with sample health records and case studies, which they individually review to determine whether the documentation meets the criteria for high-quality clinical documentation. If it does not, then the physician trainees suggest appropriate documentation. The cases are later discussed among the group, which adds to the peer-learning component of the training.

Peer learning involves instruction by a knowledgeable peer. The physician instructor is of prime importance in this component. However, it is also important for the physician trainees to learn from their peers who are also in the program. Soliciting feedback and validating (or correcting) thoughts about the CDI process is an important part of the peer-learning process.

The specific use of these components is detailed in table 8.3, which presents the complete agenda used for the CAMP Method study. This can be used as a guide when developing a CDI training program. The agenda refers to questionnaires and tests the physician trainees received during the study, but the training team can conduct the training without these data collection tools.

Table 8.3 Contents of two 2-hour CDI sessions used in the CAMP Method Training
First Session

Concept	Activity	Program Design to Incorporate Concept	Time
Peer Learning & Coaching	Introduction	Review session outline and objectives. Physician instructor shares own experience with clinical documentation and assures participants that, with the appropriate training and support, they will master this process.	10 min
Mastering	Self-assessment & test	Participants take the self-assessment and the pre-test; collect the self-assessment and the pre-test from the participants before reviewing the responses.	10 min
Peer Learning	Test review	Review test questions and correct responses with attendees.	10 min

(Continued)

Table 8.3 Contents of two 2-hour CDI sessions used in the CAMP Method Training First Session (*Continued*)

Concept	Activity	Program Design to Incorporate Concept	Time
Asking	Physician commitment to good clinical documentation	Discuss the relationship between good documentation practices and improved patient outcomes with the participants. Ask physicians to share their concerns about clinical documentation. Make a list of what the concerns are and share the list (as a way to end this portion of the session). State that we will revisit the list in the second session. Include time management if not addressed by physicians.	10 min
Peer Learning	Documentation rules	Review documentation "rules" PowerPoint with physicians. Ask for and allow questions throughout this portion of the presentation.	15 min
Asking	Break	Serve refreshments and take a 5-minute break.	10 min
Mastering	Case study examples	Review case studies 1–5 that correspond with objectives 2–5.	15 min
Mastering	Tools	Provide each physician with a CDI Handbook and a Pocket Tool for General Medicine. Review the contents of the handbook and the tool. Allow for questions throughout this portion of the presentation.	15 min
Mastering; Coaching	Case study exercises	Give physicians case study exercises 1–5 that contain documentation from actual patient records to review and provide the correct documentation to identify the patient's diagnoses. Review answers with physicians and ask participants for their responses. Provide feedback as participants share their answers.	15 min
Asking	MD concerns	Revisit list of concerns from beginning of the program.	10 min
Coaching	Conclusion	Conclude the program by assuring the physicians that they can document well. Ask them to apply the concepts they have learned during this session between now and the next session and be prepared to share their experiences during the next session.	5 min
Coaching; Peer Learning	Introduction	Review session outline and objectives. Return the pre-test results to each participant. Physician instructor asks participants to share their documentation experiences over the past week. Provide feedback to examples.	15 min

Concept	Activity	Program Design to Incorporate Concept	Time
Coaching	Videotape viewing	Have attendees view videotape of physicians. Discuss concerns about documentation. At the completion of the video, ask physicians to share their opinions of the documentation concepts shared in the video.	20 min
Mastering; Coaching	Case study examples	Review case studies 6-10 that correspond with objectives 1–6. Ask participants to comment on the examples. Provide feedback on comments.	15 min
Asking	Break	Serve refreshments and take a 5-minute break allowing participants to interact with each other.	10 min
Mastering; Coaching	Case study exercises	Give physicians case study exercises 6–10 that contain documentation from actual patient records to review and provide the correct documentation to identify the patients' diagnoses. Review answers with physicians asking participants for their responses. Provide feedback as participants share their answers.	15 min
Mastering; Asking; Coaching	Tools	Ask physicians to refer to their CDI Handbook and Pocket Tool. Ask participants to provide examples of where and when they were able to use the tools over the past week (since the first session). Provide feedback on the use of the tools as shared by the participants. Use any remaining time to review the contents of the book again.	15 min
Asking	Physician commitment	Review listing of concerns generated by residents during previous session. Identify how their dedication and commitment to medicine can be demonstrated through good documentation practices. Ask the residents to sign a "Commitment to Improved Clinical Documentation" form.	10 min
Mastering	Post-test	Have participants take the self-assessment and the post-test. Collect the self-assessments and the post-tests. Review the answers with the participants.	15 min
Coaching	Conclusion	Conclude the program by assuring the physicians that they can document well.	5 min
Coaching; Peer Learning	Evaluation	Ask participants to evaluate the educational program.	2 min

Initial Program Content

Initial program content should focus on the seven criteria for high-quality clinical documentation. Chapter 1 has detailed descriptions of these criteria (which are useful in PowerPoint presentations to review with physicians). CDI trainers should use case studies and patient examples from their own organizations to the extent possible. Physician trainees learn the most from their own documentation experiences. Table 8.4 details the objectives for the keystone training on clinical documentation. Using these objectives ensures a thorough and compliant training experience for the organization's medical staff.

The CDI physician advisor and CDI practitioner (CDIP) should conduct physician training as part of their daily process. They can provide training sessions in a one-on-one discussion, a presentation at a specialty department meeting, or a general session for a larger group. Longer presentations tend to lose audience attention, therefore it is best to keep the presentation to 10 minutes. The presenter should answer the following key questions:

- What is CDI?
- Why is CDI important to providers?
- What action does the provider need to take?

An example of a physician PowerPoint presentation is available online at http://www.ahimapress.org/hess5023/. Trainers can use this presentation as a starting point and customize it for the group attending the presentation. Trainers should be sure to use the minimal content required to make their point.

Table 8.4 Instructional objectives of CDI training program

Overall objective: Following the educational intervention, the physician will demonstrate improved skill in high-quality clinical documentation in patient health records. **Specific objectives:** The resident physician will 1. Demonstrate understanding of the relationship between physician documentation and the translation of that documentation into ICD-9-CM coded data. 2. Demonstrate an understanding that ICD-9-CM coded data is used for planning, reimbursement, quality ratings, Medicare Conditions of Participation, Joint Commission Core Measures, and research. 3. Provide documentation in the inpatient record that is timely, legible, complete, clear, consistent, reliable, and precise. 4. Document with detail and precision in the patient's principal diagnosis. 5. Document all chronic coexisting secondary diagnoses. 6. Document all acute coexisting secondary diagnoses. 7. Document the clinical significance of all abnormal diagnostic tests. 8. Document the etiology or suspected etiology of symptoms.

Conclusion

Physician training in the principles of high-quality clinical documentation is the most essential component of a CDI program. Obtaining their buy-in for the program is critical to its success and sustainability. It is important to select the proper training team that includes physician colleagues. The training team should base their selection of attendees on service lines and physician groups requiring improved clinical documentation. The team should base the program content on the seven criteria for high-quality clinical documentation. Facilities should consider using the CAMP Method given its success in the field of CDI.

Chapter Quiz

1. What theory does the scientifically validated CAMP Method for clinical documentation training draw upon?
   A. The gold standard of CDI
   B. Adult learning theory of self-efficacy
   C. Quality improvement theory
   D. Health information theory
2. What is the keystone to every CDI program?
   A. Coder staff training
   B. Installing a cost effective CDI program
   C. Physician training
   D. Creating a vision that demonstrates the goals of the organization
3. Which of these is vital to moving forward with a comprehensive physician-training program?
   A. Locating the appropriate outside resources
   B. Leading coder staff in physician-training sessions
   C. Peer leader training
   D. Executive team and physician leader support
4. Research based on the scientific method is used to demonstrate value to whom?
   A. Executive team
   B. CDI team
   C. Physicians
   D. Clinical scientific support staff
5. Which member of the CDI training team is essential for optimal training outcomes?
   A. Chief medical officer
   B. Chief information officer
   C. Director of CDI department
   D. Peer physician

6. Which CDI trainer should be well versed in clinical documentation principles, quality indicators, and coding and reimbursement methodologies?
   A. Physician trainer
   B. Nonphysician trainer
   C. Leader executive team
   D. Oversight committee leader

7. Which type of physician is often top priority for CDI training and accounts for, on average, 60 percent of hospital admissions?
   A. Hospitalist
   B. Cardiologist
   C. Endocrinologist
   D. Orthopedic surgeon

8. In the CAMP acronym, what does the M stand for?
   A. Medicine
   B. Mentoring
   C. Mastering
   D. Methodology

9. In the CAMP acronym, *asking* means:
   A. Questions students ask that the trainer needs to address
   B. Asking for feedback from physician students at the right time
   C. Asking coders which are the appropriate codes to use
   D. Querying, focusing on concurrent queries

10. A typical CAMP training program consists of:
   A. Weeks of hands-on mentoring of CDI leadership
   B. Interactive online training and materials for everyone
   C. Heavy coding-specific training for hospitalists
   D. Four hours of training for physicians to learn core concepts

REFERENCES

Bandura, A. 2000. *Handbook of Principles of Organizational Behavior.* Edited by E.A. Locke. Oxford: Blackwell.

Bandura, A. 1986. *Social Foundations of Thought and Action: A Social Cognitive Theory.* Englewood-Cliffs, NY: Prentice-Hall.

Barden, C.B., M.C. Specht, M.D. McCarter, J.M. Daly, and T.J. Fahey. 2003. Effects of limited work hours on surgical training. *Obstetrical and Gynecological Survey* 58(4):244–245.

Cascio, B.M., J.H. Wilckens, M.C. Ain, C. Toulson, and F.J. Frassica. 2005. Documentation of acute compartment syndrome at an academic healthcare center. *Journal of Bone and Joint Surgery.* 87(2):346.

Lenz, E.R. and L.M. Shortridge-Baggett. 2002. *Self-Efficacy in Nursing: Research and Measurement Perspectives.* New York: Springer Publishing.

Parochka, J. and K. Paprockas. 2001. A continuing medical education lecture and workshop, physician behavior, and barriers to change. *Journal of Continuing Education in the Health Professions.* 21(2):110-116.

Philibert, I., P. Friedmann, and W.T. Williams. 2002. New requirements for resident duty hours. *Journal of the American Medical Association.* 288(9):1112–1114.

Rifkin, W.D., A. Burger, E.S. Holmboe, and B. Sturdevant. 2007. Comparison of hospitalists and non-hospitalists regarding core measures of pneumonia care. *American Journal of Managed Care.* 13(3):129–132.

Robinson, J.C. 1998. Consolidation of medical groups into physician practice management organizations. *Journal of the American Medical Association.* 279(2):144–149.

Russo, R. and S. Fitzgerald. 2008. Physician clinical documentation: Implications for healthcare quality and cost. Academy of Management Annual Meeting, Anaheim, CA.

Chapter 9 Training Nonphysician Clinicians and CDI Program Staff

Similar to physician clinical documentation improvement (CDI) training, training for nonphysician clinicians has an impact on the sustainability of the program. Nonphysician CDI training is divided into training for program staff who may someday teach CDI sessions to clinicians and physicians, and training for nonphysician clinicians who document in patient records. This chapter begins with the training for CDI program staff, followed by the training for clinicians.

The CAMP (coaching, asking, mastering, and peer learning) Method, as described in chapter 8, incorporates the adult learning theory of self-efficacy, and it uses coaching, asking, mastering, and peer learning to ensure improved quality and sustainability. Although the CAMP Method was tested originally with physicians, CDI trainers can use it to train anyone (Bandura 2000, 120; Bandura 1986; Lasinger and Tresolini 1999). The primary difference between the format discussed in chapter 8 and the format used for training nonphysician clinicians is in the peer learning component. Peer learning means knowledgeable, respected peers teach the trainees. For instance, if nurses were the trainees, ideally, a nurse would pair with a clinical documentation expert to deliver the training. On the other hand, if nutritionists were the trainees, a nutritionist would pair with a clinical documentation expert. While it may not always be possible to find a knowledgeable peer, this training team model produces the optimal outcome for the organization.

Training CDI Program Staff

Organizations should ensure all CDI program staff members are thoroughly trained in the principles of high-quality clinical documentation as well as the review of patient records to identify possible deficiencies in documentation. Ideally, training occurs as a group. Group settings trigger the peer-learning component of training. This strengthens the sustainability of the training. Group training also ensures consistency of the presented content.

CDI staff training is a three-part process. The first part involves training the staff in the theory of high-quality clinical documentation. This is similar to the training they will someday provide to physicians and clinicians. This training also involves teaching the basics of coding and the reimbursement process. In the second part, the CDI program staff members are trained in the physician query process. Lastly, the CDI trainers train them in program data collection and analysis.

Training CDI Staff on the Theory and the Application of CDI

The initial portion of the program on the theory and application of CDI contains the same content as the physician keystone training. Exposure to this training is a good first step for the program staff. It also provides participants with the basis for the physician training program should they ever be on a training team that provides CDI education to physicians.

In addition to the basics, CDI program staff training should also include the fundamentals of coding and reimbursement systems. The content in chapter 5 related to the concurrent review process and metrics for tracking the program success is helpful in creating a more comprehensive training program for the CDI program staff. Finally, because clinical documentation determines both actual and perceived quality of care, it is important for the program staff to be trained on the basics of quality indicators and to be familiar with public quality report cards like Healthgrades (http://www.healthgrades.com), Health Compare, Leap Frog, and AQRP (Acuity Quality Review Program). Figure 9.1 contains a list of sample training objectives for CDI staff. This sample is specific to the acute care inpatient setting. Training that includes or focuses on outpatient or other inpatient settings needs modification to reflect specific objectives.

Training CDI Staff on the Record Review and Query Process

The primary operational components of the CDI program are the record review and the query process. The review process and the physician query process allow for the highest level of quality in clinical documentation. Therefore, training on both the record review and query process should be part of the CDI program staff training. Classroom training should consist of the theoretical basis for the program, the appropriate way to review a record to identify documentation deficiencies, and the parameters for querying a physician. Classroom trainers should include experienced CDI practitioners (CDIPs) (nurses and coders), inpatient coding managers, and physicians where possible. The skill set of each of these trainers provides a unique point of reference, challenges, and solutions for team building within the interdepartmental CDI team. Table 9.1 outlines suggested topics for each trainer.

CDI is a collaborative team effort between the physician, CDIPs, and the coder. It is essential to include the coders in the classroom training where possible. If coders are not available for the entire classroom program, they should attend the

Figure 9.1 Clinical documentation improvement training program objectives (for the inpatient acute care setting)

1. To adequately prepare the case manager to participate in improving inpatient clinical documentation through record review, application of official guidelines, and interaction with physicians and other clinicians
2. To understand the impact of clinical documentation on severity, mortality, and morbidity "ratings" for inpatient cases
3. To understand the relationship between clinical documentation and case mix index
4. To understand the relationship between clinical documentation and Medicare quality indicators
5. To understand the relationship between clinical documentation and healthcare quality score cards such as HealthGrades (http://www.healthgrades.com) and Joint Commission's Quality Check™ (http://www.jointcommission.org/QualityCheck/06_qc_facts.htm)
6. To identify the correct principal diagnosis statement for inpatient records in every specialty by applying official Uniform Hospital Discharge Data Set (UHDDS) guidelines
7. To understand the impact that the principal diagnosis has on determining the DRG into which the inpatient case is assigned
8. To identify accurate secondary diagnoses for inpatient records in every specialty by applying official UHDDS guidelines
9. To understand the impact that secondary diagnosis documentation has on determining the DRG for the patient's acute inpatient stay
10. To identify opportunities in the health record where clinical documentation could be further clarified to result in capturing more specific principal diagnoses
11. To identify opportunities in the health record where clinical documentation could be further clarified to result in capturing more specific or additional secondary diagnoses
12. To identify opportunities in the health record where clinical documentation could be further clarified to result in capturing more specific procedures
13. To formulate a valid concurrent physician query

case review portion discussed below in the group activity section. The combination of clinical and coding skill sets within the group provides an excellent opportunity for knowledge transfer. Those in the class with formal nursing training act as resources for clinical information during training and subsequent daily CDI and coding processes. Nurses provide insight into clinical case scenarios and clinical indicator use for the query process. Coders provide insight into accurate Medicare

Table 9.1 Suggested topics by trainer

Trainer	Topic
CDIP	Record review workflow, query process, CDI data gathering, CDI software
Coding Manager	Coding guidelines, MS-DRG assignment, inpatient record review process
Physician	Clinical criteria for query identification, best practices for communication with provider

severity diagnosis-related group (MS-DRG) assignment and coding guidelines. These two groups enhance each other's efforts when both meet daily to discuss cases. This process is especially helpful at the beginning of the program when the two groups are learning to work as a team. The buddy system works well during this early phase of CDI. Pairing a CDIP and coder together encourages one-on-one discussion and collaboration through email, phone, or in person.

The CDI training team typically conducts training in the classroom over a two-week period. Prior to the first body system presentation, the first session is an introduction to MS-DRGs, case mix index, the query process, CDI analytics, coding guidelines, and CDI workflow. Next, a trainer presents a study of major body systems using live case examples. These body systems should correlate to the MS-DRG Major Diagnostic Categories (MDC). See table 9.2 for a list of essential systems.

The body system discussion should include the following key points, which offer a comprehensive look at the most common MS-DRG groups within the body system, pertinent complications and comorbidities (CCs), associated signs, symptoms, and test results, as well as common provided treatments. The clinical documentation specialist uses this information to identify potential query opportunities and to assign the MS-DRG accurately. The key points include

- MS-DRGs with each body system, their weight, and geometric length of stay
- High-volume MS-DRG pairs and triplets
- Major CCs (MCCs) and CCs pertinent to the body system in question
- Key diagnoses and procedures within the body system
    - Signs and symptoms requiring further specificity
    - Differential diagnoses
    - Diagnosis specific clinical criteria and reference sites
    - Diagnostic testing
    - Treatment
    - Clinical documentation challenges

An example nervous system presentation is available online at http://www.ahimapress.org/hess5023/. The presentation includes a short introduction along with the key body system discussion points. The following is an outline of the presentation:

- Introduction on MS-DRGs
- Nervous system MCC/CC including some of the typical MCC/CCs found in the clinical record with a principal diagnosis categorized to the nervous system.
- Focused nervous system diagnoses including signs, symptoms, clinical indicators, diagnostic testing, and treatment
    - Mental Status Change
    - Transient Ischemic Attack (TIA)
    - Cerebrovascular Accident (CVA)
    - Encephalopathy
    - Epilepsy
- Quiz

Group Activity

Prior to the start of a CDI program, most facilities have identified high-risk or high-volume focused MS-DRGs for clinical documentation and reimbursement accuracy. A subsequent assessment of sample cases is typically performed by an outside consultant to validate the findings. Trainers can use cases with recommended MS-DRG changes in the classroom. They should copy cases for ease of use in the classroom setting and also remove the coding summaries. Each participant then reviews several cases to identify the MS-DRG, principal diagnosis, MCC/CCs, and potential queries. Participants present their case to the group and defend the MS-DRG, principal diagnosis, MCC/CCs, and potential queries. The classroom instructor guides the session, and after the discussion is complete, provides the class with the correct MS-DRG, principal diagnosis, MCC/CCs, and recommended queries. This activity provides a glimpse of the work trainees will see during the actual nursing unit training, but the environment is more conducive to the inexperienced CDIP.

Concurrent Review Training

When the classroom training is about 50 percent complete, the CDI program staff members can begin to visit the nursing units, and review health records to apply the initial information they have learned. During this initial review of records on the units, the CDI program participants should partner with an experienced CDI specialist. Ideally, a CDI staff trainee receives feedback about the review process and learns to identify query opportunities. This on-unit review progresses until the CDI staff trainee begins to query physicians. The trainer should observe and offer feedback to the CDI staff trainee until the trainer witnesses accurate record review and appropriate, consistent querying. CDI staff trainees generally need about 40 to 50 hours of observation before they can function independently.

Table 9.2 CDI classroom major diagnostic categories

Week 1	Chapters	MDC
Day 1	Introduction, Coding Guidelines, Nervous System	1
Day 2	EENT, Respiratory System	2–4
Day 3	Circulatory & Digestive Systems	5–6
Day 4	Hepatobiliary, Musculoskeletal Systems, Multiple Trauma	7–8, 24
Week 2		
Day 5	Integumentary, Endocrine Systems	9–10
Day 6	Renal, Male/Female Reproductive	11–13
Day 7	Blood Diseases, Myeloproliferative	16–17
Day 8	Infectious Disease, Injury & Poisoning	18, 21
Morning classroom lecture from 9:00 am - noon will cover training manual chapters 1-19. Afternoon classroom group activity will include case reviews for body system chapters corresponding to the morning session.		

The record review process should include addressing all components of the patient record as possible sources for query opportunities. The trainers, preferably the physician leader for CDI, should review the clinical indicators and clinical evidence in sample records with the trainees. It is important to involve the physician leader in this process, as opposed to a CDI peer because of the perspective the physician brings. CDI staff benefit from continuous exposure to the physician's perspective throughout their training. This interaction better prepares the CDI staff member for the one-on-one physician query process that is essential to the program. It is important that the CDI staff trainee can identify any documentation in a patient record that does not meet the criteria for high-quality clinical documentation. Every documentation deficiency presents a possible opportunity for a physician query.

The trainers should initially explain the physician query process in the classroom setting. Role playing between the CDI trainees and the physician leader for CDI is helpful before attempting a live query on the nursing unit. The query process can be a live verbal query or a written query. Regardless of how the CDI staff member generates a query, he or she should clearly capture it in the program documentation. Chapter 10 provides more detail about the query process.

Training CDI Staff on the Data Collection Process

Perhaps if you cannot measure a process, you cannot manage it. This includes activities related to clinical documentation. Therefore, trainers should make sure to train CDI program staff in collecting program data, entering data elements into the program database, following up on unanswered queries, and identifying trends using program data.

The collection of program data includes the identification of

- All cases reviewed
- The number of cases with queries
- The nature of the query
- The physician's response to the query

These primary data elements are the basis for reporting the key metrics of the program. The key metrics of the program, which are determined by the organization's senior management (and discussed in chapter 11), determine program success and the likelihood that the organization will continue to support a clinical documentation program.

The program staff members are responsible for entering the data elements into the program database. Several viable options are available for collecting CDI program data. Some organizations use case management software modified for CDI purposes. Most programs use software licensed from one of the consulting firms that offers clinical documentation services, like Navigant Consulting. The Navigant software, known as the CDI Monitor, allows the input of a significant amount of program data and then generates reports using these data elements. The training team must thoroughly train the CDI staff in how to use the software appropriately to ensure accurate program reporting. Once trained, a trainer should review data input during the course of the first month to ensure acceptable quality. Ideally, the CDI specialist enters this information directly into the computer. However, organizations that do not have wireless laptops available to the CDI specialists can create a manual CDI form for this purpose.

Post-training Evaluation

The entire training program for CDI staff will likely be a 60- to 80-hour process. After completing training, the training team should test all CDI specialists on their knowledge and skill level. The testing instrument serves as evidence of what the CDI specialist has learned. It also brings to light any knowledge gaps. Therefore, an organization must follow up on any knowledge or skill gaps soon after identifying them. In addition to testing, it is helpful for the CDI specialists to perform a self-evaluation. Research shows that self-evaluations such as the one in figure 9.2 are often as good an indicator of knowledge and skill gaps as testing instruments. This type of evaluation takes only a few minutes for the program staff to complete and provides information that helps improve both the program and the training process.

Figure 9.2 shows a CDI specialist self-evaluation that training staff can use to measure the improvements provided by training as well as the existing gaps in knowledge.

Figure 9. 2 CDI specialist self-evaluation

DOCUMENTATION IMPROVEMENT PROGRAM										
CDI Specialist Self-Evaluation										
Directions: Please complete the following statements by indicating your level of knowledge and familiarity with the concepts addressed BEFORE the start of the documentation improvement program as well as your knowledge CURRENTLY of the same concepts. Circle the number which best represents your level of knowledge and familiarity both before and currently. "1" signifies no knowledge and "5" represents a strong knowledge of the concept.										
	Before Training					**After Training**				
My knowledge of:	**Weak**				**Strong**	**Weak**				**Strong**
1. The relationship between documentation & coding	1	2	3	4	5	1	2	3	4	5
2. The relationship between coding & reimbursement	1	2	3	4	5	1	2	3	4	5
3. General logic of the DRG system	1	2	3	4	5	1	2	3	4	5
4. A patient's principal diagnosis	1	2	3	4	5	1	2	3	4	5
5. The role of secondary diagnoses	1	2	3	4	5	1	2	3	4	5
6. Case mix index (CMI)	1	2	3	4	5	1	2	3	4	5
7. The importance of the physician documenting a patient's condition	1	2	3	4	5	1	2	3	4	5
8. The need for physicians to document the significance of lab/other test results	1	2	3	4	5	1	2	3	4	5
9. How pneumonia is categorized in the DRG system	1	2	3	4	5	1	2	3	4	5

My knowledge of:	Before Training					After Training				
	Weak			Strong		Weak			Strong	
10. The difference between reimbursement for COPD vs. respiratory failure	1	2	3	4	5	1	2	3	4	5
11. The impact that secondary diagnoses can make on the reimbursement for acute MI patients	1	2	3	4	5	1	2	3	4	5
12. The importance of identifying the etiology for symptoms, if known	1	2	3	4	5	1	2	3	4	5
13. The importance of documenting differential diagnoses for symptoms with uncertain etiology	1	2	3	4	5	1	2	3	4	5
14. The reimbursement principle that requires the coding of any condition that a physician documents as "possible," "probable," or "questionable" as though the condition exists	1	2	3	4	5	1	2	3	4	5
15. The relationship between physician documentation and healthcare report cards (HealthGrades)	1	2	3	4	5	1	2	3	4	5
16. The relationship between physician documentation and Medicare quality indicators	1	2	3	4	5	1	2	3	4	5
17. The physician query process	1	2	3	4	5	1	2	3	4	5
I would like to know more about:										
Other comments:										

The American Health Information Management Association (AHIMA) Clinical Documentation Improvement Toolkit includes a 90-Day CDI Post-test for evaluating the CDI specialists' knowledge. A few example questions include

1. A patient is admitted through the emergency room for shortness of breath. The patient is given epinephrine and nebulizer treatments. The shortness of breath and wheezing are unabated following treatment. What diagnosis should be suspected?
   a. Acute bronchitis
   b. Acute bronchitis with COPD
   c. Asthma with status asthmaticus
   d. Chronic obstructive asthma
2. An elderly patient with a history of lung cancer is admitted from the nursing home with ataxia, syncope, and a fractured arm as the result of a fall. The patient undergoes a closed fracture reduction of the humerus in the ED, and a complete work up for metastatic carcinoma of the brain. The patient is found to have metastatic carcinoma of the brain. Which of the following is the principal diagnosis?
   a. Ataxia
   b. Fractured humerus
   c. Metastatic carcinoma of the brain
   d. Carcinoma of the lung
3. As a result of the disparity in documentation practices, queries can be made in which of the following scenarios?
   a. To clarify specificity or severity
   b. To clarify a cause and effect relationship between two conditions
   c. To clarify POA assignment
   d. Both A and B
   e. All the above
4. The following query was found in a patient's health record. Which of the answers best applies to this query?

   Dr. Smith—this patient was admitted through the ED with multi-system trauma. During surgery she was transfused with 5 units of packed red blood cells, and fresh frozen plasma. Her laboratory work indicates a 10 point drop in her hematocrit levels, and you documented anemia in her post-operative progress notes. On day two she was transfused with additional units of packed red blood cells. Please document the type of anemia you are referring to.
   a. This is a leading query
   b. This query brings in information not documented within the chart and is inappropriate
   c. This is a yes or no query
   d. This is an appropriate query

(AHIMA 2014)

Training Nonphysician Clinicians

Every clinician who documents in a patient record should receive at least initial training in CDI. Furthermore, clinicians who are well trained on the clinical documentation process may have a positive influence on physicians' documentation practices. At a minimum, trained clinicians' documentation can be used by the CDI specialist or coder to generate clinically validated queries. While this seems like a simple statement, implementing the task is difficult. The best way to accomplish this training is to communicate the basics of the CDI program to all clinical managers and with their input create a thorough schedule for training.

Who Needs to be Trained?

CDI training should be focused on nursing staff, respiratory therapists, physical therapists, and dieticians. One way to determine all of these positions in an organization is to review 10 to 20 health records and identify every clinician (by title, not by name) who documented in the records. Chances are great that this review identifies an exhaustive listing of clinicians for training purposes.

After identifying the clinicians, the program staff should schedule training. As with physician training, the best way to begin is by obtaining support from the clinicians' leader. The program staff should inform the department manager or director about the CDI education well in advance of any scheduling. Because it is important to include a peer-learning component in the training, the manager is often the best person to help identify who that peer instructor might be.

Not all training can happen concurrently due to clinicians' schedules and the organization's training capacity, therefore it is important to create a training schedule. Priorities can be set based on criteria such as training clinicians whose documentation is most likely to be essential for querying, and training clinicians who document the most in patient records.

The first criteria for clinicians whose documentation is likely to be relied upon for querying, may focus on midlevel practitioners. In fact, the program staff should give physician assistants and nurse practitioners high priority for training because of their partnership with physicians. The following is a list of clinicians who should receive training in the basics of high-quality clinical documentation.

- Physician assistants
- Nurse practitioners
- Nurses
- Nutritionists
- Respiratory therapists
- Physical therapists
- Occupational therapists
- Case managers
- Social workers and discharge planners

Who Should Do the Training?

Training should be provided by a team. The best results come from a program taught by a clinical documentation expert paired with a peer of the group in training. This may not always be feasible, but when possible, the program staff should use peer learning. Preparation for the peer-learning process includes identifying one key member from each clinical group for training. These individuals may receive some training with the CDI specialists or one-on-one training and feedback on the nursing units. They will not become documentation experts immediately, but they should know enough to explain the basic concepts to their peers. Using a peer trainer increases the sustainability of the training and is a good investment for the organization (Ford-Gilboe et al. 1997; Goldenberg et al. 2005; Opacic 2003).

What Should the Training Content Be?

The best approach is to train the clinicians using the same content as for the physician training. This is helpful because it exposes the clinicians to all of the fundamental concepts. In addition, it gives the clinicians the opportunity to become familiar with the same training process the physicians underwent (Bandura 2000, 120). If clinicians should have the opportunity to discuss a clinical documentation practice with a physician, they can refer back to the training as a common point of reference.

Conclusion

In addition to training physicians and CDI program and coding staff, it is essential to train all clinicians who document in patient records. The training staff should train clinicians and CDI program staff using the same CAMP Method concepts and basic concepts used to train physicians. The CDI program staff should participate in a three-part training process to achieve maximum results. To whatever extent possible, peer learning should be used when training nonphysician clinicians. When peer clinicians are trained initially and intensively in CDI, their assistance during the training session should result in increased sustainability of the program.

Chapter Quiz

1. The CDI staff training is recommended to be a three-part program. Which is one of the three parts?
   A. Advanced ICD-9 and ICD-10 coding process
   B. Psychology of team dynamics
   C. Program data collection and analysis
   D. Advanced use of the EHR

2. What should be done after the entire training program is complete for CDI staff?
   A. Testing and self-evaluation
   B. Begin training on Medicare Quality Indicators
   C. Recognition by program executives
   D. Training for ICD-10 CM

3. Clinical documentation determines actual and perceived quality of care which makes it important to train CDI staff on what basics of Medicare?
   A. Best-of-practice
   B. Quality indicators
   C. Medical necessity
   D. Present on admission

4. The health record review process and what other aspect allow for the highest level of quality in clinical documentation?
   A. Training on the revenue cycle
   B. Medical necessity
   C. Training on basics of coding
   D. Physician queries

5. What should the CDI program staff do after the majority of classroom basics have been discussed?
   A. Shadow the revenue cycle team
   B. Partner with leading medical staff members
   C. Conduct case review on the nursing units
   D. Independently review and analyze multiple types of records

6. The CDI specialists are partnered with the CDI trainees to discuss which aspect of the record review process?
   A. Present on admission
   B. Medical necessity
   C. Medicare claims
   D. Sources of query opportunities

7. Which tool is used by the CDI program staff to generate reports using entered data elements?
   A. LOS metrics
   B. CDI monitor
   C. Encoder
   D. Grouper

8. What can the CDI program staff generate by training the documenting clinicians on the CDI basics?
   A. Medical necessity requirements
   B. Retrospective patient satisfaction reports
   C. Clinically valid queries
   D. Revenue cycle reports

9. Which of these below should be given high-priority CDI training due to their partnership with physicians?
   A. Nurses practitioners
   B. Respiratory therapists
   C. Phlebotomists
   D. Physical therapists

10. It is vital to provide CDI training to anyone who performs _______.
   A. Collection of lab specimens
   B. Charting of vital signs
   C. Documentation in clinical records
   D. Analysis of the revenue cycle

REFERENCES

AHIMA. 2014. Clinical Documentation Toolkit. Retrieved from: http://library.ahima.org/xpedio/groups/secure/documents/ahima/bok1_050585.pdf.

Bandura, A. 2000. *Handbook of Principles of Organizational Behavior*. Edited by E.A. Locke. Oxford: Blackwell.

Bandura, A. 1986. *Social Foundations of Thought and Action: A Social Cognitive Theory.* Englewood-Cliffs, NY: Prentice-Hall.

Ford-Gilboe, M., H.S. Laschinger, Y. Laforet-Fliesser, C. Ward-Griffin, and S. Foran. 1997. The effect of a clinical practicum on undergraduate nursing students' self-efficacy for community-based family nursing practice. *Journal of Nursing Education* 36(5):212–220.

Goldenberg, D., M.A. Andrusyszyn, C. Iwasiw. 2005. The effect of classroom simulation on nursing students' self-efficacy related to health teaching. *Journal of Nursing Education* 44(7):310–314.

Laschinger, H.K., and C.P. Tresolini. 1999. An exploratory study of nursing and medical students health promotion counselling self-efficacy. *Nurse Education Today.* 19(5): 408–418.

Opacic, D.A. 2003. The relationship between self-efficacy and student physician assistant clinical performance. *Journal of Allied Health.* 32(3):158–156.

Stajkovic, A.D. and F. Luthans, "Self-Efficacy and Work-Related Performances: A Meta-Analysis," Psychological Bulletin 124, no. 2 (1998): 240–61.

Chapter 10 Documentation Review and Physician Queries

The core operational components of a clinical documentation program are concurrent documentation review and physician queries. The documentation review occurs concurrently with the patient's stay, or as close in time to the patient's treatment and care as possible. The purpose of documentation review is to identify any documentation that does not meet the criteria for high-quality clinical documentation and to ask the physician who authored the documentation to clarify the entry. Ideally, an organization should train all physicians on the principles of clinical documentation.

The activity of querying physicians has been a common practice for the past three decades. Initially, only coding professionals in the health information management (HIM) department performed physician querying. Based on the need to obtain accurate documentation for coding purposes, coding professionals would retrospectively complete a written query form and ask the physician to clarify certain documentation in the record. Accurate code assignment is a primary reason for high-quality clinical documentation in the patient health record. However, as discussed throughout the book, healthcare quality report cards, quality of care, and patient satisfaction are three additional, equally important reasons. In addition, there is an increased need for secondary data use in public health reporting. Therefore, many industry influencers count on accurate and timely documentation. This chapter addresses the concurrent documentation review and establishes metrics for this process, specific problematic documentation, and the physician query process. A key resource for the physician query process that every clinical documentation improvement (CDI) program should use is the American Health Information Management Association (AHIMA) practice brief entitled, "Guidelines for Achieving a Compliant Query Practice" (AHIMA 2013).

Setting Program Targets and Goals

In order to be both effective and efficient, every CDI operation must be guided by policies, procedures, and key metrics, which are expectations regarding productivity (Curtright et al. 2000). In a CDI program, record review and the query process need guiding and measuring. As with any decision-making process, each organization should develop specific clinical documentation policies and measures. Generic policies and measures serve as a guide. *However, to ensure alignment between the policy, procedure, measures, and the probability that staff in the organization will use them effectively, every document and decision should be customized for the organization.*

Establishing and Tracking the Concurrent Record Review Rate

While a 100 percent concurrent documentation review rate is desirable, for most organizations it is unrealistic. The reasons for this are two-fold. First, today many inpatient cases are one-day stays, which makes it difficult to perform any meaningful review. Second, most organizations do not have staffing to cover a 100 percent review of all cases, even if it excluded one-day stays from the inpatient population. *It is important to determine an achievable review rate for the organization, one the staff can work to meet.* This depends on specific organizational monitors such as service lines and documentation issues within them.

An organization determines a valid target review rate through the assessment process and some trial and error. The concurrent review portion of the assessment process, addressed in chapter 4, should have established an initial concurrent review rate. However, this rate is just a snapshot in time and the organization needs to validate the rate. Many organizations take one to three months during or after program implementation to determine a valid review rate. This requires carefully collecting data on a daily basis. The organization should collect and compare the number of records each CDI specialist reviews to determine an average valid rate. Because the program is in its beginning stages, productivity will be lower until staff members refine their skills over time. Therefore, during the first year, it is a good idea to continue to validate the review rates and to periodically "raise the bar" to ensure expectations are high enough to keep staff members motivated—but not so high as to discourage them.

Establishing and Tracking the Query Rate

The staff members should use the same process for determining an organization-specific, record-concurrent review rate to determine the query rate. Initial data from the assessment provides a good basis. Over time, program staff members continue to validate the target rates. Tracking the query rate is important because it helps determine whether the program is achieving its goals. For example, if the initial query rate is set at a 35 percent target, but by the end of the second year of the program, the query rate is 40 percent, this may be evidence that the program is not working effectively. Unless there is a specific reason for an increase, such as the addition of a new group of physicians whom the organization has yet to train in documentation principles, there is reason for concern, and the organization should consider a program reassessment by an external organization. With continued querying and follow-up training, query rates should decrease over time.

With the expected decrease in query rate, should an organization expect to decrease program staff? No, the organization should not decrease staff. Rather, it should shift its focus to more intensive follow-up training to lower the query rate even further. The focus can also move to other areas of the organization where the CDI program has not yet penetrated. Once an organization has a trained team of CDI specialists, the value of these individuals to the organization is high as long as the organization uses their skills strategically.

Both overall and individual query rates can also be used to identify potential issues with training. For example, if the overall query rate is meeting the target of 30 percent, but five staff members are querying at a 35 percent query rate and one staff member is querying at a 24 percent query rate, these numbers may show the need for additional training for one or all of the staff members. In addition, if the query rate is significantly lower than the target, and the target rate has been validated, staff members may need additional one-on-one query training on the nursing units. The process of observing staff members and providing feedback about the query process is an effective training tool.

The query rate is calculated by dividing the number of records that were queried by the total number of records reviewed. So, if a CDI specialist reviews 100 records, and 30 records contain queries, the query rate is 30 percent. Data collection can be manual or electronic, although electronic collection is preferred for reliability and preservation of CDI data over time. The process for collecting information should be well organized prior to the actual implementation of the program.

Establishing and Tracking the Query Response Rate

Establishing and tracking the query response rate is different from establishing the review and query rates because there is an additional component. The response rate depends on the physician answering the query. If the physician responds, the query response rate goes up, and if the physician does not respond, the response rate goes down. The chapter on program vision includes a discussion on the importance of an organization's executive team obtaining the initial support from physicians. Other factors that may play a role in physician cooperation include whether the physicians attended training and how they scored on post-testing (if the training included tests).

The mechanics of the CDI program and the timing of the patient's discharge also influence the query response rate. The mechanics of the program determine how to calculate a rate. The CDI manager calculates the query response rate by dividing the number of responses by the number of queries. Therefore, if a CDI specialist issues 50 queries and 25 physicians respond to them, the response rate is 50 percent. However, this number varies based on the program's definition of a "response to a query." For example, if the CDI program requires a query response within 24 hours of the query, it will have a different result than if it requires the query response within 48 hours. In addition, it is important to determine how the calculation addresses short-stay patients or queries asked the day prior to discharge.

If the program allows physicians 36 hours versus 24 hours after discharge to respond to a query, the response rate will vary.

Every organization must determine the definition of a physician response and exactly how the response rate will be calculated. AHIMA suggests considering an 80 percent physician response rate and an 80 percent agreement rate (AHIMA 2014). The documentation is essential to accurate coding, and organizations may want to consider using the same timeframe for query responses as they use for final coding. For example, if a hospital's policy is to drop bills within 72 hours of final discharge, the physician query response should be consistent with this policy. Without a standard, well-documented approach, it is impossible to compare rates over time. Physicians should be informed about the timeframe in which they have to respond.

It is the CDI program's responsibility to make sure CDI practitioners who are querying physicians just prior to the patient's discharge adequately notify those physicians in a timely manner via e-mail or an EHR messaging system (AHIMA 2013). Whatever the communication mechanism used to inform physicians about outstanding queries, it must be reliable and consistent. The physicians must be aware of how the CDI specialist will inform them of outstanding queries and what their responsibility is to respond. There are several ways to follow up on the query once submitted by the CDI specialist. Normally, the CDS continues to follow the query while the patient is in house. Once the provider discharges the patient, the responsibility remains with the CDS or is transferred to the coder. The preferred method should be based on work flow considerations within the facility. A clerical staff member can track the completion process and continue to remind the physician. After the physician answers the query and the CDI specialist adds the documentation, he or she can notify the coder for final coding.

Establishing and Tracking a Query Validation or Agreement Rate

This last key operations metric is important to establish because it measures the degree to which the physicians and the CDI program staff are synchronized in their understanding of the query and CDI process. In addition, the organization can use this metric to show it does not expect physicians to respond to every query by documenting an additional diagnosis or additional information about a patient's diagnosis in the record.

Sometimes, the documentation is valid as originally entered, but the physician just needs to confirm the documentation. For example, the physician documents the patient's diagnosis as chest pain. The CDI specialist queries the physician for a diagnosis or etiology of the chest pain. The physician may respond with documentation in the progress note, "chest pain, etiology undetermined." In this case, the physician disagrees that the symptom had an etiology (as asked by the CDI specialist).

In another example, several laboratory tests shows a patient with low potassium levels. The CDI specialist submits a query asking the physician to document the diagnosis that the abnormal test results represent. The physician documents, "K levels within normal limits for this patient with congestive heart failure (CHF)." This is another example of the physician not agreeing with the question that asks for a diagnosis to represent the abnormal laboratory values (IPRO 2005a).

It is important to collect the agreement rate because if it is too high or too low, this may represent a systemic problem with the documentation process. For example, if the agreement rate is 100 percent, the physician is agreeing with the CDI specialist on all queries. This may be evidence of either leading queries or physicians who did not receive proper training in clinical documentation practices. A query agreement rate that is too low may indicate that CDI specialists are asking unnecessary queries. It may also represent problems with physician documentation that the organization can easily correct with additional training. The organization could correct the disagreement in the chest pain and low potassium level documentation examples through focused physician follow-up education.

Table 10.1 shows an organization's key metrics. In each case, the organization sets a target. The table indicates the actual rates for the quarter as well as the percentage of achievement for that metric. Physician response rates appear to be the biggest concerns for this organization.

The Importance of Concurrent Record Reviews

Recording clinical documentation in the clinical record at the time of treatment has been shown to produce higher quality of care (Cascio et al. 2005). In addition, the physician's memory of the patient and the actual treatment interaction is clearer during the treatment as opposed to days or weeks after the physician discharged the patient. While there is no specific regulatory guideline that limits when a CDI specialist can query a physician to provide documentation clarification in a patient's record, every organization should develop a policy to address this issue. The

Table 10.1 Sample clinical documentation key measures

Key Metric	Quarter 1	Target*	% Achievement
Concurrent: Record review rate	75%	90%	83%
Concurrent: Physician **query** rate	40%	40%	100%
Physician **response** rate	50%	75%	67%
Physician **validation** rate	70%	80%	88%
Retrospective: Physician **query** rate	5%	15%	33%
Physician **response** rate	100%	60%	60%
Physician **validation** rate	65%	85%	76%

*Note: Targets are not suggested. The targets noted were created specifically by the healthcare organization using its own assessment data. All targets should be organization-specific and be validated on at least an annual basis.

primary goal for all CDI programs should be to obtain complete documentation in the patient's record prior to discharge.

The CDI staff's concurrent record review should begin on the second day after admission. Clinical documentation is normally incomplete on the first day. Review of the record at that time would have little benefit. The CDI manager should consider weekend and holiday coverage. When possible, the CDS staff should alternate schedules, working Tuesday to Saturday or Sunday to Thursday. The goal should be to cover 100 percent of the cases in the target group within 48 hours. CDI staff should assess all clinical documentation present in the patient's record to determine if there are any occurrences where the documentation is not meeting the criteria for high-quality clinical documentation. If a documentation deficiency exists, the CDI specialist should generate a query, notify the physician, and record the query in the program database. If the record does not contain any deficiencies, the CDI specialist should record the review in the program database. For every record reviewed, whether it generated a query, the CDI specialist should record the date for follow-up review in the program database (or manual tickler file if the program does not use an electronic data collection tool). The follow-up review should be one to two days from the initial review.

The CDI manager should consider an effective retrospective query process. In all cases, the coder should be aware of queries the CDS submits. This ensures the CDI specialist does not submit duplicate queries. When the coder identifies a new clarification opportunity, he or she should submit a post discharge or retrospective query. This can occur because the CDS did not review the record immediately before discharge. New information may be included that requires clarification. The coder may need additional documentation to assign the most specific code. When the coder assigns retrospective queries, he or she should share this information with the CDS for educational purposes.

Physician Queries

A physician query is a question directed to a physician to obtain clarification of documentation in a patient's record when the current documentation does not meet one or more of the criteria for high-quality clinical documentation. Therefore, the patient's record must contain clinical evidence to support any questions (or queries) the CDI specialist asks the physician regarding documentation in that record. The physician query process should be well documented by the CDI manager with a written policy and procedure for each organization. The query should clearly identify for the physician the clinical evidence in the record that is prompting the query. All staff members who are involved in querying physicians, as well as the physicians, should receive training on the query process. Some important elements found in the AHIMA practice briefs, quality improvement organization (QIO) statements regarding clinical documentation, and in the Centers for Medicare and Medicaid Services (CMS) guidelines include the following:

Queries should only be asked

- If there is valid clinical evidence that the documentation is incomplete or does not meet one of the seven criteria for high-quality clinical documentation

- By an individual with solid clinical knowledge
- In an open-ended manner (physicians must document a response and cannot just respond yes or no). The exception to this rule is the present on admission (POA) query where a yes or no answer is acceptable.
- In a non-leading manner (without pointing physicians to a specific response)
- To the individual whose documentation is in question or who is responsible for interpreting test results and other data in the patient's record

Every organization should develop a query policy and procedure that is specific to its organization and that addresses

- When to ask queries
- Who asks queries and to whom
- The hospital's responsibility in supporting the query process
- The physician's responsibility in responding to queries
- Acceptable ways to respond to queries (AHIMA 2013; CMS and NCHS 2014)

The organization also wants to ensure the physicians have access to the record. In addition, a standard format for the query form should be delineated. Finally, the organization should establish whether the form will be an approved, permanent document in the health record or require an addendum. In every case, a physician's response should be incorporated into the health record. If the form is to become a part of the health record, hospital policies and medical staff bylaws must support this practice.

While the seven criteria for high-quality clinical documentation provide an objective basis for generating a query, it is helpful for an organization to provide examples of when documentation requires a physician query. Conversely, the organization should provide examples of when documentation does not require a physician query. Often, cases where a query is unnecessary involve physician documentation of a clinical condition that is not supported by the evidence in the record. This scenario requires a peer review, not a query from the CDI specialist or a coding professional. Examples of cases that require a query may include the following:

- Documentation of reportable conditions or procedures is conflicting, ambiguous, or otherwise incomplete. An example is documentation of community-acquired pneumonia by the attending physician in the progress notes and a later consultation report specifying the pneumonia as streptococcal.
- Abnormal diagnostic test results indicate the possible addition of a secondary diagnosis or higher specificity of an already documented condition.
- The patient is receiving treatment for a condition the physician has not documented. This can occur when the physician documents medication in the medication administration record (MAR), such as Cardizem, but does not list a corresponding diagnosis of atrial fibrillation in the record.

- The physician does not document abnormal operative or procedural findings.
- It is unclear as to whether the physician ruled out a condition. An example is an acute myocardial infarction mentioned only in the emergency department (ED) record, and the discharge summary mentions that the patient had chest pain due to gastroesophageal reflux disease.
- The documentation does not identify principal diagnosis clearly (the reason, after study, for admission) (AHIMA 2013).

Figure 10.1 is an example of a query policy and procedure developed for an academic medical center. The policy is specific to the needs and processes of the organization. It makes a sufficient example, but for a policy and procedure to be effective for an organization, it should be organization specific.

Specific Problematic Documentation

Due to the compliance concerns surrounding the possible leading queries, CMS has engaged the QIOs to assist in record review of certain diagnosis-related groups (DRGs) and documentation concerns. The QIOs perform reviews as part of the Hospital Payment Monitoring Program (HPMP). CMS selects and updates them on an annual basis using historical knowledge and experience related to medically unnecessary admissions, inappropriate readmissions, and incorrect DRG coding. Some of the specific problematic documentation includes documentation for sepsis and related conditions, pneumonia, congestive heart failure, and blood loss anemia. There are more details below on documentation for sepsis and related conditions and an example of the level of detail of HPMP information that should be available to the CDI staff. Often the HIM or finance departments in the hospital conduct QIO training and communications. It is essential that these departments include the CDI function in all communications from the QIO.

Sepsis or Urosepsis?

A physician may document the terms sepsis or urosepsis when a more detailed condition is actually present and clinically supported. In most cases, if the physician had the proper training in the nuances of some of the diagnostic details, he or she would have documented the entry differently. The QIOs have created excellent tools to assist hospitals in training physicians, coding professionals, and clinical documentation staff. The definitions below for sepsis, septicemia, and related conditions are from Island Peer Review Organization (IPRO), the New York State QIO, and the Texas QIO (Texas Medical Foundation [TMF]). Each definition provides clinical information that CDI specialists can use to determine whether to query physicians. Each condition results in different ICD-9-CM coding and may result in a different DRG assignment as well. There is more information in the ICD-9-CM Official Guidelines for Coding and Reporting on the proper coding of sepsis (CMS 2014).

Figure 10.1 Sample query policy and procedure

Retrospective queries—HIM coders will query the patient's MD if opportunities to improve documentation are noted during retrospective review of the patient's record. Queries of the attending physician after discharge should be made only when there is sufficient supporting documentation within the body of the health record to warrant a query. Questions about documentation in the record may arise during the coding process or as a result of a special audit.

The physician will be queried in the following situations:

1. Documentation is inconsistent and/or ambiguous, unclear, incomplete, unspecified. or general in nature (AHIMA Standards of Ethical Coding and Compliance Guidance for Third Party Billing Companies 1999)
2. Principal diagnosis (reason for admission, after study) is not clearly identified
3. Significant CDI Specialist queries not answered prior to discharge (those which would impact severity level)
4. Abnormal diagnostic test results indicate the possible addition of a secondary diagnosis or increased specificity of an already documented condition
5. Lack of clarity as to whether a condition has been ruled out
6. Patient is receiving treatment for a condition that has not been documented
7. Significance of abnormal operative, procedural, or pathologic findings is not documented
8. Predetermined and agreed upon (with medical staff) clinical criteria are not met
9. Agreement and documentation of diagnoses documented by other members of the healthcare team (nutrition, substance abuse team [if not completed by MD member of team], wound care team) needs physician verification

Query format

The physician query form will be used for all queries, including patient identification, reason for query, directions as to how to provide the requested documentation clarification, and contact information of the person executing the query. When there are multiple questions for one case, the physician is to be alerted that there is more than one query requiring a response.

1. In completing the reason for query on the physician query form, the coder will use open-ended questions and allow the physician to render and document the clinical interpretation of the diagnosis, condition, or procedure, based on the facts of the case. Closed-ended or leading questions will be avoided.
2. Exceptions to the open-ended query, when it is appropriate to query for a specific diagnosis, include the following:
   a. Positive lab or radiology findings clinically supporting the diagnosis (*Coding Clinic*, 2nd quarter, 1998)
   b. Medication is prescribed that supports the specific diagnosis (*Coding Clinic*, 1st quarter, 1993, 2nd quarter, 1998)
3. Physicians (attending or resident) are to respond to retrospective queries within five business days and for special audits on the same day.
4. If physicians agree with the query, they are to document on a form. (All entries must be signed and dated for the date the current entry is made.)
5. If physicians disagree with the query, they are to indicate the reasons on the physician query form and return the form to the HIM department.

The form shall be documented by the physician and scanned into the hospital's imaging system, if the physician documents additional information.

Septicemia

Septicemia is a systemic disease with the presence and persistence of pathogenic micro-organisms or toxins in the blood (such as viruses, bacteria, fungus, or other organisms). Septicemia and sepsis are no longer considered synonymous (IPRO 2005b).

Systemic inflammatory response syndrome (SIRS)

SIRS is the systemic response to infection or trauma. The systemic response is manifested by a variety of clinical signs and symptoms such as

- Fever (temperature) greater than 38 degrees C (100.4 degrees F)
- Hypothermia less than 36 degrees C (96.8 degrees F)
- White blood count greater than or equal to 12000 cells/mm3 (leukocytosis)
- WBC less than or equal to 4000 cells/mm3 (leukopenia) or 10 percent immature cells (bands)
- Heart rate greater than 90 beats per minute (tachycardia)
- Respirations greater than 20 breaths per minute or a PcCO2 less than 32 milligrams of mercury
- Hypotension
- Altered mental status (comatose, confused, lethargy, obtunded) (IPRO 2005b).

Sepsis

Sepsis is SIRS due to infection. Infection can originate anywhere in the body and be triggered by a bacterial, viral, parasitic, or fungal infection (IPRO 2005b).

Severe Sepsis

Severe sepsis includes

- SIRS due to infection with organ dysfunction
- Sepsis associated with acute dysfunction in one or more organs
- Organ dysfunction that may be cardiovascular, renal, respiratory, hepatic, hematological, central nervous system, or metabolic acidosis (IPRO 2005b).

Septic Shock

Septic shock is sepsis with hypotension or a failure of the cardiovascular system. Endotoxic shock and gram negative shock are synonymous with septic shock. Septic shock also equals severe sepsis. (IPRO 2005b).

Bacteremia

Bacteremia is bacteria in the blood without an associated inflammatory response. Bacteremia also

- Denotes laboratory findings of viable bacteria in the blood with no systemic manifestations
- Progresses to septicemia only when there is a more severe infectious process or an impaired immune system (IPRO 2005b).

Urosepsis

Urosepsis is an infection confined to the urinary system. It refers to pyuria or bacteria in the urine (not in the blood). The physician should be queried to determine if the bacteria in the urine have progressed to septicemia or sepsis. (IPRO 2005b).

Other Problematic Documentation

Other diagnoses that CMS has identified as problematic for complete and accurate documentation include malnutrition, respiratory failure, sepsis, renal failure, acute blood loss anemia, congestive heart failure, and pneumonia. Another concern of CMS in some cases is when the physician documents a condition, such as blood loss anemia, when the patient's symptoms do not meet the accompanying clinical criteria for acute blood loss anemia. In these cases, the QIOs determine the diagnosis invalid and deny payment to the hospital. Every hospital can prevent this type of occurrence through proper physician training, referral of such documentation problems to peer review (or the physician CDI leader), and with close review and incorporation of all HPMP communications into the physician training and query processes.

Retrospective Review

The coding staff performs the retrospective review in most organizations during the coding process. At this time, the coding professionals can determine whether there is an opportunity for a valid physician query based on the clinical evidence in the patient's record. In addition, when there are outstanding physician queries from the concurrent review, the coding professionals can and should follow up on those queries. Retrospective review and querying serves as a safety net to the CDI program and is a process that enables a coding professional to translate physician documentation into coded data with the highest possible accuracy.

As noted in the key metric examples at the beginning of the chapter, the retrospective query rate should be much lower than the concurrent query rate: no more than 10 percent. If the retrospective query rate is higher than 10 to 15 percent, it may be evidence of the need for additional physician training and increased productivity or training for the CDI program staff. A low retrospective query rate may be due to a mature program with well-educated physicians in the CDI process or an effective concurrent review process by the CDS group. In addition, the physician response rate for retrospective queries should be 100 percent (UVA 2008). If possible, hospitals should work with the medical staff to include outstanding queries as an incomplete health record deficiency for which a physician's admission privileges can be suspended. Given the importance of the most accurate documentation, both administration and medical staff members should support such a policy.

Teaming Clinical Documentation and Coding Professionals

CDI staff and coding professionals can unite to achieve organizational CDI goals. Some of the ways organizations pair CDI staff and coding professionals include

- Involving the coding staff in the initial CDI specialist training.
- Having coding managers and staff train CDI specialists on the coding and reimbursement systems.
- Training coding and CDI staff together on the use of the CDI program database. In most cases, both groups will be entering data into the database for queries. CDI specialists will use the database to enter concurrent reviews and queries, and coding professionals will use it to enter retrospective queries.
- Having monthly meetings to discuss current QIO initiatives and communications. They can also analyze program data that may help both CDI and coding staff understand where continued documentation problems are in the record and which physicians are responsible for most significant problems.
- Inviting coding professionals to attend physician follow-up training sessions.
- Pairing each CDI specialist with a coding professional to track the final resolution of outstanding concurrent queries when the provider discharges the patient.
- Charging the coding staff with specific focus on one or two-day-stay cases where CDI program staff are unable to generate a concurrent query. CDI and coding partners can also share these cases to review for query opportunities as soon as the provider discharges the patient.

Example: Clinical Indicators and Corresponding Queries

Each facility should customize a set of frequently submitted queries and discuss them with the CDI and coding departments as well as physician representatives from specialties most likely to receive the query. For example, a CDI specialist or coding professional may frequently submit a query on metabolic encephalopathy to an endocrinologist, hospitalist, and internal medicine physician. In addition, the instruction for use of each query should include a set of facility-approved clinical indicators for the CDI and coding teams to use. Physicians representing the specialty that is likely to receive the query should review the clinical indicator sets.

Scholarly journals publish clinical indicators for specific diseases, which are available from multiple sites on the Internet. An Internet search for "clinical indicators for sepsis" gives several article results. The query and clinical criteria set examples below may be an effective beginning point for discussions with the facility medical staff, CDI, and coding teams. Each example includes a disease definition, example clinical criteria, and case scenario, as well as an example provider query specific to the disease process or procedure.

Example Queries

The following is an example query requesting clarification of the etiology of symptoms in the clinical record. Additional examples may be found in Appendix J.

Metabolic Encephalopathy

Definition:

Metabolic encephalopathy—a potentially reversible abnormality of brain function caused by processes of extracerebral origin such as acidosis, adverse reactions to medications and toxins, brain tumor, dehydration, infection, metabolic dysfunction, organ failure, or trauma.

Clinical Criteria:

- Delirium
- Confusion
- Systemic toxic states (for example, sepsis)
- Rapid presentation of fluctuating alertness (attention and concentration)
- Depressed consciousness
- Progressive loss of intellect (dementia)
- Altered mental status
- Hyper excitable states such as agitated dementia (delirium)

Note:

- May coexist with dementia
- Differential diagnosis of stroke and slowly expanding masses, such as tumor or subdural hematoma (rarely)
- The cause of the encephalopathy should be documented when known.

Citations:

Retrieved from:

NINDS. 2010. NINDS encephalopathy information page. http://www.ninds.nih.gov/disorders/encephalopathy/encephalopathy.htm.

Swenson, R. 2008. Cases: Altered mental status. http://www.dartmouth.edu/~dons/part_2/chapter_cases.html.

Clinical Scenario:

The patient presented in the ED with pneumonia, fatigue, recent altered mental status, and depressed consciousness with fluctuating levels of alertness. The family stated that the patient had no history of dementia.

Query:

Dr. Smith:

Your progress notes dated 3/5/2014 indicate the patient's symptoms include fatigue, altered mental status, depressed consciousness, and fluctuating levels of alertness. The patient's symptoms were treated with IV fluids, CT of head, and valium. Based on your medical judgment, please document the etiology of these symptoms in the clinical record:

- Altered mental status
- Toxic encephalopathy
- Metabolic encephalopathy
- Hepatic
- Septic
- Other encephalopathy
- Other (please specify)
- Clinically undetermined

Conclusion

The physician concurrent query process is one of the core operational components of every CDI program. The organization should clearly document, explain, and maintain the process in policies and procedures specific to its needs. These policies and procedures should be documented, updated by the CDI manager on at least an annual basis, and be made available for any physician, manager, or relevant staff member to review. The organization should thoroughly train both physicians and program staff on the query process. It should develop key metrics with organization-specific target rates using initial assessment and actual day-to-day operations data. In addition, the targets should be reviewed and validated by the CDI manager on at least an annual basis.

Chapter Quiz

1. Each organization should determine ______ as there is currently no benchmark for this metric.
   A. Length of stay
   B. CC capture rate
   C. Physician response rate
   D. Retrospective query response rate

2. Which is a primary reason for the demand for high-quality clinical documentation?
   A. Quality control
   B. Code assignment
   C. Medicare medical necessity
   D. Physician time demand

3. Clinical documentation policies and procedures should:
   A. Dictate the practices and procedures for medical treatment
   B. Encompass nationally recognized guidelines
   C. Meet all the requirements of physician leaders
   D. Be created by and specifically for each organization

4. Though the goal for concurrent documentation review should be 100 percent, which type of inpatient stay makes it hard for any meaningful review?
   A. One-day stays
   B. Medicare or Medicaid
   C. Same-day surgery
   D. Newborn or maternal

5. Establishing the __________ rate is determined through the assessment process and could take several months.
   A. Physician query
   B. Query response
   C. Target review
   D. Deficiency

6. If the agreement rate on retrospective queries for a physician is 100 percent, this could be a sign of:
   A. A lack of responsiveness
   B. Leading queries
   C. Cooperation
   D. Exceptionally well-written queries

7. With continued querying and follow-up training, what is the expected result?
   A. Query rate reduction
   B. Query rate increase
   C. Increased manpower needs
   D. Improved MCC capture rates

8. What has been proven to produce higher levels of patient quality of care?
   A. Increased target review rate
   B. Updated physician query process
   C. Educating leading physician in query process
   D. Concurrent clinical documentation

9. The CDI staff should perform concurrent record review on the ______ day of admission.
   A. First
   B. Second
   C. Third
   D. Final

10. Why should CDI staff be teamed up with a coding professional?
   A. To improve team morale
   B. To increase the number of CDI audits
   C. To speed up the concurrent review
   D. To achieve CDI organizational goals

REFERENCES

AHIMA. 2014. Clinical Documentation Toolkit. Retrieved from: http://library.ahima.org/xpedio/groups/secure/documents/ahima/bok1_050585.pdf.

AHIMA. 2013. Guidelines for Achieving a Compliant Query Practice. *Journal of AHIMA.* 84 no 2, 50–53.

AHIMA. 2008. Managing an effective query process. *Journal of AHIMA.* 79(10): 83–88.

Cascio, B.M., J.H. Wilckens, M.C. Ain, C. Toulson, and F.J. Frassica. 2005. Documentation of acute compartment syndrome at an academic healthcare center. *Journal of Bone and Joint Surgery* 87(2):346.

Centers for Medicare and Medicaid Services (CMS) and the National Center for Health Statistics (NCHS). 2014. ICD-9-CM Official Guidelines for Coding and Reporting. http://www.cdc.gov/nchs/data/icd/icd9cm_guidelines_2011.pdf.

Curtright, J.W., S.C. Stolp-Smith, and E.S. Edell. 2000. Strategic performance management: Development of a performance measurement system at the Mayo Clinic. *Journal of Healthcare Management* 45 (1):58–68.

IPRO. 2005a. Coding for quality: Documentation tips for the top seven DRGs. Revised 2005, Hospital Payment Monitoring Program.

IPRO. 2005b. Coding for quality: Documentation tips for the top ten denied DRGs. Hospital Payment Monitoring Program.

UVA. 2008. University of Virginia (UVA) Medical Center reduces coding errors with six sigma. Report On Medicare Compliance. http://www.isixsigma.com/industries/healthcare/uva-reduces-cpt-coding-errors-six-sigma.

Chapter 11

Collecting, Analyzing, and Reporting on Program Data

Chapter 10 discussed collecting key metrics for the query process. These metrics include the record review rate, query rate, physician response rate, and query agreement (or validation) rate. These are the core operational measures every organization must collect to ensure a smooth process. However, there are additional data the organization can gather for strategic and management purposes, as well as key metrics review and analyzation. As with all other program design elements, it is essential that an organization develop program data reporting specific to its needs. No two programs use exactly the same program data reporting. While every program uses the key metrics for querying as the base data, each program has specific nuances around the other data it collects and reviews and how it uses this data. This chapter includes examples of data from different programs.

Essential Data Elements

Table 11.1 provides the core key metric table from chapter 10 again as a review of the key data elements that form the basis for data analysis for every clinical documentation improvement (CDI) program. While the data elements of record review rate, query rate, response rate, and validation rate are the same, the targets set for each metric should be organization specific (Tangen 2003). They should also be both achievable and challenging targets.

Figure 11.1 depicts the process and timing for collecting each of the key metrics. The figure represents both the concurrent and retrospective reviews and query process. Physician response, if obtained, occurs after review and query.

Table 11.1 Sample clinical documentation key measures

Key Metric	Quarter 1	Target*	% Achievement
Concurrent: Record review rate	75%	90%	83%
Concurrent: Physician **query** rate	40%	40%	100%
Physician **response** rate	50%	75%	67%
Physician **validation** rate	70%	80%	88%
Retrospective: Physician **query** rate	5%	15%	33%
Physician **response** rate	100%	60%	60%
Physician **validation** rate	65%	85%	76%

*Note: The targets noted were created specifically by the healthcare organization using its own assessment data. All targets should be organization-specific and be validated on at least an annual basis.

Figure 11.1 Collection of operational core CDI key metrics

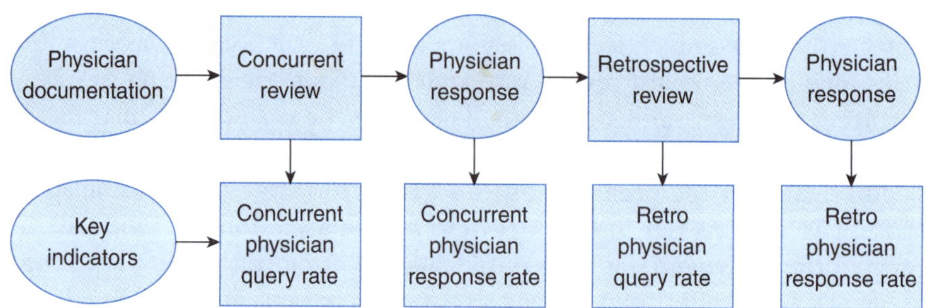

Additional Ways to Analyze Core Key Metrics

It is important to report on and analyze the CDI core key metrics in the aggregate. However, it is also helpful to generate reports that present the data in different manners. For example, the concurrent record review rate in table 11.1 is 75 percent overall. It may be helpful to report on the record review rate by CDI specialist, nursing unit, or service. Looking at the review rate by CDI specialist can identify productivity problems by individual. Review rate by nursing unit or service could identify if there are problems obtaining the patient records in certain units. If so, the units or services could be contacted by the CDI staff and appropriate problem-solving activities can follow. This analysis is only helpful for organizations with hard-copy health records because those with electronic health records (EHRs) should usually not have access problems. Access problems with an EHR indicate either a shortage of terminals or a wait time for data transfer or streaming that the information technology (IT) department should address.

Table 11.2 shows an example of the CDI core key metrics broken down by CDI specialist. The preliminary data analysis of this table shows that reviewers B, C, and E all appear to be producing results consistent with the target rates for the organization. Reviewers A, D, and F produced some outcomes that need further investigation. For example, reviewer A is reviewing many more records than the others are, but has a much lower query rate. This may represent rushed reviews. However, when viewing these data elements in light of the 98 percent agreement rate, it may actually represent more careful reviews and interactions with the physicians. The agreement rate of 98 percent may also represent leading queries or overly aggressive interactions with the physicians. In any case, individual metrics that are significantly different from the targets and the rest of the group, especially for more than a one-month period, need investigation through discussion, query reviews, possibly concurrent reviewer observation, and follow-up education to correct any gaps in skill or knowledge.

Reviewer D has the opposite problem of reviewer A. Reviewer D's review rate is much lower at 60 percent. However, the query rate is much higher at 50 percent. This may simply represent a productivity issue that, if corrected, would result in a query rate consistent with the targets. The agreement rate of 95 percent is also a concern that needs investigating. Finally, reviewer F's metrics are consistent with the exception of the agreement rate. At 29 percent, the concern is the validity of the queries reviewer F is generating, and the metric may represent a gap in skills that needs correcting (Six Sigma 2015).

Table 11.3 contains the core key metrics by specialty for concurrent queries only. If necessary, this information is sorted by individual physicians to identify who needs follow-up training. The data on this table show a problem with general surgery and orthopedic surgery. For the orthopedic service, the 55 percent query rate is much higher than the target of 40 percent (see table 11.1). Furthermore, the response rates for both services are lower than the targets. Moreover, the orthopedic surgery agreement rate is significantly lower than the target rate of 80 percent (see table 11.1). The initial follow-up to this should include a review of a sampling of these records and discussion with the chiefs of each service, followed by the appropriate follow-up education or discussions to obtain support from the physicians who respond to the queries.

Table 11.2 CDI core key metrics for concurrent queries by CDI specialist

CDI Specialist	Concurrent Review Rate	Concurrent Query Rate	Concurrent Response Rate	Concurrent Agreement Rate
A	97%	20%	67%	98%
B	80%	30%	65%	69%
C	82%	33%	68%	70%
D	60%	50%	90%	95%
E	80%	28%	63%	72%
F	85%	29%	65%	29%

Table 11.3 CDI core key metrics for concurrent queries by service

Service	Concurrent Query Rate	Concurrent Response Rate	Concurrent Agreement Rate
Internal medicine	35%	68%	65%
Cardiology	25%	80%	30%
Neurology	10%	75%	60%
Gastroenterology	35%	70%	75%
General surgery	40%	50%	60%
Orthopedic surgery	55%	35%	30%
Cardiac surgery	30%	62%	70%
Urology	36%	78%	70%
OB/GYN	25%	70%	80%

The primary purpose of collecting and reviewing core key metrics is to identify any gaps in knowledge or skills and take the appropriate corrective action. Even when the key metrics are consistent with target rates, records should be reviewed by internal or external auditors to validate the reviews and the target rates. Chapter 12 includes a more detailed discussion of these activities .

Collection and Analysis of Additional Operational Data Elements

Most programs collect operational key metrics in addition to the core metrics. These metrics are often determined as the program matures and the management team identifies additional areas of interest or concern. There are some metrics, however, that the management team reviews from the inception of the program, including the reason for the query, the types of secondary diagnoses added on review, and the types of principal diagnosis changes that were made by the CDI specialist or coders. The specialist can only review these metrics if he or she collects the appropriate data at the time of the review.

The reason for query is often focused on the type of documentation that prompted the query. For example, common ways to categorize a reason for query include

- Abnormal laboratory tests not addressed
- Abnormal radiology tests
- Medication ordered without a supporting diagnosis
- Conflicting documentation between the attending physician and the consultant

This type of information is helpful to collect because the management team can use it to focus follow-up education. For example, if the data tells us that 52 percent of all queries stemmed from abnormal laboratory tests the physician did not address, the CDI specialist can appropriately design follow-up communication and education.

It can also be helpful to analyze the type of impact produced by the physician's response. For example, in most cases, additional documentation from the physician is likely to result in either an additional diagnosis, support of a different principal diagnosis, a more refined diagnosis (either principal or secondary), or an additional or more specific procedure (IPRO 2005a; IPRO 2005b). If CDI specialists can identify trends of certain diagnoses or procedures over time, they can use this information to design follow-up education targeted at specific physicians, services, or the entire medical staff if the documentation problem appears to be a global one.

Tables 11.4 and 11.5 are examples of reports that show, over time, the types of diagnoses added and principal diagnosis changes because of query responses. Table 11.4 shows that the most significant changes in principal diagnosis were due to sepsis. This information is useful for creating follow-up training specific to documentation for sepsis and related conditions such as that discussed in chapter 9.

Table 11.5 shows the diagnoses most commonly added to patient records as a result of physician responses to queries. In this case, anemia, electrolyte imbalance, and heart arrhythmias were the top three most common conditions. CDI specialists can use this information, analyzed in conjunction with metrics about the reason for query or the location of documentation supporting a query, to design brief, focused follow-up education. For example, if coders added the arrhythmias because physicians did not document diagnoses from the electrocardiogram (EKG) into the progress notes, then CDI specialists can use copies of the EKGs during follow-up education. The EKG copies demonstrate to physicians that they cannot rely on that cardiologist's documentation (the nontreating physician) in the record to translate information into coded data (CMS and NCHS 2006a; CMS and NCHS 2006b; MedPAC 2014).

Collection and Analysis of Strategic Data Elements

Up to this point, the data elements this chapter has covered are primarily for steering program operations. However, the executive team can also use program data to make strategic decisions. In fact, to the extent that the executive team relies on data the CDI program produces, and as long as that data shows positive impact to the organization, the opportunity to continue to expand the clinical documentation function in the organization exists. The executive team has an

Table 11.4 Principal diagnosis metrics from CDI query responses

Changed to this principal diagnosis	# Times
Sepsis (from bacteremia)	7
Acute systolic/diastolic congestive heart failure (from CHF NOS)	6
Respiratory failure (from other respiratory diagnoses)	3

Table 11.5 Secondary diagnosis key metrics from CDI query responses

Diagnosis added after query	# Times added
Anemia NOS	29
Electrolyte imbalance (hypo or hypernatremia, hypo or hyperkalemia, hypo or hypercalcemia)	25
Arrhythmias (atrial fibrillation, bradycardia, tachycardia,ventricular tachycardia)	25
Intravenous drug abuse	17
Urinary tract infection	15
Pneumonia	15
Hypertension	15
Reflux esophagitis	12
Obesity	11
Loss of consciousness	11
Chronic renal failure	11
Acute renal failure	11
Tobacco abuse	10
Hypercholesterolemia	10
Dehydration	10
Blood loss anemia	10
CHF	9
Atelectasis	9
Thrombocytopenia	7
Malnourished	7
Hypotension	7

interest in reviewing data in four key areas related to strategic key metrics: quality, profitability, physician satisfaction, and patient satisfaction. The CDI team may need to demonstrate these relationships, but as the following sections show, there is a clear relationship between strategic decision making and the data obtained from a CDI program.

Case Mix Index

The case mix index (CMI), which is the average diagnosis-related group (DRG) relative weight for inpatient cases, is an indicator of average reimbursement per patient (MedPAC 2014). For example, if a hospital's CMI is 1.2 and the hospital-specific rate is $6,000, then average reimbursement is $7,200. If CMI increases, the average reimbursement increases. If CMI decreases, the average reimbursement decreases. Because of the relationship between revenue, profit, and CMI, healthcare managers have a strong interest in tracking CMI. They also have a strong interest in understanding any activity that impacts their organization's CMI, including the organization's clinical documentation practices. In particular, if documentation practices were not high quality prior to implementing the program, which would have become clear during the assessment, it is possible that improved documentation quality will have a positive impact on CMI.

Documentation and coding can impact CMI. When documentation alters CMI, it is referred to as CDI case mix change by the CDI department. However, it is important that senior executives in the organization track other indicators of CDI case mix change as well. Significant case mix change occurs when the types of patients admitted to the hospital change (Rosko and Chilingerian 1999). This is known as real patient case mix change. The following components can impact the CMI:

- Seasonal variations
- Medical and surgical mix
- Physician staffing changes
- Coding competency
- Severity of illnesses among the patient population

Below are detailed descriptions of the two types of CMI change: real patient mix change and documentation CMI change (CDI case mix).

Real Patient Mix Change

Real patient mix change is a change in CMI resulting from providers admitting and treating different types of patients at the hospital in a given time period as compared to a prior time. For example, during the month of November, a hospital discharged 100 patients, 25 of them having received a surgical procedure. During November, the CMI was 2.0. Then, in December, the hospital discharged 100 patients, but only 10 of them received a surgical procedure, and the remaining were medical patients. The CMI was 1.3. The change in CMI from November to December in this case was due to a real patient mix change caused by less demand for surgery. CDI activities do not improve this type of CMI change. It is important for executives to understand when they have fluctuations in CMI, what part of the change, if any, was due to real patient mix change, rather than CDI activities.

CDI Case Mix Change

CDI case mix change is a change in CMI resulting from documentation practice changes. For example, in the month of November, a hospital's complication and comorbidity (CC) capture rate was 85 percent and the CMI was 2.0. Then, in the month of December, the CC capture rate fell to 72 percent and the CMI was 1.5. When December cases without a CC were reviewed by the CDI or coding department retrospectively (after the period for resubmission), it was identified by the CDI or coding department that in 20 percent of these cases, the physician did not document the clinical significance (diagnosis) of abnormal test results. This same review identified that during the month of November, physicians were documenting the reason and diagnosis for abnormal test results. The change in CMI from November to December is due to documentation practices. The research behind it can be traced to link CMI with those documentation practices. This is an example of how a CDI program can improve the hospital's CMI.

It is helpful to illustrate changes in CMI with graphs. In general, all graphic illustrations shared throughout an organization should come with an explanation of the significance of the data illustrated on the graph. This practice avoids confusion and misinterpretation.

An example of a clear, simple graph appears in figure 11.2. An example of the explanation accompanying the graph reads:

> **This graph shows a decrease in surgical mix from a mean of 34 percent in 2004 to 25 percent in 2005.**

Because surgery cases are valued by the DRG system at approximately 2.25 times medical cases, this drop in surgical mix has had a significant impact on the hospital's overall case mix. This demonstrates a real patient mix change. The best possible documentation could not make up for a real change in patient mix. It is imperative that senior executives in the organization understand this concept and differentiate between the legitimate and illegitimate impacts of documentation. CDI program managers can ensure executives understand these concepts by sharing this kind of information, if they are not already.

Figure 11.2 Medical and surgical cases by month: 2004 to 2005 monthly comparison

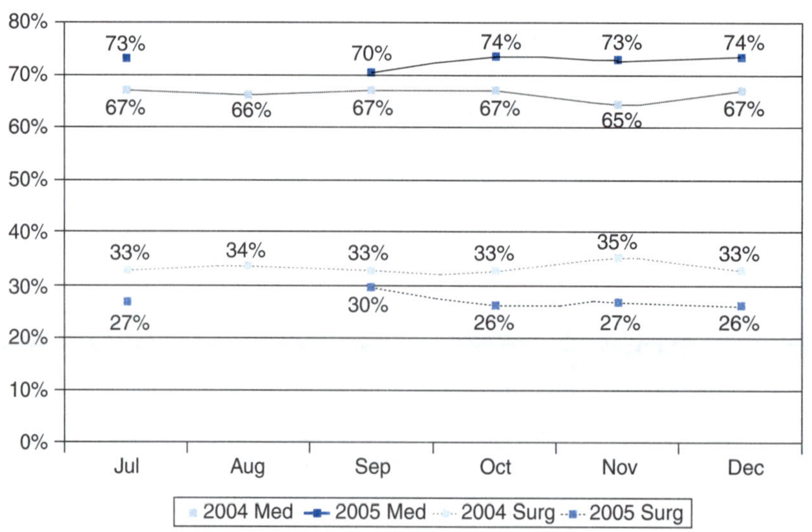

The graph in figure 11.3 links the change in medical and surgical mix to the CMI change. The following explanation can accompany this graph:

> **The Medicare CMI has shown a steady downward trend since June. This could be, in large part, due to the decline in the number of surgical cases relative to medical cases. With the exception of Blue Cross payers, all payers have shown a declining CMI since April.**

In addition to overall CMI, most hospital administrators track CMI by service and CC capture rate. Figures 11.4 and 11.5 illustrate the comparison of CMI by service and CC capture rate for the internal medicine service over time. To the extent that an increase (or decrease) in CMI or CC capture rate is not accompanied by a real patient mix change, clinical documentation changes (better or worse) may be responsible for all or part of the CMI and CC capture rate changes.

Quality Indicators and Severity of Illness Analysis

Most quality reporting systems, including Medicare quality indicators, use the all patient refined (APR) severity DRGs to calculate quality ratings. Some of the current, more visible quality measurement programs include

- The Leapfrog Group (http://www.leapfroggroup.org)
- National Quality Forum (http://www.qualityforum.org/Home.aspx)
- Agency for Healthcare Research and Quality (http://www.ahrq.gov)
- Healthgrades (http://www.healthgrades.com)
- Crimson (http://www.advisory.com/technology/crimson)
- Pay for performance or value-based purchasing (http://www.cms.gov/Medicare/Quality-Initiatives-Patient-Assessment-Instruments/hospital-value-based-purchasing/index.html?redirect=/Hospital-Value-Based-Purchasing)
- Patient Safety Indicators (http://www.qualityindicators.ahrq.gov/modules/psi_overview.aspx)
- Inpatient Quality Indicators (http://www.qualityindicators.ahrq.gov)
- Hospital Inpatient Quality Reporting Program (http://www.cms.gov/Medicare/Quality-Initiatives-Patient-Assessment-Instruments/HospitalQualityInits/HospitalRHQDAPU.html)
- University Health System Consortium Risk of Mortality Levels (https://www.uhc.edu)

APR-DRGs and other quality measurement systems require the International Classification of Diseases (ICD) code assignment for analysis and peer comparison. Integration of CDI with ICD-9, quality score management and billing, or coding risk mitigation is essential to each health information management (HIM) or CDI manager's strategic planning.

Figure 11.3 Hospital-wide CMI by month

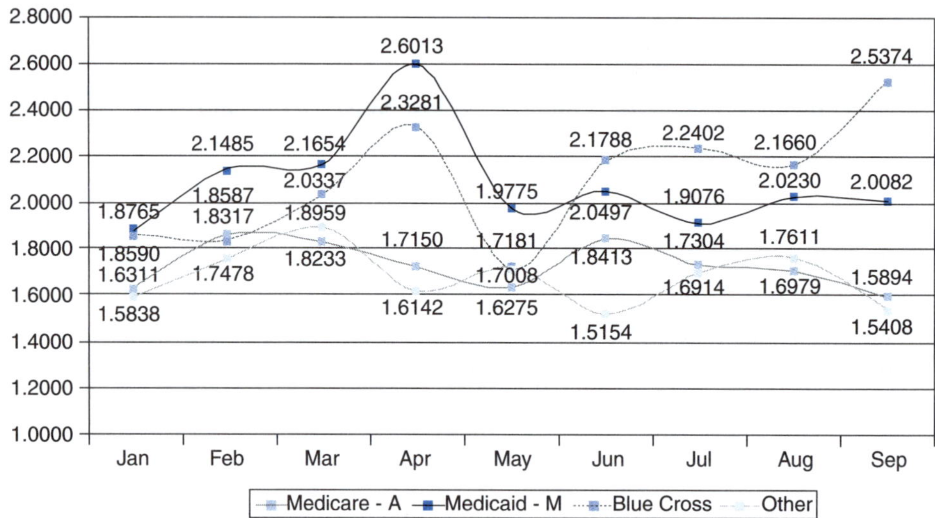

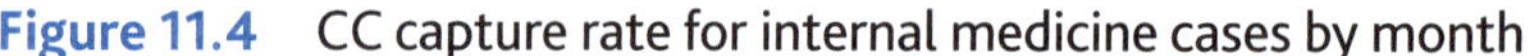

Figure 11.4 CC capture rate for internal medicine cases by month

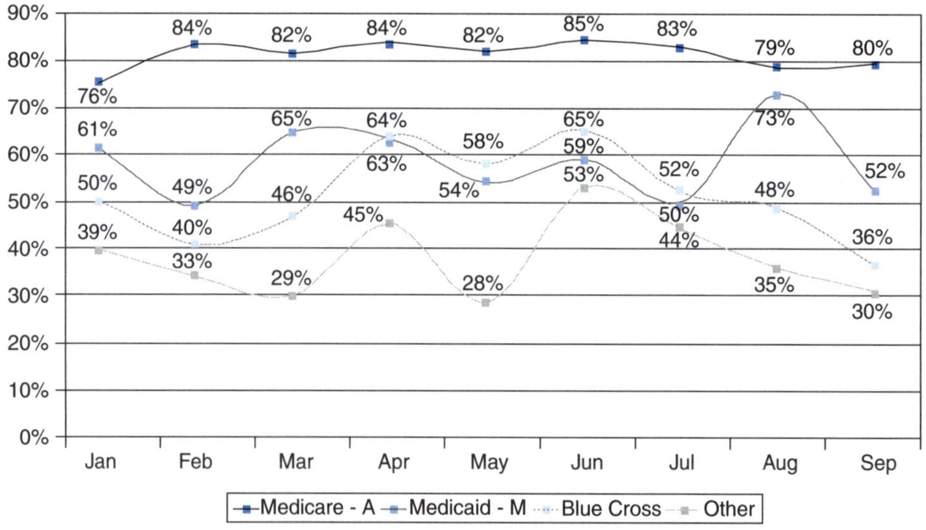

The quality landscape is complex with staff involvement at all levels. A well-thought-out work plan with timeframes and task ownership results in better program outcomes. Quality measurement and development of focused area monitoring and trending help enlist buy-in from stakeholders. Each CDI manager should consider which quality programs to integrate into the CDI program and what areas of risk each has. Next, the CDI manager should determine how the quality programs will be monitored and trended and how they will be reported.

Figure 11.5 Case Mix Index for internal medicine cases by month

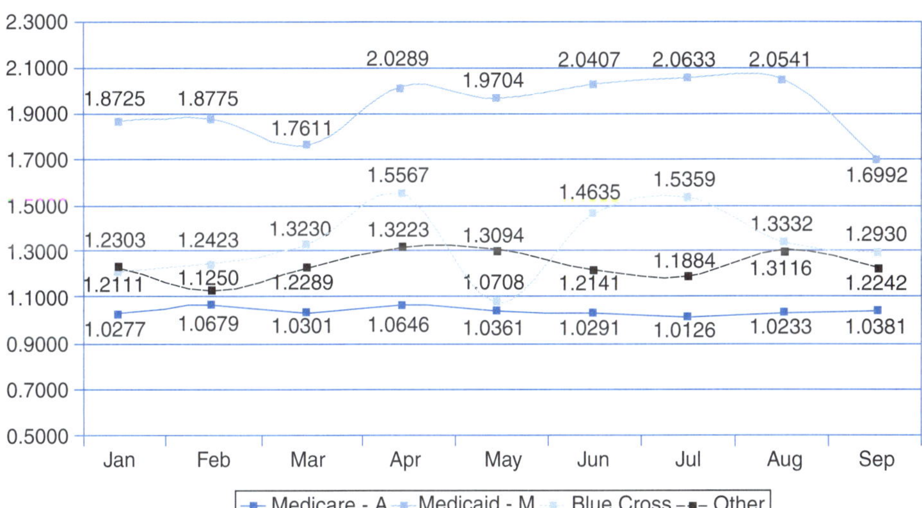

The APR system uses a four-level severity rating system for all cases (Averill et al. 2003). Severity level 1 is the lowest severity rating and severity level 4 is the highest severity rating. The four levels are

1. Minor
2. Moderate
3. Major
4. Extreme

There is no available reference (for example, a major complication or comorbidity (MCC) or CC list) to help CDI specialists and coders identify which secondary diagnoses affect the subclass. Each potential secondary diagnosis must be input into the grouper to determine the associated severity of illness or risk of mortality (SOI/ROM) score. Although the specific methodologies by private organizations are unknown, in general, hospitals can count on better quality ratings if the majority of their inpatients are in higher severity group levels. Hospitals with fewer severity level 1 cases (usually less than 20 percent) are more likely to fare better in the ratings than a peer with 30 percent of its inpatient cases grouped into severity level 1. Some of this makes basic intuitive sense. Why would an acute care hospital, whose focus is treating acute, severely ill patients, have any sizable number of severity level 1 patients? There is an argument that no inpatient cases should ever be grouped into severity level 1, which is a mild level of severity. From a medical necessity perspective, the question is whether severity level 1 patients need inpatient care at all.

Ultimately, higher quality clinical documentation in a patient record leads to more accurate severity levels. Many hospitals that implement clinical documentation programs see an initial increase in severity levels.

Figure 11.6 Severity level changes over time

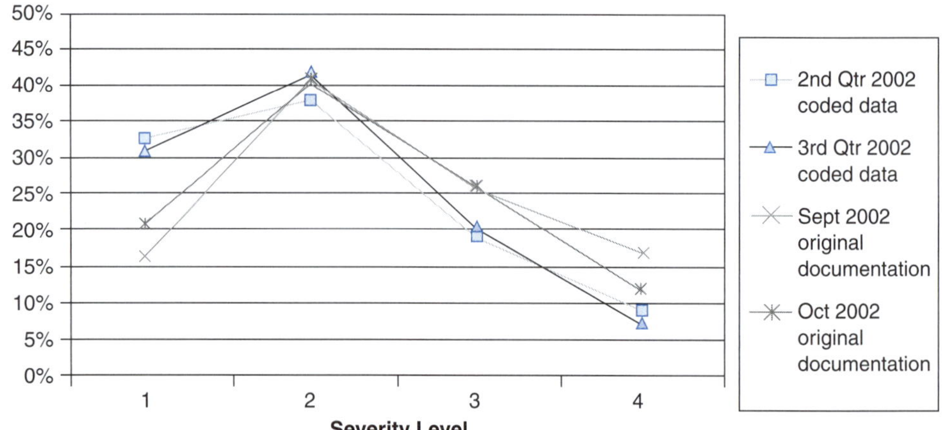

Figure 11.6 is an example of pre- and post-CDI severity level changes. The graph shows that over time the hospital's percentage of severity level 1 cases decreased from a high of 32 percent to a low of 16 percent. In addition, severity level 4 cases increased from a low of 6 percent to a high of 16 percent. Severity level 2 cases showed little change, and severity level 3 cases showed some increase. After analysis, it was clear that higher quality clinical documentation was the primary contributor to these severity level changes. Therefore, by tracking APR severity levels, an organization can predict changes in how they are represented to the public in quality ratings and healthcare report cards.

Hospitals can also track inpatient severity level differences by physician. This analysis determines if there is a particular physician or group of physicians contributing to the hospital's low severity levels through documentation or admitting patients who do not meet medical necessity criteria for an acute care admission.

Figure 11.7 shows an example of severity level tracking by physician. The table next to the graph shows that physician 09092 has a significantly lower average patient severity than the other physicians do. This information likely traces back to problems with the physician's clinical documentation practices.

The CDI program manager should implement a work plan for APR-DRG improvement. Figure 11.8 provides the basic work steps for this process. The work plan includes the initial establishment of target SOI/ROM by service line, APR-DRG, and physician. Peer facility and physician benchmarking can identify focused APR-DRGs and physicians for on-going monitoring. The CDI program manager should determine the root cause of low-level benchmark comparisons and develop an education plan for physicians, CDI specialists, and coders. It is best to also determine the reimbursement impact for on-going improvements in the SOI/ROM levels. The CDI governance committee should participate in the monitoring and stakeholder communication process.

SOI/ROM levels vary by facility. Table 11.6 shows a comparison of average SOI/ROM levels for two urban trauma providers. In this case, not only the

Figure 11.7 Severity levels by physician

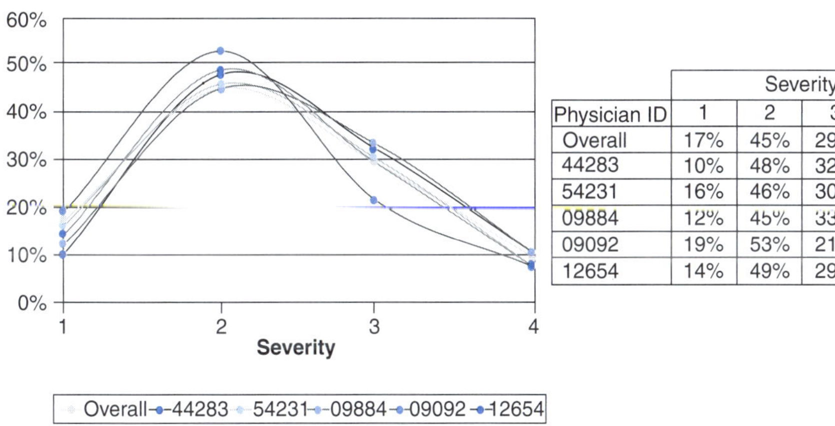

	Severity			
Physician ID	1	2	3	4
Overall	17%	45%	29%	9%
44283	10%	48%	32%	10%
54231	16%	46%	30%	7%
09884	12%	45%	33%	10%
09092	19%	53%	21%	7%
12654	14%	49%	29%	7%

Figure 11.8 High-level APR-DRG CDI program integration

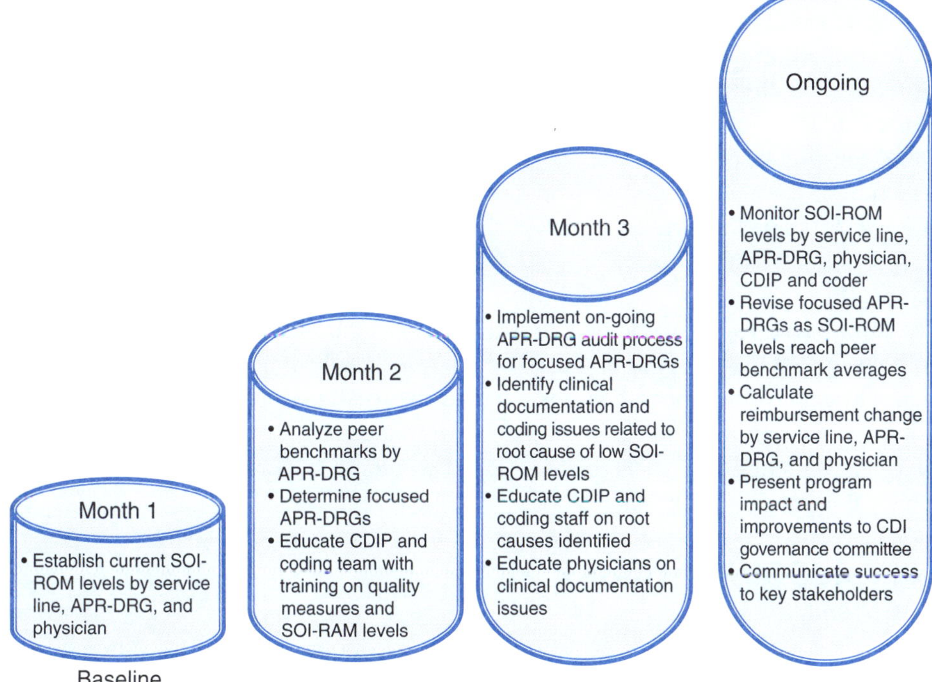

type and severity of patients affect the SOI/ROM level, but also perhaps clinical documentation issues are related to the variance.

The next step in determining a root cause for variances seen in table 11.6 is an audit of focused APR-DRGs. Cases should be selected by the CDI manager from the APR-DRGs that are below peer benchmark. During the audit, the billed

Table 11.6 SOI-ROM comparison - two urban trauma facilities

Provider	Breakout by Severity of Illness (SOI) Level									
	Total		SOI 1		SOI 2		SOI 3		SOI 4	
	FFY 2010 Cases	Case Mix	FFY 2010 Cases	Percent of Total	FFY 2010 Cases	Percent of Total	FFY 2010 Cases	Percent of Total	FFY 2010 Cases	Percent of Total
A	8,031	1.01	4,283	53%	2,652	33%	905	11%	191	2%
B	8,401	1.52	3,037	36%	3,178	38%	1,594	19%	592	7%

Prepared by Navigant for the Arizona Heath Care Cost Containment System (AHCCCS), based on preliminary analyses for demonstration purposes only. Used with permission.

SOI/ROM level should be compared to the new SOI/ROM level resulting in the addition of uncoded diagnoses or a potential level change due to provider queries. Some examples of changes that may be identified are provided below.

Example SOI/ROM Case 1

Case Scenario:

The patient presented with a perirectal abscess, diabetes, hypertension, peripheral neuropathy, and chronic kidney disease (CKD) stage III with metabolic acidosis. At the time of admission, the patient complained of inability to pass urine via the Foley catheter. The clinical record documented urinary retention and hematuria. The hematuria persisted during the admission. The patient had an incision and drainage (I&D) for the abscess and later went to the operating room for a transurethral resection of the bladder. On post-op day 1, the patient's hemoglobin value dropped from 12.7 to 8.9. The provider treated the patient with iron.

SOI/ROM:

The initial SOI/ROM would be 2/2 if the physician selected the perirectal abscess as the principal diagnosis or 2/1 if he or she selected the malignant neoplasm. The final selection would be based on the detailed circumstances of the admission. Acute blood loss anemia was not queried by the CDI specialist or coder. If there were a query agreement in this case, the SOI/ROM would be 3/2 or 3/1 depending on the principal diagnosis selection.

Example SOI/ROM Case 2

Case Scenario:

The patient presented with acute on chronic alcoholic pancreatitis. The clinical record documented alcohol dependence with symptoms of withdrawal. The patient also had metabolic acidosis. A pressure ulcer of the left buttock was noted by the physician in the history and physical exam. The wound care nurse documented the pressure ulcer as stage III but the coder did not code this. The emergency department (ED) physician noted that the patient had quadriplegia secondary to a previous motor vehicle accident. This information was not documented elsewhere in the record and was not coded.

SOI/ROM:

The initial SOI/ROM based on the acute on chronic alcoholic pancreatitis as principal diagnosis was 2/2. The addition of quadriplegia would also change the SOI/ROM score to 2/3. With the addition of the stage III pressure ulcer, the SOI/ROM moves to 3/3. Either of these two diagnoses, had coder coded them, would have improved the SOI/ROM level.

Example SOI/ROM Case 3

Case Scenario:

The patient presents in the ED with a fever and tachycardia. The lab work revealed white blood cell count (WBC) 15,000, positive for streptococcus. The attending physician diagnosed the patient with sepsis. The physician also noted diabetic peripheral neuropathy, hypertension, urinary retention, hydronephrosis, and neurogenic bladder. The patient complained of heartburn, nausea, abdominal bloating, and poor appetite. The clinical record documented a history of gastroparesis by the ED physician, but this was not documented by the providers elsewhere.

SOI/ROM:

The initial SOI/ROM based on the diagnosis of sepsis with diabetic peripheral neuropathy, hypertension, urinary retention, hydronephrosis, and neurogenic bladder was 2/1. The coder did not code the history of gastroparesis nor did he or she query the physician about the associated symptoms of gastroparesis (heartburn, nausea, abdominal bloating, and poor appetite). The addition of gastroparesis ICD-9 code 536.3 would change the SOI/ROM to 3/1.

Physician Response Rate

As well as being one of the core key metrics, physician response rate is evidence of physician-hospital alignment or lack thereof. Senior executives in the hospital should track the physician response rate for this reason. In particular, knowing which physicians are consistently unresponsive gives the organization's leadership an idea about where they need to work on relationship building. Alternatively, for those physicians who are consistent responders, the hospital should be showing its appreciation in an appropriate and regular way to these physicians.

Patient Satisfaction

Patient satisfaction is a new consideration in relationship to clinical documentation. One hypothesis is that because patients are more likely to request and review their health records today than they were a decade ago, the documentation in their record may impact their level of satisfaction with the hospital's services overall. Organizations can measure this in an indirect way through patient satisfaction surveys whenever a patient requests a health record. However, at this point, patient satisfaction related to health information is an indirect strategic measure. Patients have the right to request changes to the information in their health records because of the Health Insurance Portability and Accountability Act (HIPAA), and they are more likely to pay close attention to that information (HIPAA 1996). Today, it is most helpful for physicians to consider the role of the patient regarding documented health information, which the patient owns.

Review of Sample CDI Dashboard

Every organization needs to design its own dashboard of CDI metrics. A performance dashboard is a tool that provides timely and relevant information so organizations can measure and manage processes. Table 11.7 is an example of a CDI

Table 11.7 Sample CDI dashboard with strategic and operational metrics

		January	February	March	April	YTD 06
Concurrent Queries						
	# Queries placed	414	440	676	567	4,461
	Response rate *(Target = 90%)*	31%	32%	28%	40%	36%
Concurrent Reviews						
	# Patient reviews completed	794	826	893	864	7,946
	# Patients eligible for CDI review	1,407	1,405	1,476	1,356	14,024
	% of eligible patients reviewed *(Target = 85%)*	56%	59%	61%	64%	57%
	# 1-day LOS reviewed	94	78	70	77	834
	% Patient reviews with 1 or more queries	52%	53%	76%	66%	56%
	% CDI reviews with severity assigned	98%	98%	96%	93%	78%
Retrospective Queries by HIM						
	# Queries placed	9	18	24	88	172
	Response rate	22%	44%	21%	8%	18%
Process Flow						
	# CDI reviews accessed in CDI system by HIM	594	583	595	693	4,422
Documentation Compliance						
	Charts missing documentation at time of coding	651	572	899	886	5,463
Quarterly Change in Severity Level						
Level 1	Level 1 *(Target = <18%)*	18%	18%	15%	14%	
Level 2	Level 2	42%	42%	42%	40%	
Level 3	Level 3	28%	27%	28%	31%	
Level 4	Level 4	14%	13%	14%	15%	

dashboard that contains both strategic and operational metrics. This dashboard captures the core metrics of response and query rates. It also tracks and analyzes monthly severity levels. In this particular organization, much time was spent by the CDI staff determining which inpatient cases were eligible for CDI review based on length-of-stay criteria. To ensure that everyone in the organization had the same idea about which cases were eligible for review, this information was included with the metrics collected monthly by the CDI department. HIM querying and documentation compliance were also concerns, and they were tracked as well.

Conclusion

There is an enormous amount of information generated through a CDI program. Every organization must plan how it will capture, report, and analyze that information. Organizations can use key metrics, along with their targets, to analyze current performance and implement continuous improvements to the program. In addition, they can analyze data not only organization wide, but also by service, physician, and CDI specialist. This detailed data reporting can help identify gaps in knowledge and skill sets of specific individuals who can then participate in focused follow-up training to close the gaps.

Chapter Quiz

1. What should be organization-specific with regard to key metrics?
   A. Validation review levels
   B. Query rates
   C. Metric targets
   D. Record review rates

2. It is important to report and analyze CDI key metrics in what form?
   A. Individual
   B. Aggregate
   C. Distributive
   D. Statistical

3. Individual rates that are different from the target rates are ______.
   A. Ignored as outliers
   B. Reported to medical staff
   C. Stored for later use
   D. Investigated for significance

4. The purpose of ______________ is to identify any gaps in knowledge or skills for appropriate corrective action.
   A. Revenue cycle analysis
   B. Compiling and analyzing key metrics
   C. Physician query training
   D. Clinical documentation improvement

5. Hospitals often track the physician response rate. What could a level lower than benchmark reflect?
   A. Illegible charts
   B. Too many queries
   C. Principle diagnosis change
   D. Lack of physician-hospital alignment

6. In general, hospitals have higher quality scores when ______________.
   A. The majority of patients are severity level 2 or lower
   B. The majority of patients are severity level 1
   C. The majority of patients are grouped in the higher severity levels
   D. Quality scores are consistent with patient satisfaction

7. Which of the following is the average DRG relative weight for inpatient cases and an indicator of average reimbursement per patient?
   A. Charge capture
   B. Case mix index
   C. DRG relative weight
   D. Real patient case mix

8. What term below refers to the change in average reimbursement per patient that occurs when different types of patients are being admitted as compared to another period of time?
   A. Relative weight change
   B. CDI case mix change
   C. Capture rate change
   D. Real patient mix change

9. Which of the following occurs when a change in CMI occurs due to changes in documentation practice?
   A. CDI case mix change
   B. Real patient mix change
   C. Relative weight change
   D. Physician CDI change

10. Higher quality clinical documentation is a primary contributor to a higher level of ___________.
   A. Physician query rate
   B. Physician response rate
   C. Severity level accuracy
   D. Case mix index

REFERENCES

Averill, R.F., N. Goldfield, J.S. Hughes, J. Bonazelli, E.C. McCullough, B.A. Steinbeck, R. Mullin, and A.M. Tang. 2003. *All Patient Refined Diagnosis-Related Groups, Definitions Manual, Version 20.0, Volumes 1, 2, and 3.* Wallingford, CT: 3M Health Information

Systems Retrieved from: https://www.hcup-us.ahrq.gov/db/nation/nis/APR-DRGs V20MethodologyOverviewandBibliography.pdf.

Centers for Medicare and Medicaid Services (CMS) and the National Center for Health Statistics (NCHS). 2006a. ICD-9-CM Official Guidelines for Coding and Reporting. www.cdc.gov/nchs/datawh/ftpserv/ftpicd9/ftpicd9.htm.

Centers for Medicare and Medicaid Services (CMS) and the National Center for Health Statistics (NCHS). 2006b. ICD-9-CM Official Guidelines for Coding and Reporting—Supplement. http://www.cdc.gov/nchs/data/icd9/POAguideSep06.pdf.

IPRO. 2005a. Coding for quality: Documentation tips for the top seven DRGs, Revised 2005. Hospital Payment Monitoring Program. http://providers.ipro.org/index/hpmp

IPRO. 2005b. Coding for quality: Documentation tips for the top ten denied DRGs. Hospital Payment Monitoring Program. http://providers.ipro.org/index/hpmp

MedPAC. 2014. Payment basic: Hospital acute inpatient services payment system. http://medpac.gov/documents/payment-basics/hospital-acute-inpatient-services-payment-system-14.pdf?sfvrsn=0.

Rosko, M.D. and J.A. Chilingerian. 1999. Estimating hospital inefficiency: Does case mix matter? *Journal of Medical Systems* 23(1):57–71.

Six Sigma. 2015. University of Virginia (UVA) Medical Center reduces coding errors with Six Sigma. http://www.isixsigma.com/industries/healthcare/uva-reduces-cpt-coding-errors-six-sigma/.

Tangen, S. 2003. An overview of frequently used performance measures. *Journal of Work Study* 52(7):347–354.

Chapter 12

Ensuring CDI Program Compliance

Regulatory compliance is a concern for every healthcare organization. In particular, any activities that affect the coding and billing process are scrutinized by the Centers for Medicare and Medicaid Services (CMS) and the Department of Health and Human Services' (HHS) Office of the Inspector General (OIG) in their annual work plans for healthcare organizations. Since coding professionals translate clinical documentation into the diagnostic and procedural codes that are the basis for billing, regulatory agencies closely monitor it. Additionally, compliance investigations that involve overbilling to the federal government can result in damages and fines, as well as the possibility of exclusion from the Medicare program, not to mention significant legal and consulting fees.

Therefore, all healthcare organizations should manage their operations to ensure compliance (HHS 1999; HHS 1998). This chapter addresses the basic components of a compliance program as they relate to clinical documentation practices and discusses in detail the activities of monitoring, auditing, and follow-up education.

Overview of Compliance

An organization's compliance officer heads the development of a compliance program. The program applies to all operations throughout the organization. As discussed in previous chapters, an organization's compliance officer should be a part of the CDI oversight committee and the senior management team that works to build physician support for the program. Every organization includes the CDI function, to some degree, in its compliance plan. The CDI function is also likely to be a part of some level of annual auditing that the compliance department manages. Day-to-day monitoring, however, is the responsibility of the CDI department.

Under an organization's compliance plan, the CDI department is responsible for documenting the monitoring process and reporting the results to the compliance officer on a regular basis. Other interactions between operational units of the organization and the compliance team vary depending on the organization and the compliance department. The CDI program manager should check in with the compliance officer to make sure the officer provides the department with the necessary information to ensure the CDI program staff clearly understands all compliance-related responsibilities.

CDI programs should include a design for the day-to-day processes that include the four components of a compliance plan at the operational level. These components are

- Policy and procedure development
- Program monitoring
- Auditing
- Follow-up education (HHS 1999; HHS 1998)

Ideally, the CDI program should have documentation and processes in place that address each of these areas. Should there ever be an internal or external inquiry about possible compliance violations, not only would the data from the compliance department be available, but the CDI program's operational documentation from these four areas would be available as well.

Earlier chapters of this book discussed program policies and procedure development. Program monitoring, auditing, and follow-up education are continuous activities. However, three key components should be in place for every CDI program to ensure compliance from the outset.

Three Key Components of a Compliant CDI Program

These are the three key components an organization should include early in the implementation of a compliant clinical documentation improvement (CDI) program:

1. Documented, mandatory physician education
2. Detailed query documentation
3. CDI policies and procedures with annual sign-off from all program staff

These activities have significant synergy and interface directly with the compliance department's activities.

First, documented, mandatory physician education should be the initial step in every CDI program. The organization should implement clinical documentation through the medical staff, not around them. They are the authors of the documentation. Implementing a CDI program without first informing the physicians about their rights and responsibilities in the CDI process creates the risk for problems in the future. Comprehensive training programs attended by all physicians, preferably with follow-up testing, is the best process to follow.

Post-education testing, also discussed with follow-up education, is excellent evidence for compliance purposes. Test results serve as evidence of what the trainee retained. In the course of a compliance investigation, an organization can use follow-up education and test results, for example, to support the fact that it identified a problem and addressed it through these vehicles.

Second, every program should keep detailed query data. There should be documented evidence of all queries the CDI specialists ask, to whom they ask them, the clinical documentation or information supporting the query, and responses to queries. This documentation should even accompany every verbal query. For verbal queries, the CDI specialist may need to document the query and the response in the program database. However, in no event should a CDI specialist ask a query and receive an answer without documented evidence that the query occurred. Verbal queries and subsequent clinical record documentation should include an audit trail for future reference. CDI managers should development a practice to document all query interactions.

Detailed query documentation can also protect the hospital when physicians claim the CDI specialist asked them leading queries or forced them into documenting in a certain way. Query documentation and mandatory physician training programs both strongly support a compliant CDI process. Coupling query documentation and training with successfully completed post-training physician tests ensures a solid compliance program (HHS 1999; Russo and Fitzgerald 2008).

Lastly, it is important to develop and continuously update policies and procedures for the CDI program. It is just as important to ensure that staff members are familiar with the policies and procedures that affect them. Training sessions can be developed by the CDI manager to review key policies and procedures with staff. In these cases, testing staff members on the content of the training is the best evidence that they know how to apply the policies. Alternately, staff members can read the policies and procedures independently, but they should also be tested by the CDI staff on content, sign off on the fact that they have read the policies and procedures, and agree to them.

⊙ Monitoring the CDI Program

All CDI staff members need to have their work continuously reviewed and monitored to ensure quality. The CDI program manager or consulting team (if an outside firm is implementing the program) should begin this process in the form of shadowing during implementation. If a consulting firm is managing the implementation process, the responsibility for ongoing monitoring should be transitioned to the internal CDI program manager early in the follow-up visit. Every organization develops its own methodology for conducting regular monitoring. At a minimum, an organization can use the CDI key metrics to determine if there are any areas of concern it needs to focus on in the current reviews. Some suggestions for creating a regular monitoring process follow.

Reviews should be conducted concurrently by the CDI manager, after the CDI specialist has reviewed records on the unit. This will provide the best opportunity to provide feedback based upon the exact content of the record at the time the CDI specialist reviewed it. Targets for overall proficiency of queries should be in the 90 to 95 percent range. The quality reviews should measure the same areas the program database measures: query rate, reason for query, and location of documentation supporting the query. The organization should check productivity, and review the query rate, response rate, and agreement rate. Each of these rates plays an important role in identifying the performance level of the CDI specialist. As chapter 10 noted, if there is a low agreement rate (more than 10 percentage points below the target), it may indicate the CDI specialist is asking inappropriate queries.

During a CDI quality review, an organization should track and monitor the following elements:

- Validity of queries generated
- Validity of working DRG assignment
- Validity of CDI specialist's DRG assignment
- Missed query opportunity

Table 12.1 shows a form used for concurrent CDI reviews. The form focuses on validating queries or missed query opportunities. An organization can modify data elements to fit its specific needs. Ideally, the data elements would be entered by the CDI specialist directly into a program's database for analysis and reporting. The organization should collect and review monitoring data at least quarterly. However, some organizations may want to collect and review data weekly and monthly. It is important to review and analyze results on a regular basis so organizations can correct any gaps in skills or knowledge the review reveals through education or program modifications.

Every program should include regular observation of the query process. For example, a CDI program manager may select one day a month to visit the units and observe verbal queries posed directly to physicians by the CDI specialists. The CDI program manager may also listen to discussions between physicians and the CDI specialists about previous queries. During the observation, the CDI program manager should document the interaction between the CDI specialist and the physician. In particular, the manager should note whether the query was

- Supported by clinical evidence and what the evidence consisted of
- Asked in a non-leading manner
- Responded to by the physician through appropriate documentation in the patient record

The organization can design a simple form to record this information. The form should allow the CDI program manager to assess whether the interaction was leading, the demeanor of the physician, the outcome of the discussion, and any other comments. The manager should file a copy of the form with other program data, and give a copy to the CDI specialist with the appropriate feedback. The CDI

Table 12.1 Sample CDI monitoring form

MR#/ Name	Admit Date	Working DRG	Agree? Y/N	If no, Audit DRG	CDS DRG	Agree? Y/N	If no, Audit DRG	Concurrent Query Type	Agree? Y/N	If no, Audit query	Missed Query Opportunities
99999	2/1/06	90	Y		89	Y		Dehydration	Y		
99998	2/3/06	320	Y		320	Y		None	N		Abn Labs
Totals											

program manager should schedule observations to assess all CDI specialists on their interaction with physicians at least twice a year.

Auditing the CDI Program

CDI program query opportunities should undergo a comprehensive review retrospectively at least once a year. An organization can perform the audit internally, however, it will likely benefit from bringing in an outside firm to perform the annual audit. Primary focus of the CDI audit is to ensure the program is operating compliantly and achieving program goals. The quality component assesses whether the reviews generated appropriate queries, whether the query forms were completed accurately, and whether the physician's documentation in response to a query was appropriate. The CDI manager should identify and report any of these issues and follow up with education or changes in the program process. Focused follow-up education is the key to keeping a CDI program in compliance.

Sample Selection

The CDI manager selects a sample from the population, which is all records that CDI staff concurrently reviewed for CDI purposes, regardless of whether someone asked a query. The sample size may be a judgmental sample of focused DRGs or codes, or a statistical sample size using confidence levels. Refer to RAT-STATS statistical software for more information on sample size selection from the OIG (OIG 2014). There are many other decisions to make regarding the sample selection process. One of the most important considerations is that sample-selection decisions made for the first review must remain constant in all future reviews to compare results among different reviews. Since organizations prefer audit result comparison, it is important to make good initial decisions about sample selection (and even the review and data collection process). The more carefully thought out the initial decisions are, the greater the chance that the program will have useful historical data for comparison over time. The reviewer should carefully document sample-selection decisions so future reviewers can reproduce the methodology in the future.

The reviewer must also determine whether to select records for concurrent or retrospective review. Each method has its own pros and cons and every organization has different needs. The decisions should be based on each organization's specific needs and capabilities. It is both easier to obtain a random sample and more efficient to audit using a retrospective review. A retrospective documentation review minimizes the issue of bias that may exist when reviewers know they are being audited (as they do during a concurrent audit). However, with a retrospective audit, it is more difficult to recreate the actual situation that existed at the time the CDI specialist was reviewing the patient record. One commonly used option consists of auditing the majority of records retrospectively and then including 10 to 20 cases concurrently. The reviewer needs to report on cases differently, but the process often reveals issues in the concurrent practice that a retrospective review would not uncover.

The reviewer must also determine the number of records for review. As noted initially, 30 is the minimum. The size of the organization may require more record reviews to obtain a representative sample. For outpatient cases, 100 or more cases may be necessary to obtain a representative sampling. For inpatient cases, one methodology to use is the number of beds in the hospital involved in the CDI process. For example, a hospital has 150 beds. Obstetrics and newborn, which represent 20 beds, are currently excluded from the program. Furthermore, about 10 percent of hospital admissions are one-day stays, which represents 15 beds. The total beds involved in the program then is 115 (150 – (20 + 15) = 115). Auditing 25 percent of the beds means reviewing 30 records. However, the organization may want to audit 50 percent, which is 60 records. There is no magic number in this process. What is important is that the organization maintains decisions for future audits.

Random sampling versus focused sampling is another issue to address. It is almost impossible to select a truly random sample in a concurrent CDI review because of the nature of the review process. For a retrospective review, the reviewer can select cases randomly. However, the compliance department may have a concern about random reviews because a problem that affects reimbursement may trigger a payback process. When this is the case, a convenience sampling may be preferable. With convenience sampling, the reviewer pulls the last 30 discharges that had a concurrent CDI review, or 10 discharges from three different time periods in the last quarter to ensure seasonality representation. Essentially, a convenience sample is just what the word states: selecting cases that are convenient to retrieve. As long as the organization uses the same methodology in the future, it can compare results of different audits (Babbie 1999).

Retrospective Record Audit

Qualified individuals who are not involved in the day-to-day operations of the CDI program should conduct the retrospective record audit. The methodology for review should be consistent among all reviewers and for each audit conducted. For example, at the time of review, the record should be in as close as possible a condition to the way it was when the CDI specialist reviewed it. For a retrospective review, this is particularly challenging. However, it is helpful to document how the auditors view the record. For instance, for all retrospective reviews, it is important that the auditor not refer to the discharge summary or any documentation that was unavailable to the CDI specialist at the time of the concurrent review.

Data Collection and Analysis

It is also important to determine what data elements the reviewer will collect and how the reviewer will collect them. Some data elements to consider include

- The CDI reviewer's name
- Whether a query was asked (yes or no)
- If a query was asked:
  - Does the auditor agree with it?
  - Where was the location of the documentation supporting the query?
  - What type of documentation and coding changes resulted from the query (IPRO 2005a; IPRO 2005b; CMS and NCHS 2006a; CMS and NCHS 2006b)?
- If a query was not asked:
  - Was there a lost query opportunity? If yes, what was it?
  - Can a retrospective query be asked at this time?
- If the physician responded
- If the physician did not respond
- DRG assignment
- Severity assignment

Figure 12.1 presents an example of a data collection form the reviewer can use or modify for a clinical documentation audit. The reviewer would complete one audit form for each record reviewed. He or she could also use the form to collect information about retrospective queries, if desired.

Presentation of key performance indicators (KPI) to the governance committee and CDI task force keeps the program highly visible in the organization. Visibility is essential to a sustainable program. KPIs should also be presented by the CDI and HIM managers to the CDI specialists and coding staff as a performance enhancing measure as well as a congratulation for work well done. Table 12.2 and 12.3 are graphical depictions of KPIs importance in maintaining an effective CDI program.

The CDI specialist KPI scorecard in table 12.2 reflects below target productivity throughout the first quarter, but an increase beginning in the second quarter. Capture, query, response, and agreement rates all improve beginning in April. This could be the result of a CDI program refresh in March, which revitalized the program and provided additional CDI skills for the department.

The scorecard in table 12.3 depicts a provider with an above normal query rate both concurrently and retrospectively. This is an indicator of less specific clinical documentation. The response and agreement rates trend lower than the target. A major complication and comorbidity (MCC) capture rate of 20 percent in January is below the target of 35 percent and continues below target for the remainder of the fiscal year. As expected, the provider's case mix index (CMI) is consistently below peers at 1.89. This provider is a good candidate for one-on-one discussions with the physician advisor and close monitoring by the CDI staff.

Figure 12.1. Sample data collection form

Medical Record			
Account Number #:		Coder ID:	
APR-DRG/SOI Assignment			
CDS Name	**Admit Date**	**CDS Review Date**	**Working APR-DRG/SOI**
CDS (target) Severity DRG/SOI	Coder DRG/ APR-DRG/SOI	Final DRG/ APR-DRG/ SOI	Coder Relative Weight Variance (coder & final)
Concurrent Query Response Verification			
Concurrent Query	**Recorded Response**	**Audited Response**	**If "y" condition coded?**
	Y N NR A	Y N NR A	Y N
	Y N NR A	Y N NR A	Y N
	Y N NR A	Y N NR A	Y N
	Y N NR A	Y N NR A	Y N
	Y N NR A	Y N NR A	Y N
	Y N NR A	Y N NR A	Y N
	Y N NR A	Y N NR A	Y N

"N" "NR" or "A" Retrospective Queries				
Concurrent Query	**Response**	**Condition Documented in Record (not coded)**	**Impacting Query**	**Re-Queried?**
	N NR A	Y N	Y N	Y N
	N NR A	Y N	Y N	Y N
	N NR A	Y N	Y N	Y N
	N NR A	Y N	Y N	Y N
	N NR A	Y N	Y N	Y N
	N NR A	Y N	Y N	Y N
	N NR A	Y N	Y N	Y N

Missed Coder or CDS Query Impact		
Missed Query	**APR-DRG Impact**	**Relative Weight Impact**

Developing a Corrective Action Plan

Most audits should identify some issues, either operational or compliance, in the CDI process, even if they are minor issues. Some organizations use an issue rating system for every issue identified on an audit. The system may be from 1 through 5 with a level 1 issue being minor and only operational in nature and a level 5 being significant or potentially significant and compliant in nature. The organization needs to develop a corrective action plan for any identified issues.

Table 12.2 CDIP individual key performance indicator scorecard

CDI Key Performance Indicator Scorecard — Allen&Shariff HEALTHCARE CONSULTING

General Hospital
CDIP: #2413
FY 2014

	Target	Jan	Feb	Mar	Apr	May	Jun	Jul	Aug	Sep	Oct	Nov	Dec	Annual
Initial Reviews	195	176	171	174	190	194	201	196	199	194	200	203	198	191
Subsequent Reviews	325	315	321	318	330	329	340	335	341	345	340	344	347	333
Total Reviews	520	491	492	492	520	523	541	531	540	539	540	547	545	524
Productivity/ day	100%	94%	91%	93%	95%	95%	96%	95%	96%	95%	96%	97%	95%	95%
MCC capture Rate	35%	31%	30%	29%	32%	34%	33%	33%	34%	35%	35%	36%	35%	33%
CC capture Rate	25%	19%	18%	18%	20%	21%	23%	25%	24%	26%	25%	27%	26%	23%
Query Rate	30%	26%	25%	24%	27%	29%	27%	28%	29%	31%	29%	32%	30%	28%
Response Rate	85%	25%	28%	35%	71%	79%	81%	82%	85%	83%	86%	87%	85%	69%
Agreement Rate	80%	70%	69%	68%	79%	78%	80%	81%	82%	79%	82%	84%	81%	78%

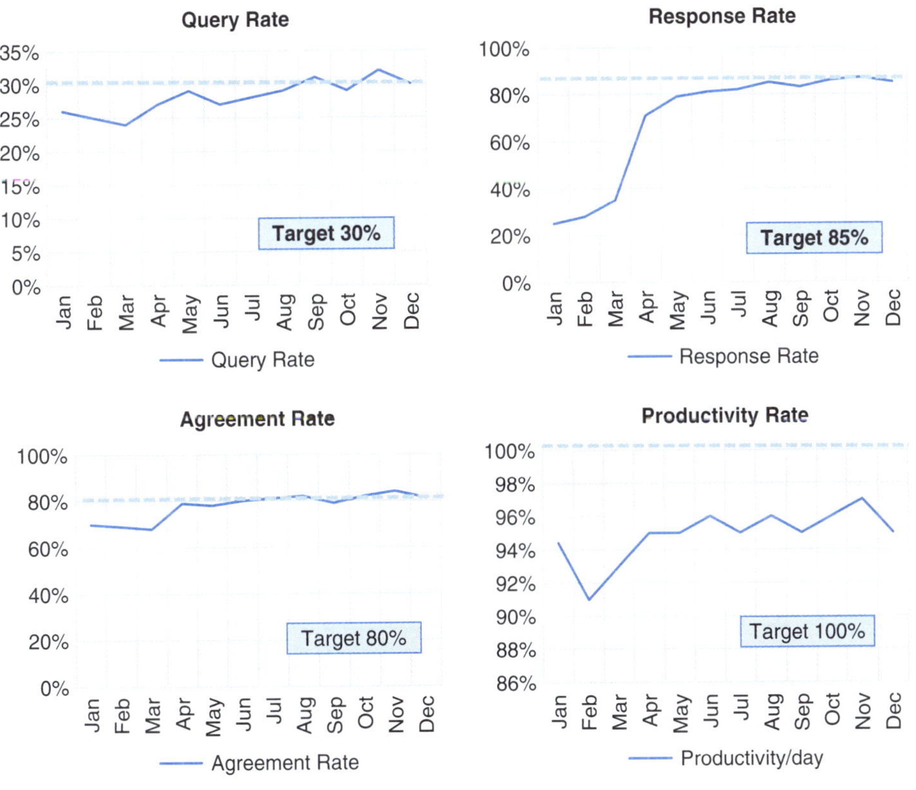

(Continued)

Table 12.2 CDIP individual key performance indicator scorecard (*Continued*)

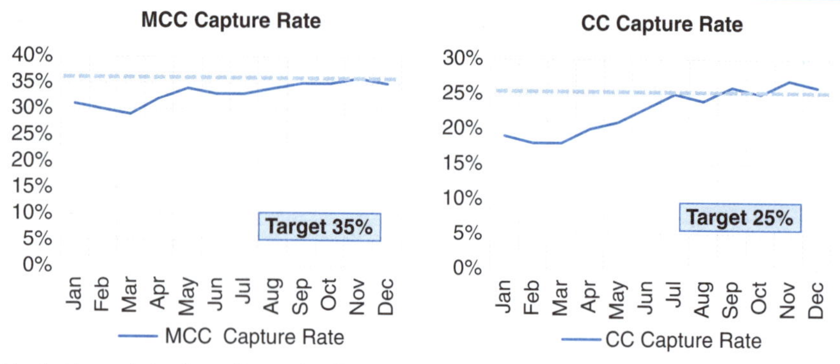

Used with permission from Allen & Shariff, Inc.

Table 12.3 Internal medicine provider CDI scorecard

CDI Key Performance Indicators — Allen&Shariff HEALTHCARE CONSULTING

General Hospital
Provider: #xxxx
FY 2014

	Target	Jan	Feb	Mar	Apr	May	Jun	Jul	Aug	Sep	Oct	Nov	Dec	Annual
Concurrent Query Rate	40%	15%	16%	20%	18%	24%	28%	34%	31%	39%	43%	42%	45%	30%
Concurrent Response Rate	100%	90%	89%	92%	93%	95%	91%	89%	94%	95%	93%	94%	95%	93%
Concurrent Agreement Rate	85%	80%	81%	81%	83%	85%	84%	86%	84%	86%	87%	86%	88%	84%
Retrospective Query Rate	20%	10%	11%	13%	18%	17%	19%	21%	23%	21%	24%	25%	25%	19%
Retrospective Response Rate	100%	75%	77%	76%	78%	80%	78%	84%	83%	85%	84%	85%	86%	81%
Retrospective Agreement Rate	85%	70%	67%	72%	74%	78%	76%	80%	79%	77%	79%	80%	82%	76%
MCC Capture Rate	35%	20%	21%	20%	22%	24%	23%	25%	26%	28%	27%	27%	28%	24%
CC Capture Rate	25%	10%	15%	18%	25%	21%	28%	30%	34%	36%	42%	38%	41%	28%
DRG Validation Denial Rate	0%	50%	52%	56%	53%	55%	50%	53%	55%	50%	54%	55%	56%	53%
DRG Validation Appeal Win Rate	100%	25%	28%	23%	38%	45%	49%	52%	50%	48%	65%	62%	67%	46%
CMI	1.89	1.53	1.55	1.59	1.57	1.59	1.61	1.60	1.66	1.71	1.79	1.84	1.88	1.66

(Continued)

Table 12.3 Internal medicine provider CDI scorecard (*Continued*)

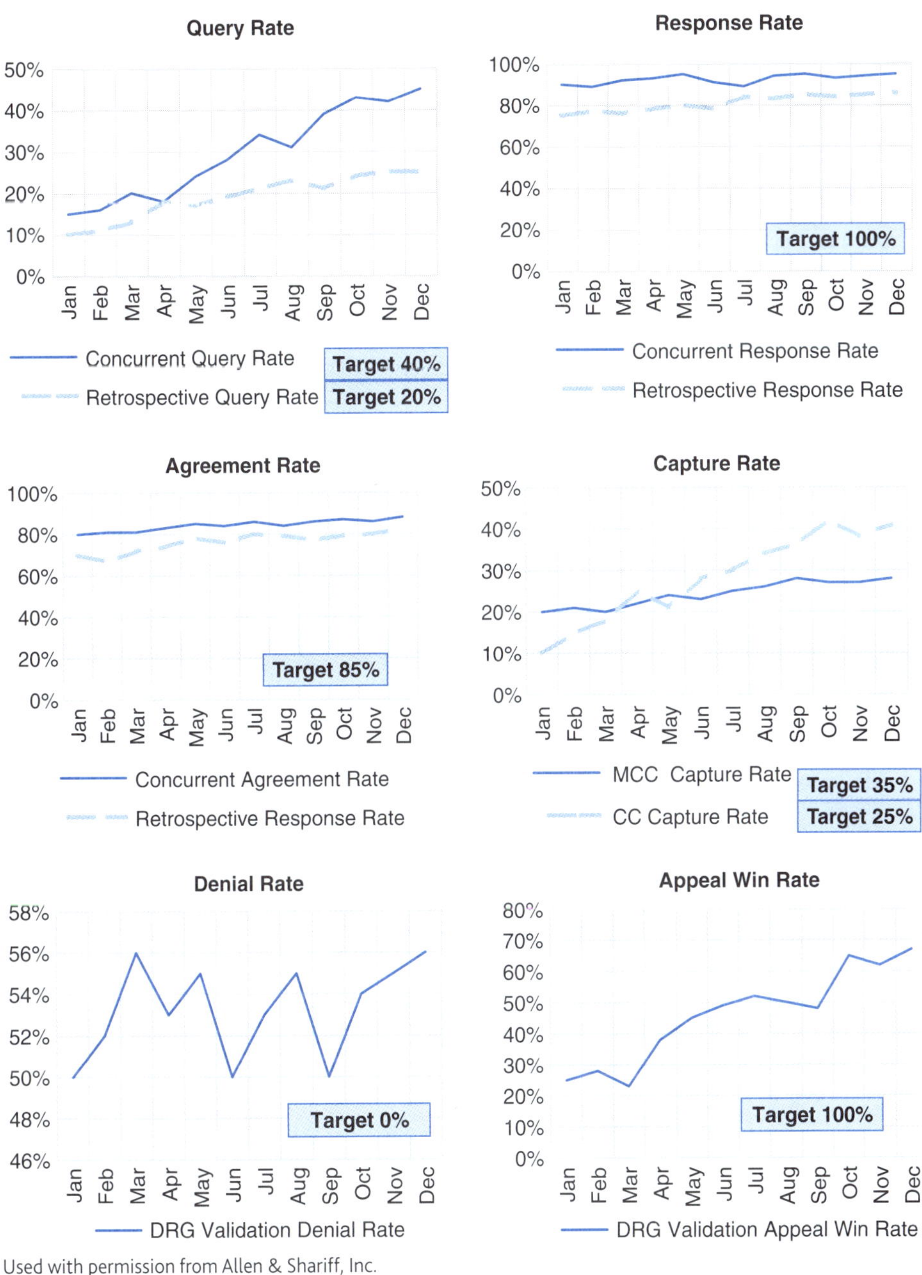

Used with permission from Allen & Shariff, Inc.

The corrective action plan should include individual communications, training, testing, and operational changes. The plan should include dates for completion and a checklist that needs to be completed and filed by the CDI manager with program documentation when all of the corrective actions have been completed. Table 12.4 contains an example corrective action plan. This plan includes the identification of two high-risk issues. Item 1.a points out an error in Medicare

Table 12.4 Corrective action work plan

CDI Audit Corrective Action Plan						Allen&Shariff HEALTHCARE CONSULTING
Task #	**Task**	**Risk Level (1-5)**	**Responsible Party**	**Due Date**	**Target Date**	**Status**
1	Conduct detailed review of audit results for each case including MS-DRG changes, appropriateness of physician queries, coding changes including PDX assignment and identification of MCC/CCs, and physician response and agreement.		CDIP Manager/Coding Manager	Mar 2014	Mar 2014	Complete
1.a	30% error rate identified for MS-DRG assignment of sepsis cases. CDIP/coding staff requires further training on sepsis indicators and query submission. High risk for RAC audit. Train and monitor.	5		May 2014		Pending
1.b	Low rate of complex pneumonia MS-DRG 177-179 as compared to peer hospitals. Audit reveals low query response rate from physicians. Potential lost reimbursement. Increase audit sample of MS-DRG 193-195 Simple Pneumonia. Trend by provider, communicate with provider through physician advisor and attending physician.	4		May 2014		Pending
2	Analyze the data for trends by MS-DRG and coding accuracy rate, physician query, response and agreement rates, and MCC/CC capture rates.		CDIP Manager/Coding Manager	Mar 2014	Mar 2014	Complete
3	Where unfavorable trends are identified, identify root cause of each and categorize by CDIP and physician.		CDIP Manager	Apr 2014	Apr 2014	Complete
4	Identify compliance issues and discuss with compliance department.		CDIP Manager/ Compliance Officer	Apr 2014	Apr 2014	Complete
5	Identify trends requiring training, develop training materials, and conduct training sessions for all issues identified for the entire CDIP/coding staff.		CDIP Manager/Coding Manager	Apr 2014	Apr 2014	Complete
6	Identify trends requiring workflow and process changes. Develop new process, implement, and monitor until resolved.		CDIP Manager/ Department Manager			
7	Identify trends related to physician/provider response and discuss with physician advisor and medical staff department chair.		CDIP Manager/ Physician Advisor/ Medical Staff Chair	Apr 2014	Apr 2014	Complete
8	Establish monitoring process for issues identified in tasks 1 & 2 above. Identify root cause and conduct required training and/or process/workflow change. Continue until issue is resolved.		CDIP Manager/ Department Manager	May 2014	May 2014	Complete
9	Report results of audit, root cause assessment, monitoring, and resolution to CDI Taskforce and Governance Committee.		CDIP Manager	May 2014		In Progress

Used with permission from Allen & Shariff, Inc.

severity diagnosis-related group (MS-DRG) assignment of sepsis as the principal diagnosis. After further investigation, the CDI program manager identified a training deficit related to sepsis clinical indicators. Because this is a recovery audit contractor (RAC) issue, the manager assigned a risk level of 5 and discussed this information with the compliance officer. Item 1.b identifies an issue with MS-DRG assignment for pneumonia. The rate for assignment of complex pneumonia was much lower than peer facilities. After further investigation, the CDI program manager identified the root cause as a lack of response to queries for bacterial pneumonia. The physician advisor and attending physician will discuss this issue.

Reporting on Results

Reviewers should summarize every audit in a report. The design of the report format should be specific to the needs of the organization, as should how the reviewer presents the audit results and to whom. For example, will the reviewer present the results at a CDI committee meeting? Will he or she forward copies of the results to the compliance department in every case or only if he or she finds compliance concerns? If possible, the reviewer should design reports to enable easy results comparison over time. The first page of the report can contain an executive summary that lists the basic data findings. For each audit, the report can include the findings from the previous two reviews to show changes over time.

Follow-up Education and Testing

The goal of any compliance review is to determine whether query generation and physician responses to the queries are compliant. If either activity is determined to be noncompliant, then the organization must develop a corrective action plan. The most common and generally useful corrective action plan uses focused follow-up education. Earlier chapters addressed details around ensuring physician attendance at educational programs and program content design. This chapter concentrates on the design and use of post-education testing as a tool for compliance.

Focused follow-up education should address every issue identified in an audit or during monitoring. Reviewers should clearly document all issues in the audit or monitoring report. The report should also include a general plan for educational follow-up to correct these issues. Organizations should create and maintain detailed documentation for every training program. The CDI program manager should maintain the program content, session attendance, and results of any post-training tests. Ideally, the documentation should be electronic and any hard copy documents should be imaged by the HIM department into the electronic filing system. Every training program should include the following components:

- **Objectives:** The program materials should clearly state the objectives that attendees should achieve through the training. If the organization is to provide continuing education credits, most professional associations require a list of educational objectives. The organization should use these objectives to create the content of the program and to design any post-training tests.

- **Training method:** Using the CAMP Method (coaching, asking, mastering, and peer learning) leads to optimal outcomes. The CAMP Method is a structured methodology for educating adults. Using this method not only improves skills, it also increases the sustainability of the training. Chapter 8 contains an overview of the CAMP Method's four components and how to incorporate them into the training program (Russo and Fitzgerald 2008).
- **The right trainers:** The CAMP method requires both trainers to be experts in the subject matter and peer trainers. In most cases, CDI training requires pairing a CDI expert with a peer of the trainees, if possible.
- **Resolution of concerns:** After a review of the objectives, trainers should begin every training program by asking the attendees for their concerns and addressing these concerns as best as possible before proceeding with the training.
- **Delivery of information:** Trainers deliver the information in a manner that follows the program's objectives. They provide attendees with a handout of the PowerPoint slides or other reference tools, involve trainees in discussions about their own experiences, and encourage questions and concerns throughout the program.
- **A mastering component:** To ensure sustainability of the training and obtain the best results, the organization should design the training program so the trainees have an opportunity to apply the information during the training session. There should be at least one opportunity for the trainees to practice during the training session.
- **Coaching:** Trainers end the session with encouraging statements regarding the trainees' ability to internalize and apply the information they learned during the training session.
- **Evaluation and feedback:** The trainers ask the attendees to evaluate the program. The trainers can use the evaluations to improve future sessions and identify other opportunities for training program topics.
- **Testing:** To the extent possible, trainers should test trainees on the information they learned during the session.

Post-training Tests

Requiring program attendees to successfully pass a test following a training program has compliance, operational, and even personal benefits.

First, from a compliance perspective, having documented evidence of what the organization's staff and the physicians know can be helpful in demonstrating that the management team provided the correct direction, support, and tools to these individuals.

Second, because a test is more likely to guarantee that program attendees retain and use the information, the CDI function benefits from the operational improvements likely to result.

Third, when trainees know they need to complete a test after training, they are more likely to focus on the information. At the very least, the trainees benefit personally from learning a new skill or adding to their information base.

The easiest tests to administer are multiple choice. Since the organization is accountable for acting on poor test results, it is best to use an online testing system that allows continuous retakes until the test-taker passes the test. These tests, which are embedded in most e-learning systems, generate subsequent tests with different questions in a different order.

Organizations can use data from test results in overall program management. Minimally, the trainer should share the results of the test with the test taker. However, CDI program managers can also calculate mean scores for trainees overall or by subgroup and use this information in their program reporting. They may want to set targets for mean scores. For example, they may want to set a mean test score at 90 percent and continue to require staff to either retake the random testing instruments (if they have a web-based testing instrument) or continue to participate in follow-up training until the mean score reaches the minimum target.

Tables 12.5 and 12.6 provide examples of mean test score reporting together with operational and compliance measures for both CDI staff members and physicians. These tables are presented in a report card format and can be used by the CDI manager to inform senior management, the compliance department, and the medical staff of the current strengths of the program as well as areas that need improvement.

⊙ Compliance versus Operations as the Reason for Review and Education

Not every issue identified during CDI program monitoring or during an audit is a compliance issue. In many cases, problems or concerns are operational in nature. If not corrected, it is possible for some operational issues to become compliance

Table 12.5 CDI specialist report card

Key Indicator	Grade	Achievement	Target	Variance
Doc Spec Fitness Test™ results	◆◆◆◆◆	92%	90%	102%
Concurrent review productivity	◆◆◆	98%	100%	98%
Documentation review accuracy	◆	87%	98%	89%
Concurrent query rate (records w/queries)	◆◆◆	26%	35%	74%
Total number of queries placed	◆◆◆◆◆	350	325	108%
Concurrent response rate	◆	25%	60%	42%

◆◆◆◆◆ —key indicator results better than expected
◆◆◆ —key indicator results within 10% of expected
◆ —key indicator results

Table 12.6 Medical staff CDI report card

Key Indicator	Grade	Achievement	Target	Variance
Physician CDI knowledge assessment	◆	75%	90%	83%
Concurrent query rate	◆◆◆	26%	35%	74%
Concurrent response rate	◆	25%	60%	42%
Retrospective query rate	◆◆◆	7%	12%	58%
Retrospective response rate	◆	50%	85%	59%
Documentation legibility	◆	72%	98%	73%
Documentation accuracy	◆	50%	90%	56%

◆◆◆◆◆ —key indicator results better than expected

◆◆◆ —key indicator results within 10% of expected

◆ —key indicator results

issues. Ultimately, the organization wants the CDI program running smoothly from both an operational and a compliance perspective. It also wants the program and its review processes to be as efficient as possible. There is no reason, for example, to conduct CDI department-specific operational reviews differently from reviews used to validate compliance. The organization's compliance department is focused on auditing for compliance purposes. However, it makes the most sense for CDI reviews not conducted by the compliance department to look at any potential issues with the CDI function: compliance, operational, or other. The same is true for educational follow-up. Both operational and compliance issues can be addressed by the CDI staff in the same educational session. For example, the same educational program can train the staff or the physicians on how to query in a more compliant manner as well as how to increase the productivity of reviews.

Conclusion

Clinical documentation is the basis of the coding and billing activity in every organization, therefore CDI should be a part of the organizational compliance program. CDI program managers can and should organize their internal operations to include policies and procedures, regular monitoring, annual audits, and targeted follow-up education that address both compliance and operational issues. The lines of communication between the CDI program manager and the compliance team should continuously remain open. The compliance department should be informed by the CDI manager of any possible compliance problems identified within the CDI department. Education that focuses on addressing issues identified during monitoring or auditing should include a follow-up test. Reviewers should create and maintain detailed documentation for all CDI monitoring, audits, and educational program content and attendance.

⊙ Chapter Quiz

1. Which is an important component of follow-up education?
   - A. Review of key metrics
   - B. DTM (Direct teaching method)
   - C. Compliance officer attendance
   - D. Testing
2. A convenience sampling methodology implies:
   - A. Selecting every fifth case by discharge date
   - B. Selecting cases that are convenient to retrieve
   - C. Selecting 30 cases randomly from discharges the same month
   - D. Selecting one in five cases for each physician
3. What type of testing is best taken post-training?
   - A. Multiple choice
   - B. Verbal
   - C. Fill-in the blank
   - D. Pass-fail
4. What is one key component of a compliant CDI program?
   - A. Detailed review of Joint Commission findings
   - B. Documented, mandatory physician education
   - C. Revenue cycle team involvement
   - D. Exceeding query response targets
5. Detailed query documentation can be used to:
   - A. Protect the hospital from law suits
   - B. Protect the hospital against claims from physicians about leading queries
   - C. Show the effects of follow-up training
   - D. Protect the auditor from corrective action
6. A comprehensive retrospective review should be conducted at least once a year on what aspect of the CDI program?
   - A. Proficiency statistics
   - B. Compliance issues
   - C. All query opportunities
   - D. Core key measures
7. Qualified individuals who are not involved in the day-to-day operations of the CDI program should conduct a:
   - A. Retrospective record audit
   - B. Quality improvement review
   - C. Key metric review
   - D. Retrospective query process

8. Which plan should be devised to respond to issues arising from the CDI compliance and operational audit process?
- **A.** CDI response plan
- **B.** Quality assurance plan
- **C.** CDI plan
- **D.** Corrective action plan

9. What is the goal of the CDI compliance review?
- **A.** To ensure adequate CDI improvement
- **B.** To monitor compliant query generation and physician responses
- **C.** To ensure corrective action for any compliance concerns
- **D.** To ensure compliance between CDI program staff

10. When conducting an audit review of records for CDI, what would the minimum number of records to pull be?
- **A.** 10
- **B.** 150
- **C.** 30
- **D.** 1 percent of retrospective reviews

REFERENCES

Babbie, E.R. 1999. *The Basics of Social Research.* Albany, NY: Wadsworth Publishing Company.

Centers for Medicare and Medicaid Services (CMS) and the National Center for Health Statistics (NCHS). 2006a. ICD-9-CM Official Guidelines for Coding and Reporting. http://www.cdc.gov/nchs/icd.htm.

Centers for Medicare and Medicaid Services (CMS) and the National Center for Health Statistics (NCHS). 2006b. ICD-9-CM Official Guidelines for Coding and Reporting—Supplement. 2006. http://www.cms.gov/Medicare/Medicare-Fee-for-Service-Payment/HospitalAcqCond/Coding.html.

Healthgrades. 2015. Healthgrades. http://www.healthgrades.com/.

IPRO. 2005a. Coding for quality: Documentation tips for the top seven DRGs, Revised 2005. Hospital Payment Monitoring Program.

IPRO. 2005b. Coding for quality: Documentation tips for the top ten denied DRGs. Hospital Payment Monitoring Program.

RAT-Stats- Statistical Software. 2014. Office of Inspector General. Retrieved from: http://oig.hhs.gov/compliance/rat-stats/.

Russo, R. and S. Fitzgerald. 2008. Physician clinical documentation: Implications for healthcare quality and cost. Academy of Management Annual Meeting, Anaheim, CA.

Part III
Growing and Refining the Clinical Documentation Program

Chapter 13

Continual CDI Program Renewal

Clinical documentation improvement (CDI) should be a dynamic function in every organization. The healthcare environment supports continuous renewal of the clinical documentation program. Moreover, CDI is an expanding function in most organizations. Therefore, changes are likely to occur because of the program's natural development. Examples of activities that create an environment ripe for continuous renewal include

- Regulatory changes
- Training for new medical staff, house staff, and other clinicians
- Evolution of quality initiatives
- Expansion of the CDI program into new areas
- Ongoing refinement of the program with the assistance of the medical staff

Business and personal growth experts have found that the most effective organizations and individuals practice continuous renewal, also known as "sharpening the saw" (Covey 2014). This chapter discusses clinical documentation renewal efforts in terms of how the programs are likely to grow organically. The chapter also covers the development of the physician training function and the refinement of program measures.

Growing the CDI Function

Organizations focus all CDI program implementation, at least initially, on one patient care area. The patient care area depends on the organization, specialty services, or preferences. Most CDI programs begin in the inpatient setting. The reasons for this are threefold.

- The organization is taking a risk by investing in a new program. Focusing on one area minimizes the risk of failure.
- The organization will want to measure return on investment (ROI) in some meaningful way. Focusing on one area makes this initial measurement more efficient and reliable.
- Targeting one area for CDI allows an organization to develop a successful model it can replicate or modify to fit the needs of other patient care areas. It also allows the organization to create the building blocks for CDI to develop other functions such as training and patient education that are synergistic with CDI.

Where an organization takes the CDI function after the initial implementation depends on the organization. However, allowing a program to stagnate at its original level of implementation usually results in less support over time from the medical staff (Russo 2008). If continued, a lack of medical staff support eventually leads to an inability to reach program targets and the potential program dissolution. Table 13.1 is an example of various growth and renewal patterns that a CDI program can take. These are only suggestions; it is essential for every organization to grow the function based on what makes sense for that organization. Basic suggestions about program renewal include

- Waiting until the program has a complete year of stable, successful operations before attempting to expand it.
- Planning the initial expansion in small steps so as not to detract from the core program. In table 13.1, the initial year of implementation shows the only expansion being the addition of specialty-specific training for physicians as a follow-up to the initial base education all physicians receive.
- Adding services and activities in the initial growth years that are most likely to add value to the organization. Pilot studies performed prior to the expansion can help determine these services and activities.

While riskier expansion often results in big payoffs, this activity should wait. In table 13.1, some of the less traditional expansions include providing community education to healthcare consumers to train them on the content and use of their health records. The ultimate purpose is to show the direct relationship between clinical documentation and quality patient care. Natural benefits of this activity might include improved patient satisfaction and even improved alignment with the medical staff, especially if the hospital involves physicians in training the community about their health records.

Enlisting Physician Buy-in

Initially, the medical staff may not look forward to the mandatory documentation training sessions provided by the CDI function. However, it should be the goal of every CDI program to develop a rapport with the physicians so that eventually, the medical staff views CDI as a valuable resource they can access for their own benefit

Table 13.1 CDI program growth and renewal possibilities

Program Timeline	Operational Activities
Initial Implementation	Inpatient review and querying Obtain support and cooperation of the medical staff Provide specialty-specific education
Year 2	Add ED and clinic concurrent reviews Add quality measures review into annual audit results for inpatients All attending physicians trained in documentation principles by end of the year
Year 3	Add ambulatory surgery concurrent reviews Begin CDI training for every clinician who documents in a patient record
Year 4	Continue CDI training for every clinician Add outpatient testing concurrent reviews Create synergy between current clinical education processes (grand rounds, mortality and morbidity review) and clinical documentation principles
Year 5	Offer community training to healthcare consumers to understand their health records; recruit physicians to assist in the process Develop a predictive measure between clinical documentation practices and quality measures using first three years of program data
Year 6	Develop a tracking system to measure patients' satisfaction with their health information Incorporate patient satisfaction and predictive quality measures into regular program reporting

Position CDI as Value-added

It is important to position the CDI function in a way that the physicians view the services offered by the clinical documentation staff as a value-added service for them (Russo 2008). The following six activities are ways to develop a better understanding of how the CDI function can better serve physicians.

1. Obtain Feedback from Physicians

The best way to find out how to better serve a customer is to ask. And physicians are a customer of the clinical documentation function. They also serve as a provider of raw material in the clinical documentation supply chain. However, thinking of them as customers helps develop the right approach to the ongoing relationship between CDI staff and the medical staff. CDI staff should ask physicians for feedback—verbally, with web-based surveys, and through service chiefs. They should ask what the physicians do and do not like about the CDI function, what CDI staff can do to facilitate the process for physicians, and how CDI staff can better serve physicians to improve their documentation skills overall.

2. Listen and Observe Physicians

When asking, it is important to listen. CDI staff may obtain a significant amount of information from physicians by simply listening to the physicians talk at training functions, during staff meetings, and on the units. The CDI function is not designed to be a panacea for all physician problems with the hospital. However, if CDI staff learn about a physician issue and determine how CDI training or support can help, they should act on it. For example, they may have heard a physician mention a problem with a certain payer rejecting office bills for medical necessity issues, and neither the physician nor the office staff have been able to manage the situation effectively. While the CDI staff cannot offer their services to analyze and fix the problem for the physician, they can offer education and training that benefits both the physician's practice and the hospital. The CDI staff may even develop tools that provide the physician with a takeaway during the training.

3. Demonstrate How the Health Record is Common Ground

The health record is the common ground between the medical staff and the hospital. The medical staff needs the record to treat the patient and communicate with other caregivers. The hospital needs the record to translate its contents into coded data for billing, quality indicators, research, and planning. Explaining this to physicians will not make them see their responsibility in clinical documentation any differently. However, taking the opportunity to interject the health record topic into physician encounters such as mortality reviews, department meetings, grand rounds, and training programs helps to convey the message. Using the health record as a tool to accomplish goals in the hospital encourages the physicians to begin to incorporate the same tools in their day-to-day activities. As the electronic health record (EHR) becomes more prevalent, this concept grows in popularity with physicians. Since many physicians are enamored with technology, pulling together the CDI opportunity with the EHR may increase their curiosities.

4. Provide Web-based Training and Web-based Resources

Web-based training provides advantages for all staff, not just physicians. Increased productivity, less cost, and greater compliance justify the initial investment (Chung et al. 2004). Organizations that already provide web-based training should ask physicians for feedback about their experience with the tool. If possible, CDI staff should improve the tool to increase physician satisfaction. They can also develop a web-based resource that provides physicians and their office personnel with information about billing issues related to clinical documentation practices. If an organization owns physician practices, chances are it already has these resources for use by the billing staff. Making this type of resource available to physicians offers another way for them to see the importance of clinical documentation, especially for billing purpose.

5. Create Codevelopment Opportunities

Some hospital CDI staff members have begun to partner with their physicians to present the success of their CDI program at local, state, and even national association meetings. This type of codevelopment opportunity can improve relationships with physicians, using the CDI program as a common ground. CDI staff can also work with physicians to design research projects (or even pilots to expand the CDI program) or write papers for publication in academic journals. Physicians, especially those in academic medical centers, have a great interest in publishing their work. Any of these activities benefit both the physician and the organization (Flamholtz and Lacey 1981). The fact that CDI is used as the basis of the activity is likely to make physicians more responsible and accountable for their documentation practices.

6. Establish a Clinical Documentation Advisory Board (and Pay for Their Time)

This may be a long stretch for many organizations. However, considering the minimal cost to an organization for paying a physician to serve on a board for clinical documentation planning, the benefits far outweigh the expenses. If the organization has an interest in this type of venture, it needs to be explicit about the responsibilities of the physician advisors. The advisory board cannot be like every other committee that physicians serve on in the hospital, since the organization does not pay them for those activities. The physicians would have additional responsibilities. Perhaps CDI staff can train them to be peer reviewers or trainers for physician CDI training. If the advisory board member service time can be limited to six months or a year, not only would it potentially appeal more to the members, it would also give the organization the opportunity to intensively train several physicians a year in CDI principles. With the right planning, the right physician participants, and the right process, the results could prove to be mutually beneficial to the organization and to the physicians.

CDI staff should consult their compliance officer for specific guidance on how to create the advisory board and work with physicians compliantly. There are certain Medicare antitrust laws that prohibit hospitals from giving physicians anything of value that appears to be an inducement to the physician for admitting patients to the hospital. However, if the hospital is paying the physicians fair market value for actual work performed outside of normal hospital duties, this should not be a problem. The organization's compliance team or general counsel should oversee this activity.

Providing Specialty-specific Training Following Implementation

After training all physicians (or some acceptable target percentage of physicians) in baseline CDI education, it is important to begin developing specialty-specific training. A physician CDI advisory board is the perfect place to begin creating the programs with the assistance of the physicians on the board. In creating the sessions, CDI staff should obtain feedback from physicians in each specialty. They should also consider using service-specific patient records from the hospital in all educational programs. Creating ongoing educational programs that use the case study method will make it easier for physicians to learn because they are accustomed to this technique.

Professional Fee Training

Training physicians about how their documentation in patient records affects their professional fee reimbursement is a key benefit to the physician. In addition, this training is a prime benefit to the hospital if additional physicians cooperate because they appreciate the hospital providing them with this information (Russo 2001). Figures 13.1 and 13.2 show examples of hospital progress notes that demonstrate how documentation added to the hospital record to bring notes into compliance for high-quality clinical documentation also affects the physician's professional fee billing for the hospital visit. During these training sessions, it is best to have a physician's professional fee coding and billing expert available to answer specific questions physicians may pose. Providing this expert resource for the physicians during the training benefits them, and hopefully results in higher levels of support and cooperation from the physicians for the CDI program.

Refining Program Measures

A final consideration for continuous program renewal is the refinement of program measures. The core CDI metrics described in prior chapters will always remain in place. However, the CDI staff can add other metrics or modify current ones to spark renewed interest. To the extent that CDI staff can continue to develop measures that show the value CDI brings to the organization, they will want to implement these measures. Some specific ways to think differently about program metrics include

- How can CDI staff use the metrics to develop physician report cards?
- Where has CDI had an integrative impact with other functions in the organization and how can CDI staff report those to show greater value to the organization?
- How does CDI influence quality measures?
- How has CDI positively affected physician satisfaction?
- How has CDI positively affected patient satisfaction?

Figure 13.1 Sample hospital progress note (also used for physician professional fee billing)

Progress Note: Admitted through ED for generalized abd pain, dehydration
Old records: Requested, reviewed
    Heart: RRR, carotid pulses
    Lungs: CTA
    ABD: soft, NT, BS normal, no hemorrhoids
RLQ tenderness, guarding
A/P: RLQ abd, pain, dehydration

Additional "query" diagnosis: ETOH abuse or intoxication on admission based on blood alcohol levels upon admission, but not documented.

Figure 13.2 Sample hospital progress note (also used for physician professional fee billing)

Progress Note: No complaints, Hx bleeding ulcer 2 yrs. ago
Labs: WBC-10.5 Hemoglobin-10.5 Hematocrit-30.6
Heart: RRR
Lungs: CTA
ABD: soft, NT, No HSM, BS normal, CVAT, no hemorrhoids
Small umbilical hernia, easily reducible stools for ⊕ occult blood
A/P: GI bleed, umbilical hernia

Additional "queried" diagnosis: blood loss anemia based on lab values

Physician Report Cards

One of the easiest measures to create from CDI data is an individual physician report card. The CDI staff can use the same measures they collect and report on regularly for the program to create a measurement tool for physicians. CDI staff should only take on this activity with the support of the medical staff. Otherwise, creating and distributing physician report cards could harm the hospital-physician relationship. Table 13.2 shows an example of a physician report card that includes measures for testing (knowledge assessment), query rates, response rates, documentation legibility (assessed separately at this hospital), and documentation accuracy (determined through an auditing process). The diamonds, which mimic the Healthgrades' graphics, allow the viewer to determine at a glance the documentation quality for each physician. This report card represents poor quality documentation practice as the majority of the grades are lower than expected.

Figure 13.3 is a graph containing a different version of a physician report card. In this example, severity is measured by physician against the average length of stay. As previously discussed, lower severity levels are likely to receive lower quality indicators and lower scores on Healthgrades' quality reports since severity is a key indicator of quality for these measures. One feature of this report card is that it compares several different physicians. Here, there are identification numbers for each physician. The CDI staff can assign these numbers so only the individual physician knows the number, thus preserving anonymity. This type of reporting system may be preferred by some medical staffs.

Integrative Impact of CDI

How much the CDI function interfaces with other functions may determine that the synergies create added benefits to the organization. If this is the case, CDI staff should report on that phenomenon. For example, CDI may influence the work of health information management (HIM), quality, compliance, patient accounting, and case management functions. When CDI staff suspect this, they must work

Table 13.2 Sample physician CDI report card

Key Indicator	Grade	Achievement	Target	Variance
Physician CDI knowledge assessment	◆	75%	90%	83%
Concurrent query rate	◆◆◆	26%	35%	74%
Concurrent response rate	◆	25%	60%	42%
Retrospective query rate	◆◆◆	7%	12%	58%
Retrospective response rate	◆	50%	85%	59%
Documentation legibility	◆	72%	98%	73%
Documentation accuracy	◆	50%	90%	56%

◆◆◆◆◆ —key indicator results better than expected
◆◆◆ —key indicator results within 10% of expected
◆ —key indicator results less than expected

together as a team with the managers of these departments to demonstrate that the improved results are coming from synergies that would not exist if either department was acting independently. For example, the CDI specialists may interact with the coding staff on a regular basis. In some organizations, CDI specialists and coders team up to discuss cases and follow retrospective queries. The team may find that the retrospective query response rate prior to the teamwork was 50 percent but has now risen to 90 percent. This is a good example of a measure CDI staff should report.

Quality Impact

As the Centers for Medicare and Medicaid Services (CMS) continue to refine Medicare quality indicators and other quality measures, it is important to clarify the CDI program and the program measures that accompany the quality component. Today, severity of illness is the measure of CDI that most closely impacts severity. As CDI staff identify additional relationships and demonstrate a positive impact between CDI activities and the quality outcome, they should collect the data and report on the measures. An example is to define further the present on admission (POA) status of hospital-acquired conditions such as vascular catheter-associated infection. It is import for the provider to document if this infection was POA. A CDI query may be necessary to clarify the POA status further.

Physician Satisfaction

As CDI staff position CDI as a value-added service to physicians on the medical staff, it is important to collect information from them about their attitudes and

Figure 13.3 Severity of illness and length of stay measures by individual physicians

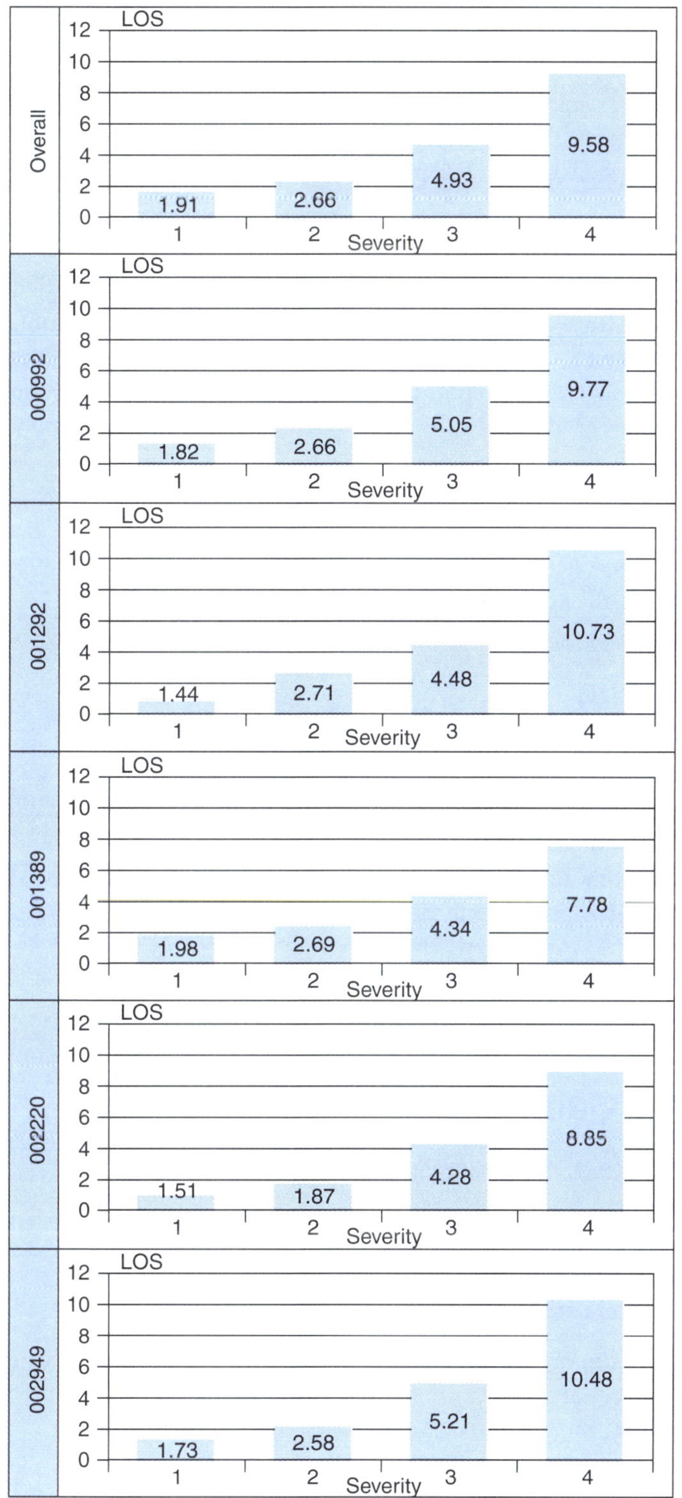

opinions regarding the program, documentation practices, and the other services they offer. They need to track these responses internally on an ongoing basis. Once the CDI program has reached the point where it is able to show consistently high levels of physician satisfaction with the services provided by the CDI function, CDI staff should share this information with the appropriate managers in the organization. If possible, the physician satisfaction measure should be included on the organization's dashboard (Carroll and Tansey 2000).

Patient Satisfaction

Today, thinking about the relationship between CDI activities and patient satisfaction is a long stretch. However, as CDI initiatives are able to engage in continuous program renewal, they may have the opportunity to bring documentation to the patients. By providing individuals in the community with training on how to request, use, and read their health records, CDI programs are educating them on their documentation. One way to show the impact that CDI has on patient satisfaction is to ask patients how the training helped them read and interpret their health records. This activity is an important community service, and it can demonstrate to physicians that their documentation practices directly impact not only the care the patient receives, but the patient's overall satisfaction with the healthcare experience.

Conclusion

The healthcare organization should spend a full year implementing a clinical documentation program. At the end of the second year of operations and beyond, it is important to begin refining and renewing the program. Renewal efforts begin with subtle refinements that include physician-specialty training and progress to larger activities that involve expanding CDI into outpatient treatment arenas. The renewal of the program should be viewed by the CDI staff as an opportunity to build better relationships with the physicians. Program renewal should include refining program measures, expanding physician training, and positioning the program as a value-added service by the medical staff.

Chapter Quiz

1. Generally, initial CDI implementation programs should:
   A. Conduct reviews for all payers
   B. Plan expansion in small steps
   C. Be expanded in large steps
   D. Focus on patient satisfaction
2. Why is it important to obtain support of the medical staff when creating a physician report card?
   A. They will have to provide all the inputs.
   B. There could be compliance issues.
   C. It may impact their quality-of-care metrics.
   D. It could harm hospital-physician relationships.

3. The initial focus of a CDI implementation program in one patient care setting is often due to what reason?
   A. Profit is often focused in one area.
   B. Implementation is must faster.
   C. Targeting one area is less risky.
   D. Investment measurement becomes more difficult.

4. Treating these people as customers often develops a positive ongoing relationship with CDI staff.
   A. Patients
   B. Executive staff
   C. Coding and billing staff
   D. Medical staff

5. What is considered common ground between medical staff and the hospital?
   A. Healthcare reimbursement
   B. Health records
   C. Physician query process
   D. Clinical documentation improvement

6. When developing CDI training for physicians, you should:
   A. Position CDI as value-added
   B. Train emergency department staff first
   C. Develop a patient satisfaction survey
   D. Create physician report cards

7. Which of the following might create an environment ripe for continuous program renewal?
   A. Physician report cards
   B. Medical staff dissatisfaction
   C. Evolution of quality initiatives
   D. Lower staff turnover

8. A benefit to the CDI program comes with the reporting of what phenomenon?
   A. Severity-of-illness outcomes
   B. CDI interfaces with other functions
   C. CDI program improvement
   D. Physician disapproval

9. What information should be collected as a measure of physician satisfaction?
   A. Metrics on professional fee reimbursement
   B. Attitudes and opinions on documentation practices
   C. Physician score cards
   D. Peer review

10. What should the CDI program be adding after the first year of implementation?
    A. Outpatient treatment areas
    B. Subtle refinements
    C. Community health education
    D. Comprehensive key measures

REFERENCES

Carroll, R.F. and R R. Tansey. 2000. Intellectual capital in the new internet economy—its meaning, measurement and management for enhancing quality. *Journal of Intellectual Capital* 1(4):296.

Chung, S., K.D. Mandl, M. Shannon, and G.R. Fleisher. 2004. Efficacy of an educational website for educating physicians about bioterrorism. *Academic Emergency Medicine.* 11(2): 143–148.

Covey, S.R. 2014. *The 7 Habits of Highly Effective People.* New York: Simon & Schuster. Retrieved from: https://www.stephencovey.com/7habits/7habits-habit7.php.

Flamholtz, E.G. and J.M. Lacey. 1981. Personnel management: Human capital theory and human resource accounting. Institute of Industrial Relations, University of California.

Russo, R. 2008. *A Compelling Case for Clinical Documentation: Use Clinical Documentation to Achieve Strategic Alignment with Your Medical Staff.* Bethlehem, PA: DJ Iber Publishing.

Russo, R. 2001. The application of knowledge management principles to compliant coding activities. *Topics in Health Information Management* 21(3):18–22.

Chapter 14 CDI Best Practices: Operational and Financial

Clinical documentation improvement (CDI) programs worthy of benchmarking use the best practices available. To maintain a top notch program, CDI staff must manage them proactively. However, the term "best practices" is subjective in nature and extremely dynamic. By their very nature, best practices change and evolve as other organizations find a better way. There are portions of best practice descriptions, however, that remain constant over time. This chapter uses four criteria that require best practices to

- Remain constant over time
- Be supported by research or actual application by more than one healthcare system
- Affect at least two out of three management areas (operations, strategy, and compliance)
- Provide some measurable value to the organization

Ten Best CDI Operational Practices

Listed below are ten best CDI operational practices that enhance CDI programs and encourage sustainability. These practices relate to the program's vision, physician education, policies and procedures, query process, management tools, and collaboration between denials management, compliance, and health information management (HIM). The ten best CDI operational practices are

- Designing CDI as a patient-centered process
- Creating a vision

- Implementing initial, compulsory physician education
- Creating policies and procedures and requiring sign-off
- Maintaining complete query documentation
- Operationalizing a feedback loop between denials, management, and CDI
- Operationalizing a feedback loop between CDI and compliance
- Operationalizing a feedback loop between HIM and CDI
- Conducting continuous targeted physician education and relationship building
- Using rigorous management tools

Design CDI as a Patient-centered Process

The primary reason for the existence of every healthcare system is the patient. Organizations that design their systems around the patient are often more successful than organizations that do not (Penfield et al. 2009). Because CDI focuses on ensuring the best possible documentation in a patient's health record, it is easy to draw some initial analogies between the function and its direct impact on patients, namely quality of patient care.

However, there are additional areas that CDI programs can take advantage of to expand the patient focus of their function. These include increasing the patient's awareness of the health record, assisting the patient to obtain that record, and showing the patient how to read the information in that record. CDI departments have an opportunity to provide information to the community with training or other programs about their health records. This is also an opportunity for the CDI program to work with HIM and members of the medical staff. All three functions together are likely to deliver a better result to patients than just one.

Create a Vision

Every CDI program needs a strong vision that is both compelling and consistent with the organization's overall values, vision, and mission statement. Research has shown that organizations that develop meaningful vision statements are more likely to achieve their goals and be profitable (Covey 1989; Collins and Porras 1994; Collins 2001). While a vision statement is strategic in nature, it is also operational when CDI managers and staff create it.

The vision statement is an affirmation of where the CDI program is going. Additional details about developing a viable vision statement for CDI are in chapter 6. The vision statement explains in a brief sentence why the organization is willing to dedicate resources to support the clinical documentation effort. The statement may be as simple as, "The CDI program will ensure our data is of the highest possible quality and, as a result, our healthcare system will have accurate reimbursement, quality measures, and high patient satisfaction with health information." Organizations usually pair the vision statement with a mission statement that explains how they will achieve the vision. In the case of a CDI program, some of the means used to achieve the vision include obtaining physician support and involvement in the program, and using the best technology including electronic health record (EHR) implementation. As with the organizational vision and mission statement, the CDI vision must be specific to the organization.

Implement Initial Compulsory Physician Education

Compulsory physician education in CDI using a model like the CAMP (coaching, asking, mastering, and peer learning) Method discussed in chapter 8 is probably the single most important activity to ensure the success of the CDI program. Experience shows that organizations that believe they can move forward and be successful implementing a clinical documentation program without full support from the medical staff have significantly underestimated the impact physicians have on CDI. In every case, the organizations either abandoned their program or went back to the drawing board and recreated the program from the ground up with physician support.

Physician documentation is the issue at hand in the CDI program. Not only do physicians need training on the principles of clinical documentation, they also need to take a leadership role in the function. Through training, physicians develop the skills and confidence to document accurately (Bandura 2000; Cascio et al. 2005). More importantly, they become active participants in the CDI process. This may mean they attend follow-up training sessions, respond more quickly to queries, and are willing to assist with the training of new physicians.

Training staff using an effective adult learning model has had a positive impact on organizational efficiency and sustainability over time (Bandura 2000; Cascio et al. 2005; Mulvehill et al. 2005). In addition to increasing operational efficiency, education and training also reduce compliance risk.

Create Policies and Procedures and Require Sign-off

Policy and procedure development may seem mundane, but programs that develop them, even in their most simple and straightforward form, have consistently been more efficient in their processes and more consistent in their data reporting. Not only is it essential to develop the policies and procedures, it is just as important to require program staff to sign off on them. This shows they understand the documents and agree to abide by them. Creation of policies and procedures requires the authors, who are usually the managers and staff of the CDI program, to think through their processes thoroughly. In essence, writing the process down validates it. Written policies and procedures support operational efficiency and reduce compliance risk.

Maintain Complete Query Documentation

Every organization should apply the same criteria for high-quality clinical documentation to the recording of CDI program activities (queries and case notes) as it does to the review of clinical documentation. Query documentation is important because it not only serves as an audit trail for clinical documentation revisions, but also as a teaching opportunity for physicians, CDI specialists, and coders. Complete query documentation is maintained for three reasons.

First, thorough documentation of program activities engages the staff members more and holds them responsible for their work. In a program that maintains excellent documentation on the query process, staff is involved in maintaining the documentation. They also know that every step they take in the CDI process is traceable, so they are more likely to act consistently and compliantly.

Second, the documentation makes physicians more accountable for their responsibilities to the hospital. Physicians know they cannot slip through the cracks in an efficiently run program. For example, if the CDI program generates regular reports showing outstanding physician queries, the reason for each query, and the query rate by physician or by service, it sends the message that program documentation is impeccable.

The third reason for keeping thorough query documentation is for compliance purposes. Because CDI is the raw material for coding and billing, government and private payers often closely scrutinize activity around the function.

In every instance, the program must have the ability to recreate every query it generates. The query paper trail serves the organization well in the event of an investigation or during regular auditing activities. Assuming that CDI activities are compliant, the query paper trail supports why a CDI specialist asked the query (there was clinical evidence to support it), how he or she asked it (not in a leading manner), and how the physician responded.

Without the query paper trail, the government will hold the lack of evidence and documentation against the organization. The organization can protect itself and minimize compliance risk by maintaining complete documentation on all queries (IPRO 2005a; IPRO 2005b; CMS and NCHS 2006a; CMS and NCHS 2006b).

Operationalize a Feedback Loop between Denials, Management, and CDI

CDI is an integrative function in every organization. Most organizations embrace this concept in the initial implementation phase. During implementation, members of the organization responsible for functions that should continuously integrate with CDI generally serve on the CDI committee. This usually includes compliance, finance, HIM, case management, medical staff, data analysts, case mix managers, and EHR staff. However, often after a successful implementation, formal committees dissolve, and the managers and representatives retreat to their respective areas.

It is the responsibility of the CDI manager to ensure continuous communication with many of these managers. Specifically, the CDI manager should coordinate a feedback loop with each of these functional managers that involves reporting data from the department to CDI and then from CDI back to the department. The three areas for CDI best practices include operationalizing feedback loops with denials management, compliance, and HIM.

Every organization has a denials management process in place. Ideally, an organization wants the insurance company to pay its bills without a denial. In some organizations, denial rates are higher than 50 percent (Johnson 2008; Robertson and Dore 2005). Therefore, the need for a function dedicated to managing the process is necessary in most organizations. Denials management may be part of the finance and patient accounting function, or it may be its own function. The CDI manager should seek out the denials manager to discuss how they can help each other. In particular, denials managers should be collecting the reasons for denials, and one of those reasons is, or should be, documentation issues. In these cases, the denials manager should inform the CDI manager of the documentation-related reasons for denials, so the CDI manager can develop a process that helps prevent those types of denials.

At a minimum, the CDI manager can use the information to educate the staff and even develop follow-up education for the physicians to clarify what types of documentation issues are causing denials and what strategies they need to take to prevent future denials. The CDI manager can then provide the denials manager with information about the training. This illustrates one possible synergistic opportunity between CDI and denials management. In tracking the cause for denials, the managers should expect to see a decrease in denials due to documentation.

Payment denials are an increasing challenge for healthcare facilities with 1 to 3 percent of their net revenue at risk. Industry studies report that facility billing departments do not rebill 50 percent of denied claims, 90 percent of denials are preventable, and 67 percent are recoverable (MedAssets 2014). Payers face financial challenges operationalizing the Affordable Care Act, which requires them to carefully screen claims for possible errors. The Department of Health and Human Services (HHS) requires the initial validation auditors to perform an internal review of claims, and HHS performs a second level audit (CMS Risk Adjustment Program 2014). With so much at stake, healthcare facilities need a clear understanding of the magnitude of their denials and effective action steps to prevent them in the future. The CDI team can be an asset to this process by improving clinical documentation specificity needed to appeal denials and to prevent them altogether.

CDI managers should be proactive to assist using these ten steps:

1. Contact the department manager responsible for the denial process
2. Identify analytics available on denials by payer, root cause, financial impact, trends over the past twelve months, percent appealed, and percent overturned
3. Focus on and quantify lost revenue for those denials that improved clinical documentation will affect: medical necessity (pre-authorization, authorization, and continued stay), diagnosis-related group (DRG) validation, present-on-admission (POA), and pre-existing conditions
4. Establish a taskforce to include the CDI, HIM, and denials managers
5. Identify the high-dollar categories in step 3 and prioritize
6. Select the top category, review the denial letters, and audit a sample of 50 records to determine the root cause of the denials
7. Develop a plan for mitigation of the root cause (physician, CDI, and care management education, denials and appeal process workflow, care management staffing, and ineffective denial letters)
8. Evaluate the appeal letter process, review samples of the letters, and develop a template for level I, II and III appeals for the care managers and HIM departments to use
9. Implement the mitigation plan and track progress until denials are at target for a category
10. Discuss payer contract issues with the contract department so further negotiations with the payer can move forward

These steps provide a starting point for the taskforce to identify the problem and develop a short-term solution. Medical necessity denials outweigh those from other categories. Improved clinical documentation can prevent many of those claim denials. Most hospitals experience this familiar scenario:

> The patient presents with an acute exacerbation of congestive heart failure. Clinical circumstances warranted the admission using Interqual criteria (McKesson's level of care criteria). The care manager reviewed the case daily and discussed the need for continued stay with the providers. They decided to continue the patient's stay four days after admission. Several months after the patient's discharge, the facility received a denial letter for the last two days of the stay. The denials taskforce reviewed the case and found that on days three, four, and five the provider progress notes stated "patient doing well, ready for discharge." The provider did not document any details regarding the need for the continued stay. The medical decision-making process was not evident within the clinical record. The patient appeared to be stable. Further discussion with the care manager on the case revealed the patient had a stage III pressure ulcer requiring excisional debridement and intravenous (IV) antibiotics on day three. The provider did not document the stage of the ulcer in the record, nor did he use the word "excisional" for the debridement. The case manager said the physician was concerned about the possibility of cellulitis, but did not document this "possible" diagnosis in the record.

The denials taskforce uncovers many similar scenarios during the root cause investigation. It is important to categorize these findings to identify trends and solutions. The taskforce should report these trends to the appropriate stakeholders for further root cause identification and solution development.

Operationalize a Feedback Loop between CDI and Compliance

A second feedback loop that organizations should put into place is between CDI and the compliance function. As previously discussed, CDI can present a significant compliance risk to an organization that does not manage the process correctly. One way to keep CDI on track is to keep a regular, open feedback loop between the function and the compliance manager. For example, the CDI program manager should ask for recommendations from the compliance manager that relate to the current OIG workplan or other compliance activities of the organization. In addition, the CDI manager should report audits and monitoring results to the compliance department regularly. The CDI manager should also see the compliance function as an opportunity to discuss concerns about physicians who may not be cooperating with program staff or who are ignoring queries. If not managed appropriately, these physicians may become disgruntled with the CDI process and file complaints with CMS, the state's attorney general, or even the OIG. The CDI manager should run the program proactively. Identifying the potential for compliance issues and resolving them before they turn into actual issues is a smart idea for CDI program managers, the organization, and the medical staff. Keeping a close liaison with the compliance department through a formal feedback loop is a good way to manage this risk.

Operationalize a Feedback Loop between HIM and CDI

The last feedback loop that should be in place for a best practice CDI program is between HIM and the CDI program. In some cases, CDI may report to the HIM manager. However, even a formal reporting structure does not guarantee the right individuals will share the right information. Therefore, it is necessary to ensure the CDI manager works directly with the HIM manager to obtain data about retrospective physician queries. This includes retrospective queries made both by the coding professionals and by the CDI specialists on the unit that no one responded to before the patient's discharge. This should be a formal reporting loop.

In some CDI databases, the coding professionals have the ability to record retrospective queries (IPRO 2005a; IPRO 2005b; CMS and NCHS 2006a; CMS and NCHS 2006b). This is ideal, but in the absence of such a computer program, the CDI manager and the HIM or coding manager need to determine a methodology to ensure the sharing of this information. Another informal feedback loop that organizations should put into place between the departments is joint educational sessions for the CDI specialists and the coding staff. Joint training cannot take the place of formal reporting, but it provides a strong support for the staff, especially around common frustrations with the query process.

Figure 14.1 demonstrates the feedback loop that should be in place between the CDI function and other integrated functions within the organization. Depending on the organization, other functions may share data with CDI, but denials management, the HIM department, and compliance have the greatest synergy and are likely to produce the most significant value to the organization if teamed with CDI.

Figure 14.1 The clinical documentation integrated feedback loop

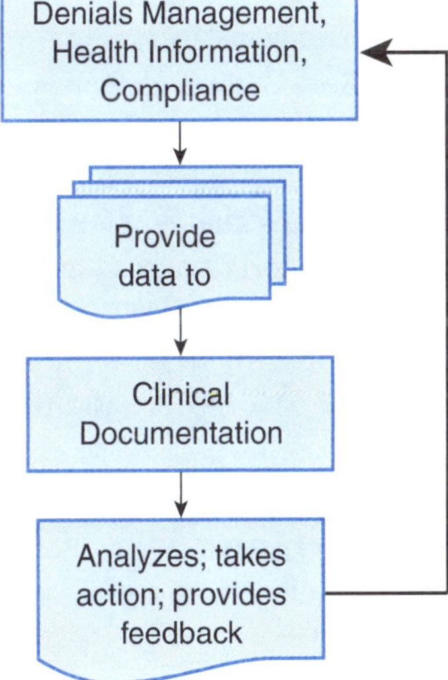

Conduct Continuous Targeted Physician Education and Relationship Building

Basic physician education, as noted earlier, is essential to the initial success of a CDI program. However, follow-up education and relationship building are just as essential to the continued success and sustainability of a CDI program. The key to this activity is that the department is not just conducting follow-up education, but doing it in a way that engages the medical staff. The ultimate outcome of physician involvement in the CDI process should be the physicians' perception of CDI as a value-added service to them. Over time, physicians are likely to align themselves naturally with the effort because they see it is in their own best interest and their patients' best interest to practice high-quality clinical documentation.

Use Rigorous Measurement Tools

As mentioned before, an unmeasured activity is unmanageable. CDI practices are no exception. As noted in earlier chapters, first the organization develops baseline measures for clinical documentation practices through assessment. Then, during the course of implementation, the program develops CDI core key metric targets. Finally, the organization begins to track additional measures as part of its program renewal process. The CDI manager must diligently track this data, accurately and carefully analyze it, and report it to senior management on a regular basis. The CDI manager must also compare current data against data from an earlier time to determine whether the program is making progress.

In later stages of the life of the CDI program, the organization may want to consider using a Six Sigma process to track and measure program outcomes. Six Sigma is a highly disciplined process that helps to focus on developing and delivering near-perfect products and services. In an organization that practices Six Sigma quality, the goal is to attain a 99.99999 percent accuracy rate. By way of example, the Six Sigma goal in coding is 3.4 defects per one million records coded.

Today, it is common for organizations to set a 95 percent proficiency rate for coding. This standard would allow 50,000 defects per million occurrences, far outside the acceptable range for Six Sigma. Although the manufacturing industry first practiced Six Sigma, the service industry has been successfully applying it (UVA 2008). Healthcare organizations that implement Six Sigma methodologies for improving efficiencies in many different areas have all seen significant financial benefits because of the Six Sigma activities (UVA 2008). While a Six Sigma program is likely not part of the initial CDI implementation for every organization, excellent tracking and measuring should be. Moreover, attaining Six Sigma-level quality should be the goal for the future.

Denials Management Workplan

The denials taskforce should establish a workplan to guide the group during the initial stages of the project. The workplan should be a team effort to foster acceptance by all stakeholders. The workplan in table 14.1 is a starting point for

Table 14.1 Denials management workplan

Allen&Shariff HEALTHCARE CONSULTING

CLIENT Payer Denials & Appeals Project Workplan pg 1

Task ID	Task Description	Responsible Party	Due Date	Date Complete	Week 1	2	3	4	5	6	7	8	9	10	11	12	13	14
1	**Taskforce Development and Assessment**																	
1.2	Kick-off meeting with Denials Taskforce	Denials Taskforce																
1.3	Interview and job shadow appeals coordinators separately	Denials Taskforce																
1.4	Review currently available metrics/reporting	Denials Taskforce																
1.5	Review denials and appeal letters	Denials Taskforce																
1.6	Review current state software support	Denials Taskforce																
1.7	Interview and job shadow appeals support staff	Denials Mgr																
2	**Appeals Department Workflow**																	
2.1	Review policies and procedures	Denials Mgr																
2.4	Prepare current and future state workflow charts	Denials Mgr																
2 3	Compile supporting industry standards & guidelines for policies and procedures	Denials Mgr																
2.5	Prepare revised draft policies and procedures	Denials Mgr																
3	**Reporting and Metrics**																	
3.1	Conduct root cause analysis and payer contract opportunities report	Denials Taskforce																
3.2	Prepare future state reporting requirements	Denials Taskforce																
4	**Implementation Plan Development**																	
4.1	Complete assessment report, implementation schedule, and timeline	Denials Taskforce																

On Task
At Risk
Blocked
Complete

CLIENT Payer Denials & Appeals Project Workplan pg 2

Task ID	Task Description	Responsible Party	Due Date	Date Complete	Week 1	2	3	4	5	6	7	8	9	10	11	12	13	14
5	**Implement Recommendations**																	
5.1	a. Implement improvements to denial letters	Denials Mgr																
5.2	b. For each root cause identified during the assessment, establish process improvement solutions:																	
5.21	1. Denial response	Denials Mgr																
5.22	2. Utilization review	Case Mgmt																
5.23	3. Case management process	Case Mgmt																
5.24	4. Insurance verification and authorizations	Revenue Integrity																
5.25	5. Payer contract negotiations	Contracts Mgr																
5.26	6. Clinical documentation	CDI Mgr																
5.27	7. Coding	HI Mgr																
5.3	c. Develop revised policies and procedures	Denials Taskforce																
5.4	d. Work with IT to ensure software is in place for appeals tracking, and recommend a tracking report set and report distribution process utilizing current software where possible	Denials Mgr																
5.5	e. Establish milestones for each root cause identified in Phase II.I.b. above and create method for oversight and monitoring of progress	Denials Taskforce																
6	**Stakeholder Training**																	
6.1	a. Develop training materials around solutions identified in Phase II.I.b. above	Denials Mgr																
6.2	b. Provide training for solutions identified in Phase II.I.b. above (utilization review, case managers, HIM, CDI, physicians)	Denials Taskforce																
7	**On-Going Program Monitoring**																	
7.1	Taskforce meets monthly to evaluate trends, identify items resolved, and establish new focus areas	Denials Taskforce																
7.2	Taskforce communications project successes and challenges to executive sponsors																	
				Total														

On Task
At Risk
Blocked
Complete

Used with permission from Allen & Shariff, Inc.

the group. The taskforce should revise it to allow for inclusion of specific facility challenges. The workplan includes seven steps:

1. Taskforce development and assessment
2. Appeals department workflow
3. Reporting and metrics
4. Implementation plan development
5. Recommendations implementation
6. Stakeholder training
7. On-going program monitoring

The taskforce should modify each step to include sub-steps required to complete each task. Excel is useful for setting up the workplan. Colors are helpful to identify task status. However, if paper copies are black and white, symbols or patterns are more practical. Each team member should update the workplan prior to the taskforce meeting. The group can then discuss the updated plan.

Effective Appeal Letters

The turnaround of payer denials requires an effective appeal letter. Each facility should develop a template for the various types of appeals. This makes the letters more effective and decreases time requirements for the authors. The most common types of appeal letters are

- Preauthorization
- Authorization
- Admission medical necessity
- Continued-stay medical necessity
- DRG validation

Each payer has a specific process; facilities should be familiar with the detailed requirements. Most payers allow for a first and second appeal. Some payers allow for a third-level appeal. For government payers, the last appeal is through the administrative law judge and is usually in person or via conference call. Industry experience suggests payers deny most first-level appeals. Facilities should submit second-level appeal letters for all first-level denials. An example of an appeal letter template follows:

> Hospital Name and Address:
> Patient Demographics, Policy, and Numbers
>
> To Appeal Reconsideration Department
>
> General Hospital received your letter dated October 20, 2014, denying the inpatient patient stay, (*dates of service*), based on the medical necessity of the admission. Your review of Mr. Jones's clinical record suggests the documentation provided does not support the billed level of care (acute inpatient admission).

We have completed a thorough review of the clinical record on this case, and our opinion is that the services Mr. Jones received are medically necessary in the acute inpatient setting where he received them.

Dr. Johnson, the attending physician and a board certified cardiologist with the American Board of Cardiologists, provided the treatment in the acute inpatient setting. In addition, consulting physicians Dr. Andrews, a board certified internal medicine physician, and Dr. Ellis, a board certified infectious disease physician both agreed with Dr. Johnson that the appropriate level of care was the acute inpatient setting.

Case Scenario: Mr. Jones presented in the emergency department with a history of congestive heart failure, hypertension, coronary bypass surgery, and diabetic peripheral neuropathy. His routine medications included (*enter medications here*). His chief complaint was shortness of breath, pitting edema, recent weight gain of 15 pounds, fatigue, and chest pain. His vital signs upon arrival to the ED were (*enter vitals, oxygen saturation, and so on, here*). His pertinent physical findings upon examination were (*enter positive findings here*). Diagnostic tests performed were (*enter tests performed and positive findings for electrocardiogram [EKG], x-ray, Doppler, and so on*). The provider treated Mr. Jones with (*enter medications including IV fluids, respiratory therapy, and such*).

Dr. Williams, an ED physician, referred Mr. Jones to Dr. Johnson, who evaluated him. His clinical impression was acute systolic congestive heart failure. The patient had a past medical history of (*enter findings here*). Positive findings upon physical exam were (*enter here*). Dr. Johnson ordered (*enter diagnostic tests, consultations, monitoring, and treatments, including medications*)

The attending physician based his determination of the need for an acute inpatient setting on his comprehensive evaluation of the patient's severity of illness at the time of admission and of the patient's risk of mortality and comorbidity. Dr. Johnson perceived Mr. Jones to be at risk for (*enter risks discussed in scholarly articles on congestive heart failure*). Because of these risks, Mr. Jones required close monitoring provided in the acute inpatient setting.

In addition, CMS uses McKesson's Interqual criteria for quality evaluation and utilization review decisions. In this case, the admission met the criteria using Interqual's (*enter specific criteria set used*) criteria, specifically, Mr. Jones's clinical record documents (*enter documentation specific to Interqual criteria used*).

Medicare Benefit Policy Manual Chapter 1 Section 10.1, states:

An **inpatient** is a person who has been admitted to a hospital for bed occupancy for purposes of receiving inpatient hospital services. Generally, a patient is considered an inpatient if formally admitted as inpatient with the expectation that he or she will remain at least overnight and occupy a bed even though it later develops that the patient can be discharged or transferred to another hospital and not actually use a hospital bed overnight.

The physician or other practitioner responsible for a patient's care at the hospital is also responsible for deciding whether the patient should be admitted as an inpatient. Physicians should use a 24-hour period as a benchmark, [in other words], they should order admission for patients who are expected to need hospital care for 24 hours or more, and treat other patients on an outpatient basis. However, the decision to admit a patient is a complex medical judgment, which can be made only after the physician has considered a number of factors. Some factors include the patient's medical history and current medical needs, the types of facilities available to inpatients and to outpatients, the hospital's by-laws and admissions policies, and the relative appropriateness of treatment in each setting. Factors to be considered when making the decision to admit include such things as

- The severity of the signs and symptoms exhibited by the patient
- The medical predictability of something adverse happening to the patient
- The need for diagnostic studies that appropriately are outpatient services (in other words, their performance does not ordinarily require the patient to remain at the hospital for 24 hours or more) to assist in assessing whether the patient should be admitted
- The availability of diagnostic procedures at the time when and at the location where the patient presents.

In this case, Dr. Johnson expected Mr. Jones to be in the hospital at least 24 hours as he documented in his progress note dated October 23, 2014. Dr. Johnson was also concerned about a possible adverse event based on the risk identified above for congestive heart failure patients, cited in (*name scholarly article cited*).

The final determination of this case should be based on the complex judgment made by Dr. Johnson, the risks to the patient, and in accordance with the regulations in the Medicare Benefit Policy Manual Chapter 1 Section 10.1. General Hospital respectfully requests your consideration of the adverse admission determination on Mr. Jones. Thank you for your further consideration of this case.

Respectfully submitted,

Dr. Andersen
General Hospital, Physician Advisor

Note that the appeal letter includes information from scholarly articles on specific disease processes. These are available via Google Scholar (http://scholar.google.com/). The appeal letter author should add enough detail from the article to outline clearly the risks of comorbidity and mortality for the diagnosis or procedure discussed in the letter. Statistics on risk of mortality and comorbidity are beneficial when explaining the reason for admission or continued stay. Educating attending physicians on the appeal letter process can enlighten them on necessary clinical documentation to prevent future denials. Physicians should clearly state in the clinical record the

- Reason for admission to the level of service ordered, specifying clinical indications
- Risks of treating the patient in a lower level of care
- Risks of comorbidities and mortality related to the diagnosis or treatment scheduled

Five Best Practices for Management of Financial Measures

Because the financial impact of a CDI program is important and because many programs may lose their continued funding without the ability to demonstrate economic value, every organization should have a best practices approach to managing the financial measurement of its CDI program.

Hospital management teams often express concerns related to clinical documentation and case mix index (CMI) management that invoke a compliance, ethics, quality improvement organization (QIO), or fiscal intermediary-related reason as the cause for non-action. While apprehension is understandable given the nature and size of some compliance, fraud, and abuse settlements, it is essential for hospitals to manage their financial affairs accurately and proactively. The five best practices follow:

- ***Track CMI closely and identify real patient mix change.*** The CDI program manager should know and understand the organization's patient base and the true value of the services the organization is providing to them. Reporting where possible, for patient admissions, increases accountability of both the physician and the organization.
- ***Track and report on MCC and CC capture rates across the organization and by service.*** Concurrent intervention through a clinical documentation program ensures documentation is reflective of care provided. The resulting complete and accurate documentation will result in good information to be translated into coded data by the hospital's coding staff. If the hospital is confident in its data, because monitoring and auditing of the process is in place, then complication and comorbidity (CC) capture rates that exceed the mean or norms should not be a concern.
- ***Know the benchmarks and validate the data regularly.*** Benchmarks for CMI, major complications and comorbidity (MCC) and complications and comorbidity (CC) capture rate, and DRG pairs are published nationally by the RAC (recovery audit contractors) and by regional quality improvement organizations (QIOs). These benchmarks are generalized guides to data reporting outcomes. Each hospital's outcomes may be different. The CDI manager should conduct regular internal or external audits to validate documentation and coding. If the hospital's outcomes are higher or lower than the benchmarks, then the program may modify the internal targets to fit the severity and service line patterns of their patient population.

- ***Do the right thing for the most accurate data outcome.*** A concurrent process ensures completeness and quality but if, through an audit process, any inaccuracies in documentation or coding are discovered, the CDI program manager should consider the pros and cons of retrospective rebilling and decide along with the right people on the CDI team what approach to take. Proactive management of the hospital's relationship with the QIO and Medicare Administrative Contractors (MACs) will likely pave the way to address any legitimate retrospective rebilling issues the hospital may encounter.
- ***Create a concurrent documentation process with physician leadership.*** Ensuring accurate clinical documentation is a specific practice just as is the practice of medicine. Physicians do not currently learn how to document accurately in medical school or residency. They do not learn the seven criteria for high-quality clinical documentation, nor do they learn the "language of medicine" as it relates to coded data, reimbursement, or quality measures. It is the hospital's responsibility to teach and monitor clinical documentation practices.

Table 14.2 summarizes the best practices for management of clinical documentation financial measures.

Best Practices in Relationship Building for Financial Managers Concerning CDI

The five best practices discussed in the previous section are essential to managing a hospital's clinical documentation and CMI. The relationships the hospital financial management team builds inside and outside of the organization will have just as much impact on the success of the hospital's fiscal management driven by clinical documentation practices. The hospital's financial management team should ensure proactive management of relationships with the following:

- The QIOs
- MACs
- Primary insurers

The hospital should manage relationships with all payers proactively, not just when the payer, MAC, or QIO shows up for an audit or questions a bill. Building relationships and sharing necessary information also strengthens the credibility of the hospital in the eyes of these organizations. The hospital management

Table 14.2 Best practices for managing clinical documentation

Best Practices Approach to Management
Track CMI closely and identify real patient mix change
Track and report on CC rates overall and by service
Know the benchmarks and validate the data regularly
Do the right thing for the most accurate data outcome
Create a concurrent process with physician leadership

team should delegate a specific individual in the hospital to be responsible and accountable for each entity relationship.

Conclusion

This chapter outlined the 10 best CDI operational practices and five best financial management measures for healthcare organizations to consider. In order to be a best practice for CDI, it needed to be timeless, bring value, and be performed by at least a few organizations that operate successful and sustainable CDI programs. The practice also had to benefit the system in at least two of the following three areas: operations, strategy, and compliance.

Chapter Quiz

1. Which of the following is one of the four criteria describing the basics of best of practice CDI programs?
   A. Intangible best practices in middle revenue cycle
   B. Practices must be central to only one area
   C. Practices supported by research and actual application by multiple healthcare systems
   D. Best practices with high validity are included
2. When a meaningful ____________ is developed, an organization is more likely to achieve its goals and be profitable.
   A. Physician education
   B. Organizational value statement
   C. Vision statement
   D. CDI mission statement
3. Which item below is one of the three management areas that a best practice must affect?
   A. Medical staff
   B. Human resources
   C. Strategy
   D. Medical necessity
4. The CDI program must keep high-quality records of the query process for:
   A. Revenue cycle analysis
   B. Compliance issues
   C. Chart deficiency tracking
   D. Reducing the workload on HIM
5. Which of the following groups are included in the feedback loop between denials, management, and CDI program staff?
   A. Compliance
   B. OIG
   C. CMS
   D. Payers

6. The CDI staff might create a feedback loop with which department to prevent disgruntled physicians from filing claims against them?
   A. Billing or finance
   B. Health information management
   C. Compliance
   D. Case management

7. CDI staff members must work directly with this department to obtain data about retrospective physician queries.
   A. Coding
   B. Health information management
   C. Compliance
   D. Case management

8. Organizations that design their systems around this have been proven to be more successful.
   A. Physician queries
   B. Compliance
   C. Patients
   D. Utilization review

9. Which of the following is one of the five best practices for management of financial measures in the CDI program?
   A. Track and report on CC capture rates across the organization and by service
   B. Build relationships with QIO and primary insurers
   C. Publish data to benchmarking organizations
   D. Document corrective actions

10. A future goal for any CDI program should be to implement:
   A. A train-the-trainer program
   B. Real case mix index
   C. Relationship management with patients
   D. Six Sigma

REFERENCES

Bandura, A. 2000. *Handbook of Principles of Organizational Behavior.* Edited by E.A. Locke. Oxford: Blackwell.

Cascio, B.M., J.H. Wilckens, M.C. Ain, C. Toulson, and F.J. Frassica. 2005. Documentation of acute compartment syndrome at an academic healthcare center. *Journal of Bone and Joint Surgery* 87 (2):346–350.

Centers for Medicare and Medicaid Services (CMS). 2014. Risk Adjustment Program: HHS Operations. Retrieved from https://www.cms.gov/CCIIO/Resources/Presentations/Downloads/hie-risk-adjustment-operations.pdf.

Centers for Medicare and Medicaid Services (CMS) and the National Center for Health Statistics (NCHS). 2006a. ICD-9-CM Official Guidelines for Coding and Reporting. http://www.cdc.gov/nchs/data/icd/icd10cm_guidelines_2014.pdf.

Centers for Medicare and Medicaid Services (CMS) and the National Center for Health Statistics (NCHS). 2006b. ICD-9-CM Official Guidelines for Coding and Reporting—Supplement. http://www.cdc.gov/nchs/data/icd/icd10cm_guidelines_2014.pdf.

Collins, J. 2001. *Good to Great: Why Some Companies Make the Leap and Others Don't.* New York: HarperCollins Publishers.

Collins, J., and G. Porras. 1994. *Built to Last: Successful Habits of Visionary Companies.* New York: HarperCollins Publishers.

Covey, S. 1989. *The 7 Habits of Highly Effective People.* New York: Free Press.

Healthgrades. 2015. Healthgrades. http://www.healthgrades.com/.

IPRO. 2005a. Coding for Quality: Documentation tips for the top seven DRGs, revised 2005. Hospital Payment Monitoring Program.

IPRO. 2005b. Coding for quality: Documentation tips for the top ten denied DRGs. Hospital Payment Monitoring Program.

Johnson, R.M. 2008. Denial management in a clinical laboratory setting. *Clinical Leadership and Management Review.* 22(3).

MedAssets. 2014. Denials management: Key assessment steps to prevent and recover repetitive revenue leakage. Retrieved from: www.rncasemanager.com/articles/DenialsMgmtKeyAssessment.pdf.

Mulvehill, S., G. Schneider, C.M. Cullen, S. Roaten, B. Foster, and A. Porter. 2005. Template-guided versus undirected written medical documentation: A prospective, randomized trial in a family medicine residency clinic. *Journal of the American Board of Family Practice* 18(6): 464–469.

Penfield, S., K.M. Anderson, M. Edmund, and M. Belanger. 2009. Toward health information liquidity: Realization of better, more efficient care from the free flow of information. http://www.boozallen.com/insights/insight-detail/40808278.

Robertson, B., and A. Dore. 2005. Six steps to an effective denials management program. *Journal of the Healthcare Financial Management Association.* 59(9):82–86, 88.

UVA 2008. University of Virginia (UVA) Medical Center reduces coding errors with Six Sigma. Report on Medicare compliance.

Chapter 15 Synergies with the Electronic Health Record

Introduction

The majority of US hospitals have implemented an electronic health record (EHR) system to replace the manual clinical record. The Healthcare Information Management and Systems Society (HIMSS) divides EHR transformation into eight stages with Stage 0 being the lowest level of transformation and Stage 7 being the highest level. These stages correspond to the logical sequence of activities that healthcare organizations are most likely to undertake when implementing an EHR. The steps include

1. Assess your facility readiness
2. Plan your approach
3. Select or upgrade to a certified EHR
4. Conduct training and implement an EHR system
5. Achieve meaningful use
6. Continue quality improvement (HealthIT.gov 2015)

HIMSS estimates that as of the third quarter of 2014, 4.4 percent of US hospitals were at Stage 0 (HIMSS 2015b).

A hospital in Stage 0 has implemented some clinical automation, but not in all three of the major ancillary department systems: laboratory, pharmacy, and radiology. At the end of the fourth quarter 2014, 3.6 percent of hospitals in the HIMSS analytics database were at Stage 7 (HIMSS 2015b). In stage 7, the hospital maintains a paperless shared electronic health record (SEHR) environment with a mixture of discreet data, document images, and medical images (HIMSS 2008).

Figure 15.1 provides a graphical depiction of the EHR implementation stages and the percentage of hospitals that have completed each stage.

The criteria for each stage builds upon the activities for the prior stages. An analysis of the stages of EHR implementation reveals several opportunities for synergies between EHR implementation and clinical documentation improvement (CDI). This chapter identifies these synergies, which are likely to add value to the organization. Stage 2 is the foundation stage for implementing more sophisticated EHRs. The analysis in this chapter begins with Stage 3 and continues through Stage 7, since the focus is on the opportunities for CDI synergies during EHR implementation. Hospitals with 101 to 200 beds have median scores of 5.1185, which means they have implemented an EHR system through Stage 3 (HIMSS 2015a).

In order to reach Stage 4, a hospital needs to achieve all requirements for Stages 0 through 3 first, or concurrently with the Stage 4 transformation activities. HIMSS suggests that there is a strong correlation between higher quality indicators and hospitals that have achieved at least Stage 4 of an EHR implementation (HIMSS 2006). A Stage 4 EHR means hospitals have the following in place:

- The physicians have access to retrieve and review data from a central data repository (CDR) that houses data from all three of the major ancillary clinical systems (pharmacy, laboratory, and radiology).
- The CDR contains a controlled medical vocabulary and the clinical decision support and rules engine for rudimentary conflict checking.
- The clinicians must document electronically clinical information such as vital signs and flow sheets. At least one service or one unit in the hospital uses electronic nursing notes, care plan charting, and the electronic medication administration record (eMAR) system. The hospital has added computerized practitioner or physician order entry (CPOE) to the nursing

Figure 15.1 Stages of EHR implementation (2nd Quarter 2014)

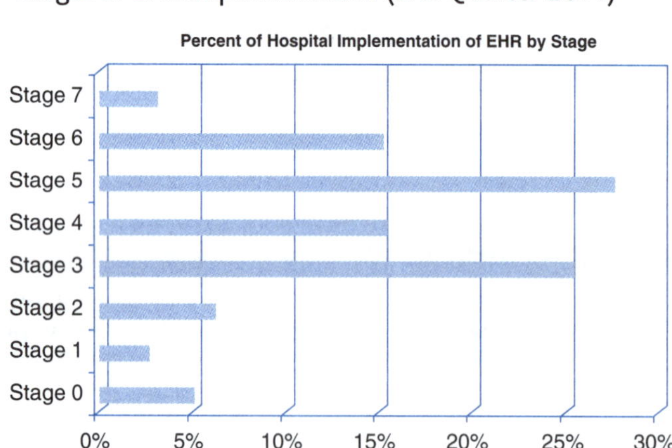

HIMSS 2014

and CDR environment along with the second level of clinical decision support capabilities related to evidence-based medicine protocols. If one patient service area has implemented CPOE and has completed the previous stages, then that area has achieved this stage (HIMSS 2006).

The biggest challenge with clinical documentation and the EHR is achieving a balance between technology demands and the necessary physician input to ensure the system produces useful, high-quality information (Fichman and Moses 1999; Goldberg 2000). The only way to accomplish this goal operationally is to involve the medical staff in the process from the beginning. In addition, strategically, it is important to understand what is most critical to the physicians for patient care and their own practices, and combine this information with the hospital's needs regarding care, reimbursement, research, and planning. Everyone, including the patient, the physician, and the healthcare organization, benefits from these collaborations.

Meaningful Use Incentive Programs

The Centers for Medicare and Medicaid Services (CMS) established objectives for meaningful use incentive programs requiring providers to prove they are using their EHR system meaningfully to receive an EHR incentive payment. CMS defines meaningful use as a healthcare organization positively affecting the care of its patients, and meeting the required thresholds for a number of objectives (CMS 2015). Hospitals and providers demonstrate their EHR meaningful use by progressing through a series of eight stages. "Regardless of the payment year, the Medicare hospital incentive payment is the product of three factors:

- An initial amount
- The Medicare share
- A transition factor applicable to the payment year

This payment methodology will be utilized to calculate Medicare hospital-based EHR incentive payments for eligible hospitals participating under both the Medicare fee for service and [Medicare Advantage (MA)] incentive programs" (CMS 2015).

CMS uses the following formula to calculate the Initial Amount:

Initial Amount = a base amount of $2 million + a discharge-related amount (CMS 2015).

Table 15.1 provides an example of the Initial Amount calculation for three hospitals of varying size.

CMS bases the Medicare Share portion of the meaningful use incentive on the following calculation:

Number of inpatient (IP) Part A Bed Days + Number of IP Part C Days
Total IP Bed Days × [Total Charges – Charges Attributable to Charity Care
Total Charges] IP = inpatient Medicare share (CMS 2013).

Table 15.1 Initial amount calculation

Type of Hospital	Hospitals with 1,149 or fewer discharges during the payment year	Hospitals with at least 1,150 but no more than 23,000 discharges during the payment year	Hospitals with 23,001 or more discharges during the payment year
Base Amount	\$2,000,000	\$2,000,000	\$2,000,000
Discharge-Related Amount	\$0	\$200 ×(n – 1,149) (n is the number of discharges during the payment year)	\$200 × (23,001 – 1,149)
Total Initial Amount	\$2,000,000	Between \$2M and \$6,370,400 depending on the number of discharges	Limited by law to \$6,370,400

CMS 2015

The latest filed 12-month Medicare cost report is used by the facility to identify the number of bed days and total charges.

CMS uses the Transition Factor to calculate the incentive payments over time. If hospitals demonstrated meaningful use beginning in 2011 and continued through 2013, they could receive payment for up to four years. Table 15.2 "shows the possible years an eligible hospital could receive an incentive payment and the Transition Factor applicable to each year" (CMS 2015)

Table 15.2 Transition factor

	Fiscal Year				
	2011	**2012**	**2013**	**2014**	**2015**
2011	1.00				
2012	0.75	1.00			
2013	0.50	0.75	1,00		
2014	0.25	0.50	0.75	0.75	
2015		0.25	0.50	0.50	0.50
2016			0.25	0.25	0.25

CMS 2014

The example below illustrates how CMS calculates the Medicare incentive payment for an acute care hospital with 1,000 annual discharges:

> The hospital becomes a meaningful user and is eligible for incentive payments beginning in [fiscal year] FY 2011. The hospital had 1,000 acute care inpatient discharges in FY 2010 (the latest filed 12-month cost report). Also, in FY 2010 it had 3,000 Part A acute care inpatient-bed-days and 4,000 Part C acute care inpatient-bed-days. Its total acute care inpatient bed-days in FY 2010 were 10,000. Hospital A's total charges excluding charity care were $2,700,000, and its total charges for the period were $3,000,000. Based on this information, Hospital A received a preliminary incentive payment of $1,560,000 for being a meaningful user of certified EHR technology in FY 2011. Its incentive payment was calculated as follows:
>
> **Initial Amount – $2,000,000 (Hospital A did not have more than 1,149 discharges)**
> **Medicare Share – 0.78 = ([3,000 + 4,000] divided by [10,000 × (2,700,000/3,000,000)])**
> **Transition Factor – 1**
> **Preliminary Incentive Payment – $2,000,000 × 0.78 × 1 = $1,560,000**
>
> The hospital's final payments would be based on hospital discharge data and Medicare Share data from the cost report that begins after the beginning of the payment year and determined at the time of settlement for that cost reporting period (CMS 2015).

CDI Opportunities at Stage 1 EHR Implementation

Stage 1 transformation implies that the hospital demonstrates the following criteria:

- Electronic capture of health information is in a standardized format
- Uses health information to track key clinical conditions
- Communicates information for care coordination processes
- Reports clinical quality measures and public health information
- Uses information to engage patients and their families in their care (Butler 2013)

Because one of the key criteria for Stage 1 relates to engaging patients by making their health information more accessible, CDI practitioners can assist by ensuring clinical documentation is professional, clear, concise, and ready for patient access and that providers are aware that patients are increasingly scrutinizing their records. "Patient-centered health [information technology] IT allows providers to look at an individual holistically and treat them through the coordination of other providers." (Dimick 2011). Through improvements in the quality of clinical documentation, CDI practitioners support care coordination between providers by educating them about the need for completeness and accuracy in EHR documentation. CDI practitioners should collaborate with the quality and health information management (HIM) departments to ensure clinical documentation needed for quality measures and public health information is accurate and specific, reflecting the quality of care provided within the facility. The CDI task force charged with governing the quality of clinical documentation should focus keenly on reviewing analytics, monitoring queries, and coding.

CDI Opportunities at Stage 2 EHR Implementation

Stage 2 transformation implies that the hospital demonstrates the following criteria:

- More rigorous health information exchange (HIE)
- Increased requirements for e-prescribing and incorporating lab results
- Electronic transmission of patient care summaries and across multiple settings
- More patient-controlled data (Butler 2013)

Stage 2 increases the amount of patient-centric measures providers require (Dimick 2011). Much of the Stage 2 requirements focus on additional patient access to their own clinical record. Patients must be able to receive a log recording any release of their medical information, in addition to increased encryption requirements for the security of data (Heubusch 2012).

The *Journal of AHIMA* states:

> Once accomplished, the widespread adoption of EHRs will represent a fundamental change in how providers use, collect, and document clinical information. This paradigm shift will transform not only how medicine is practiced, but also how patients interact with the healthcare system. The promise of interoperable electronic health record systems promotes an environment where complete documentation and timely access to patient information facilitates sound clinical decision making, improved outcomes, and lower costs (Rhodes 2013).

This statement reflects the reasons for the EHR meaningful use requirements and the goal behind the plans that will improve clinical documentation and make it more available for patient care. With increased patient access in Stage 2, the CDI program should further evaluate the clinical record as a tool for communication with providers, patients, and payers that will improve the quality of care and reimbursement accuracy. Cases with high-volume practitioners, service lines, diagnoses, and treatments should be part of focused audits by CDI practitioners to identify any need for improvements. For example, CDI practitioners could evaluate cases with a principal diagnosis of acute respiratory failure for completeness, accuracy, and specificity in diagnostic lab results, respiratory treatments, ventilator time flow sheets, physician progress notes, and discharge summaries. The documentation should clearly reflect improvements in the patient's status backed by clinical indicators and the reasons for the improvements based on treatments and patient response. Providers should also document clearly a lack of response to treatment. Physician documentation should clearly state the reasons for level of service decisions such as admission to intensive care units and reasons for planned discharge dates based on patient clinical status. This information is important to justify the medical necessity of the patient's level of service and to ensure payment by the payer.

CDI Opportunities at Stage 3 EHR Implementation

Stage 3 transformation implies that clinical documentation (vital signs, flow sheets) is present. The hospital should equip at least one service or one unit in the hospital with the CDR, which should integrate nursing notes, care-plan charting, and the eMAR system scored with extra points. The first level of clinical decision support checks for errors with order entries like drug/drug, drug/food, and drug/lab conflicts normally found in the pharmacy. Physicians should have access to some level of medical images from a picture archive and communication systems (PACS) via the organization's intranet or other secure networks outside of the radiology department confines (HIMSS 2007).

It is essential to involve CDI in the initial stages of CPOE. One of the most common reasons documentation fails to meet the criteria for high quality is incompleteness or a lack of precision when an order is placed by a provider without a diagnosis or other reasons documented for the order. This applies to orders for diagnostic testing as well as medication. In every instance, the hospital requires the physician to enter a reason for the order. Depending on what the physician knows at the time of the order, the reason may be a symptom, a condition listed as ruled out, or an established diagnosis (Pepper 1994).

It is important that healthcare organizations consider documentation practices prior to implementing CPOE. For example, this may mean including a drop-down menu in the EHR that provides physicians with choices as well as the ability to enter free text. Alternatively, an organization may decide to permit only free text. The healthcare system's compliance department as well as the CDI department should be involved in the EHR implementation. Involving both functions not only ensures the documentation meets the criteria for high-quality clinical documentation, but also that providers use compliant methodology. There are many opportunities to pull forward, copy, or check off information in the EHR, so the system needs to include specific built-in checks as well as training protocols.

CDI Opportunities at Stage 4 EHR Implementation

Stage 4 implies the hospital has a CPOE system in place for clinicians to use, along with the second level of clinical decision support capabilities related to evidence-based medicine protocols. If one patient service area has implemented CPOE and completed the previous stages, then it has reached Stage 4. (HIMSS 2007)

Stage 4 involves both full CPOE implementation and decision support related to evidence-based medicine protocols. The organization should continue to work with CDI and CPOE implementation in the same manner as described in the Stage 3 transformation. Computerized evidence-based medicine protocols present additional opportunities for value-added synergies between EHR implementation and the CDI department. There are a few ways to accomplish this.

Educational Programs

First, organizations can develop educational programs that explain the relationship between evidence-based medicine and clinical documentation. Trainers can emphasize examples of how practicing high-quality clinical documentation helps achieve evidence-based medicine, or at least the legitimate documentation of it. Evidence-based medicine is a concept that appeals to most physicians because they are trained scientists. Showing a relationship between evidence-based medicine and clinical documentation practices strengthens physician support for the CDI program (Brown et al. 2005; Timmermans and Berg 2003). More importantly, if physicians believe their clinical documentation practices can affect the practice of medicine through evidence-based medicine protocols, they are more likely to incorporate high-quality criteria into their clinical documentation practices.

CDI Staff Work with Software Vendor

Second, the CDI department should work closely with the organization's protocol management software vendor, if present. There are several software programs available to ensure the provider abides by established evidence-based medicine practices. Evidence-based medicine software provides medical practitioners access to the latest treatment guidelines and protocols at the point-of-service. By centralizing this information and automating its delivery, the software enables healthcare institutions to comply with the demanding requirements of evidence-based medicine and achieve high standards of consistency and quality in dispensing patient treatment (Donaldson and Lohr 1994). In cases where it is possible to create organization-specific queries, the CDI function should be involved. Here, the CDI staff can identify, for example, documentation issues that lead to frequent queries for certain diagnoses and incorporate these into the program as reminders for the physicians. If the organization properly designs this process and trains its physicians, it will see an improved quality of documentation as well as a compliant process.

Ensure Criteria Included in Clinical Guidelines

Third, the CDI program manager should include criteria for high-quality clinical documentation and on-going updates or revisions in any clinical guidelines the organization uses, even if it is not currently using a software program. Clinical documentation and international classification of diseases (ICD) coding guidance revisions become effective throughout the year. The organization should consider and include these guideline changes in the facility criteria. Some of the purposes of evidence-based medicine include informing medical staff of current treatment guidelines and procedures as well as ensuring protocol adherence and regulatory compliance. The treatment guidelines are a convenient place to include the seven criteria for high-quality clinical documentation as a constant reminder for physicians. It is a good idea to reinforce high-quality clinical documentation criteria with the physicians beginning with the CDI physician training, follow-up training, and key metrics reporting, and extending into as many day-to-day encounters the physicians have with the patient record. The CDI program manager should identify every possible opportunity to build the criteria for high-quality clinical documentation into existing and new systems, such as the EHR.

Finally, by the time an organization has achieved Stage 4 transformation, the CDI function should have worked with the EHR team to design a methodology to alert the attending physicians whenever an abnormal test result is reported by the clinical department into the system. This process can be cumbersome if not managed appropriately. In teaching hospitals, residents are responsible for reviewing and documenting abnormal test results. In other organizations, the CDI specialists may be responsible for determining whether physicians documented the clinical significance of an abnormal test result, and query accordingly. This can be achieved through a template designed by the IT team specifically for this purpose. Figure 15.2 demonstrates the importance of documenting the clinical significance of abnormal test results as well as the EHR's opportunity to alert physicians during Stage 4 transformation. Using this methodology, the EHR could flag pertinent treatment-based protocols for the provider when he or she documents abnormal test results or designated key phrases. These flags could assist in gathering additional specificity in the record as well as improve the quality of patient care. Query alerts could be added to the EHR functionality to request additional specificity in the clinical documentation for key focused diagnoses or diagnosis-related groups (DRGs).

CDI Opportunities at Stage 5 EHR Implementation

Stage 5 transformation implies the organization has fully implemented the closed-loop, eMAR environment in at least one patient care area. The data flows of the CPOE, pharmacy, and the eMAR applications utilize bar coding technology (or radio-frequency identification [RFID] technology) for the nurse, patient, and medication to support the five rights of medication administration, thereby maximizing point-of-service patient safety processes (HIMSS 2007).

Figure 15.2 Relationship between abnormal test results and the EHR

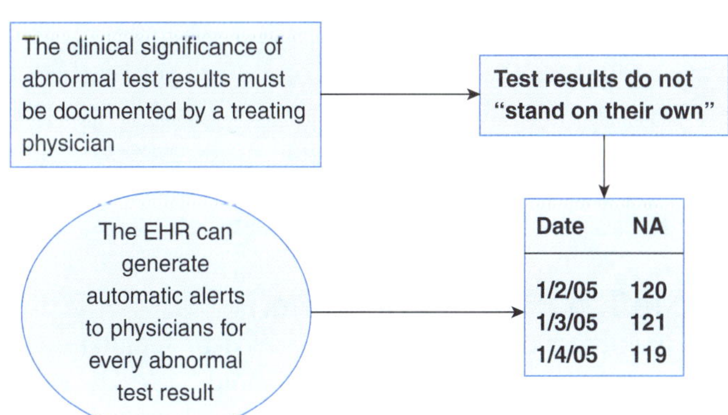

The five rights of medication administration are

- Right patient
- Right route
- Right dose
- Right time
- Right medication (Pepper 1994)

It is interesting to note that in one state health department's description of the five rights of medication administration, the sentence subsequent to the statement of rights read, "Ultimately, the appropriate *documentation* should occur as well" (DORA 2008). This is just one example of how medication administration is tied closely to high-quality documentation. Some of the documentation is the physician's, but much of the documentation responsibility belongs to the nursing staff. As noted earlier in the book, organizations should train every clinician who adds documents in the patient record in the principles of high-quality clinical documentation. Synergies with the EHR create the perfect opportunity to get CDI in front of every clinician in the organization.

The closed-loop medication administration includes CPOE plus bar coding, automated dispensing cabinets and robots, and smart infusion pumps. In each step of this process, there are several documentation requirements. For example, step 1 in the CPOE process is to obtain the patient's medication-related history. Steps in closed-loop medication administration related to CDI include educating both staff and patient regarding the medication, and documenting the administration and the patient's response to medication.

CDI Opportunities at Stage 6 EHR Implementation

Stage 6 transformation implies the organization has implemented full physician documentation and charting (using structured templates) for at least one patient care area. Level three of clinical decision support provides guidance for all clinician activities related to protocols and outcomes in the form of variance and compliance alerts. A full complement of radiology PACS systems provides medical images to physicians through the intranet and displaces all film-based images (HIMSS 2007).

Stage 6 transformation of the EHR provides a huge opportunity to solidify CDI concepts in ways and places the program may not have yet reached. For example, facilities may design a template for documenting clinical information related to congestive heart failure. This template could pull in the echocardiogram and heart cath ejection fraction values and ask for clarification on the specificity of congestive heart failure (CHF) (acute, chronic, systolic, or diastolic).

CDI Involved in Template Development

First, the CDI function should be closely involved in template development as well as education on usage. Template design should include requirements for documentation that are clear, consistent, complete, reliable, and where possible, precise. There may be some boilerplate criteria, which are common in all template development. However, each organization should use data from its CDI program reporting to determine specific edits and checks it may need to build in to electronic templates.

Add Documentation for Quality Indicators and Develop Alerts

Second, Stage 6 transformation incorporates documentation for quality indicators in templates for the physician. This could be a cost saving initiative for the organization as it decreases the need for manual reviews for missed indicators or documentation. The organization can also work with the EHR vendor to develop alerts for missing documentation used for quality indicators. This is also a time to revisit the alerts for abnormal test results discussed during Stage 4 transformation. If additional alerts are desired or if any are not working correctly, they should be repaired by the EHR vendor by the time the organization achieves Stage 6.

Intensive Focus on Documentation Practices of Diagnostician

Third, Stage 6 transformation may be a perfect time for intensive focus on the documentation practices of diagnostic medicine physicians, like radiologists, nuclear medicine physicians, pathologists, and even cardiologists and neurologists involved in interpreting tests like electrocardiograms (EKGs) and electroencephalograms (EEGs). The impact of improved documentation practices in these areas and the value to the organization extends into almost every patient care setting. At a minimum, this includes not only the inpatient environment, but also the emergency department, ambulatory surgery, outpatient diagnostic testing, and clinics. Simply training the physician diagnosticians on the definition of high-quality clinical documentation may have an impact on the content of radiology, magnetic resonance imaging (MRI), nuclear medicine, and other diagnostic reports.

When educating diagnostic physicians on CDI practices, it is necessary for the CDI staff to stay in the realm of clinical documentation practices only. It is not the role of CDI to judge or make recommendations for diagnosing; this remains the diagnostician's responsibility. However, it is essential to train these diagnosticians using examples of their diagnostic reports that were inconsistent with the attending physician's documentation or that lacked diagnostic precision. This type of training helps diagnosticians understand the significance of high-quality documentation and how much others rely on it (Bandura 2000; Lenz and Shortridge-Baggett 2002, 143).

In all training, the CDI staff's role is to give physicians the criteria with examples and allow them to apply those criteria to their thought process as they are viewing results and dictating reports. It is particularly important for the CDI staff to be cautious with diagnosticians because most do not actually see the patient, so for them, the test results and documentation are the sum total of the encounter. It is even more important that the CDI training for diagnosticians remains focused on the criteria for high-quality clinical documentation because the coding staff cannot rely on the diagnostician's documentation for coding. However, it is important to inform diagnosticians that CDI professionals can and should use their documentation as essential evidence for queries in relation to the attending physician's documentation.

CDI Opportunities at Stage 7 EHR Implementation

Stage 7 transformation implies the hospital has a paperless SEHR environment with a mixture of discreet data, document images, and medical images. All entities within a regional health information network (other hospitals, ambulatory clinics, sub-acute environments, employers, payers, and patients) can readily share clinical information via electronic transactions or electronic records exchange to access healthcare data. This stage allows the healthcare organization to support the true integrated care EHR (ICEHR) as envisioned in the ideal model (HIMSS 2007).

Stage 7 transformation supports the extension of CDI into areas beyond inpatient, if that has not already occurred. Many of the documentation rules created for templates and CPOE should remain fixed to the clinical documentation modules for outpatient and long-term care service areas. As a result, the means for achieving high-quality clinical documentation in these settings is already in place with the EHR. However, it is still necessary to provide basic education and training to physicians and clinicians in patient care settings where the EHR is migrating. At a minimum, these practitioners should receive training on the principles of clinical documentation and the criteria for high-quality clinical documentation. This training, coupled with documentation rules already in the EHR system, should produce good documentation outcomes for the organization.

A second benefit of Stage 7 transformation is that it makes health information available to the patient. Prior chapters discussed improved patient satisfaction as an outcome measure for clinical documentation, particularly once more patients begin reviewing the content of their health records. The percentage of patients who review the content of their records is likely to increase after a Stage 7 EHR transformation is complete because patients will have access to their EHR without needing to request the information (Tang and Newcomb 1998, 563). Patient satisfaction with their health information brings CDI to a whole new level. It opens the door for the CDI staff to train the community about how to use and understand the EHR. It also makes healthcare providers more accountable to patients for the content of the EHR. The EHR places the hospital, the medical staff, and the patients all behind the need for high-quality clinical documentation, and its achievement appears likely in all patient care settings, with the EHR as the catalyst, as long as healthcare organizations seize the opportunity to incorporate clinical documentation rules into the EHR as described in this chapter.

EHR, Documentation, and Compliance

The focus in this chapter has been on the strategic opportunities to synergize the CDI workflow with each stage of an organization's EHR implementation. Any change brings risks if the HCO does not manage it appropriately. In the EHR environment, it is essential to disconnect documentation from coding and change events that can otherwise present compliance risks to the organization (Trites 2008). In particular, because of compliance concerns, such as cutting and pasting documentation in an EHR, it is essential to ensure that a member of the compliance team is involved in the entire EHR implementation process, as well as the part of the process involving clinical documentation practices.

Conclusion

Significant opportunities exist for synergies between the EHR and improving clinical documentation practices. Different opportunities exist at each of the eight stages of implementation. Most hospitals and healthcare systems have reached Stage 3 EHR transformation. Therefore, the activities with the most impact and value for the organization are in Stages 4 through 7 of the EHR transformation. Each stage provides the possibility for education to all clinicians. However, an organization's CDI experts can also identify CDI opportunities in template development, CPOE design, closed-loop medication administration, and extension of the EHR to ancillary services such as radiology, as well as to the patients themselves.

Chapter Quiz

1. What stage of EHR transformation does the SEHR system benchmark with a mixture of discreet data, document imaging, and medical imaging?
   A. Stage 2
   B. Stage 6
   C. Stage 7
   D. Stage 3
2. Which stage shows the strongest correlation between higher quality indicators and the hospital's EHR scores?
   A. Stage 6
   B. Stage 4
   C. Stage 5
   D. Stage 2
3. Which stage are vital signs and flow sheets required as electronic documentation?
   A. Stage 6
   B. Stage 7
   C. Stage 2
   D. Stage 3
4. What is one of the key benefits of a Stage 7 transformation?
   A. Makes health information available to the patient
   B. Reduces implementation cost
   C. Fulfills compliance requirements with the Joint Commission
   D. Reduces HIPAA risks

5. What is the earliest stage in which the HCO fully implements the closed-loop medication administration environment in at least one patient care area?
   A. Stage 5
   B. Stage 4
   C. Stage 6
   D. Stage 3

6. Which of the following is one of the five rights of medication administration?
   A. Place
   B. Privacy
   C. Provider
   D. Time

7. What stage of transformation does full closed-loop medication administration implementation in at least one patient care area represent?
   A. Stage 3
   B. Stage 4
   C. Stage 5
   D. Stage 2

8. Stage 6 transformation includes implementing full physician documentation and what other item in at least one patient care area of the hospital?
   A. ICEHR
   B. Charting using structured templates
   C. RFID
   D. CDR

9. What median stage have most acute care facilities reached?
   A. Stage 1
   B. Stage 2
   C. Stage 3
   D. Stage 4

10. Why is it essential for members of the compliance team to be involved in the entire EHR implementation process?
    A. To ensure HIPAA compliance
    B. To meet evolving regulatory guidelines
    C. To monitor cut and paste documentation
    D. To reduce reimbursement risk

REFERENCES

Bandura, A. 2000. *Handbook of Principles of Organizational Behavior*. Edited by E.A. Locke. Oxford, UK: Blackwell.

Brown, M.M., G.C. Brown, and S. Sharma. 2005. *Evidence-Based to Value-Based Medicine*. Chicago: American Medical Association Press.

Butler, M. Meaningful use opens up its deep end. 2013. *Journal of AHIMA* 84(10): 24–29.

Centers for Medicare and Medicaid Services. 2015. An Introduction to the Medicare EHR Incentive Program for Eligible Professionals. http://www.cms.gov/Regulations-and-Guidance/Legislation/EHRIncentivePrograms/downloads/Beginners_Guide.pdf.

Centers for Medicare and Medicaid Services. 2013. EHR Incentive Program for Medicare Hospitals: Calculating Payments. http://www.cms.gov/Regulations-and-Guidance/Legislation/EHRIncentivePrograms/Downloads/MLN_TipSheet_MedicareHospitals.pdf.

Department of Regulatory Agencies (DORA). 2008. The five rights of medication administration. Colorado Department of Regulatory Agencies. Retrieved from: http://cdn.colorado.gov/cs/Satellite/DORA-OPRRR/CBON/DORA/1251624516078.

Dimick, C. First steps to patient-centered care: Meaningful use focuses industry on baby steps. 2011. *Journal of AHIMA* 82(2): 20–24.

Donaldson, M.S. and K.N. Lohr., eds. 1994. *Health Data in the Information Age.* Washington, DC: National Academy Press.

Fichman, R.G. and S.A. Moses. 1999. An incremental process for software implementation. *Sloan Management Review.* 40(2):39–52.

Goldberg, I.V. 2000. Electronic medical records and patient privacy. *The Health Care Manager.* 18(3):63–69.

HealthIT.gov. 2015. How to Implement EHRs. Retrieved from: http://www.healthit.gov/providers-professionals/ehr-implementation-steps.

Heubusch, K. 2012. EHR 2014: Highlights of the proposed Stage 2 certification rule. *Journal of AHIMA* 83(5): 38–39.

HIMSS. 2015a. Current EMRAM Scores. Retrieved from: http://www.himssanalytics.org/emram/scoreTrends.aspx.

HIMSS. 2015b. HIMSS Analytics. Retrieved from: http://www.himssanalytics.org/home/index.aspx.

HIMSS. 2008. HIMSS Analytics Essentials of the US Hospital IT Market (derived from the Dorenfest IHDS+ Database). http://www.himssanalytics.org/docs/iIntro.pdf.

HIMSS. 2006. EMR Sophistication Correlates to Hospital Quality Data: Comparing EMR Adoption to Care Outcomes at UHC Hospitals, including Davies Award Winners, using HIMSS Analytics' EMR Adoption Model Scores. http://www.himssanalytics.org/docs/UHC25.pdf.

HIMSS. 2005. EMR Sophistication Correlates to Hospital Quality Date: Comparing EMR Adoption to Care Outcomes at UHC Hospitals, Including Davies Award Winners, Using HIMSS Analytics' EMR Adoption Model Scores. HIMSS Analytics White Paper. http:www.himsanalytics.org.

Lenz, E.R., and L.M. Shortridge-Baggett. 2002. *Self-Efficacy in Nursing: Research and Measurement Perspectives.* New York: Springer Publishing.

Pepper, G.A. 1994. Understanding and preventing drug misadventures: Errors in drug administration by nurses. *American Journal of Health-System Pharmacy* 52(4):369–373.

Rhodes, H. Meaningful use program faces audits, scrutiny. 2013. *Journal of AHIMA* 84(2): 40–41; 72. Retrieved from: http://www.ashpfoundation.org/drugmisadventures.

Tang, P.C. and C. Newcomb. 1998. Informing patients: A guide for providing patient health information. *Journal of the American Medical Informatics Association.* 5(6):563–570.

Timmermans, S., and M. Berg. 2003. *The Gold Standard: The Challenge of Evidence-Based Medicine and Standardization in Health Care.* Philadelphia: Temple University Press.

Trites, P. 2008. *How to Evaluate Electronic Health Record (EHR) Systems.* Chicago: American Health Information Management Association.

Chapter 16

Clinical Documentation Improvement Technology

CDI Program Software—Functionality for Success

Rapidly changing technology offers a variety of options for maximizing clinical documentation improvement (CDI) program efficiency. CDI tasks have evolved from a manual paper process used for case review and data analytics. The current state includes health information systems using natural language processing (NLP) to identify cases and provide analytics in a graphical format. The advent of the electronic health record (EHR) encouraged the latest technology using NLP to identify key words and phrases making it easier for the CDI specialist and coders to determine query opportunities. Considering that half of the target CDI cases reviewed concurrently require no further action, CDI teams can leverage technology for rapid analysis to determine cases needing clarification. The CDI practitioner can use this saved time to clarify concurrent cases directly with providers, expand the program to include other payers, and for critical one-on-one education with providers. The result is an increase in concurrent query response and a chronological case scenario that supports the true sequence of provider decision making.

Natural Language Processing

Advances in computer technology in the last century have resulted in scientific inventions only dreamed of before. Work in the field of natural language processing began in the 1950s with a focus on machine translation. The history of NLP includes four phases:

- 1940–1960: Machine translation (MT) with automatic translation from Russian to English using punch cards and batch processing that took seven minutes to analyze a long sentence.
- 1960–1970: Artificial intelligence (AI) focused on data construction and knowledge bases with work on interactive dialogue.
- 1970–1989: Grammatico-logical phase using a range of grammar types and logic programming growth dealing with user's beliefs and intentions. The period includes an expanding community of commercial systems using database query for information extraction.
- 1990–2000: Statistical language processing for data analysis, semantic classification, and powerful machines to handle the data. There was significant progress made in web architecture for managing the flood of text found on the World Wide Web.

The present offers computing power to find, digest, package, and represent speech with a large variety of systems including highly modular architecture and conceptual tools for developers (Jones 2001).

Building upon the historical base, modern day advances in health information technology provide a platform for CDI using a core set of technologies for efficient data capture. These technologies allow for and support our existing NLP applications including CDI tracking and analytic software:

- Speech-understanding technology converts natural speech into a structured clinical note. This computer-aided process provides real-time clinical documentation and is the next generation of speech recognition systems.
- Natural language understanding is a sophisticated technology used to read and understand a clinical narrative. This allows structured information to be produced by the technology automatically from narrative content. Using speech and NLP technology, a highly accurate context-aware clinical content can be codified by the technology to classifications such as Systemized Nomenclature of Medicine-Clinical Terms (SNOMED-CT).
- Semantic clinical reasoning uses a structured narrative in a workflow-friendly mode. The technology allows the user to abstract and summarize relevant clinical data across millions of documents. The result is relevant data for one particular patient without a structured form requirement.
- Real-time deficiency tracking provides mined information from a narrative content combined with structured EHR data to identify deficiencies in clinical documentation. This ensures immediate documentation of specificity needed for the CDI and coding processes.
- Machine learning algorithms offer technology that allows prediction of future outcomes using human-verified samples. The technology learns through observing scenarios and becomes more efficient over time. The result is improved machine understanding of the dictated word (M*Modal 2014b).

NLP offers a solution to the problem of data mining within textual information. Historically, most data retrieved for the purposes of analysis and reporting was identified by the technology from a discrete data field within the software. For example, the patient's blood pressure reading could be identified by the technolgy from a discrete field in the vital signs flowsheet. Data mining within narrative text presents a problem with interpreting the data due to contextual concerns. For example, there are various meanings to phrases using the word pneumonia:

- Evidence of pneumonia
- Pneumonia cannot be excluded
- Rule out pneumonia
- Pneumonia is not appreciated
- Pneumonia in 1985

The number of pneumonia cases cannot be discerned by the CDI specialist from the documentation above. NLP technology offers a solution by extracting individual words and determining the relationships among them. The technology uses modifiers and relational assigned values to determine actual incidences of pneumonia (Friedman et al. 2013). This is a giant step for data analytics and application functionality.

Healthcare professionals use NLP to complete the patient story in the clinical record by facilitating workflows, enabling collaboration, and providing insight for improved care delivery. Medical transcription professionals have used it extensively to provide automatic provider dictation translation. For example, M*Modal, a healthcare technology firm, offers cloud-based technology to convert a physician narrative into a customized EHR. This results in a more detailed clinical record that improves the quality of data and enhances provider efficiency by automating clinical documentation. Through a process called collaborative intelligence, NLP has several solutions to improve clinical documentation:

- Search and discovery based on semantic indexing and ontological reasoning
- Real-time CDI
- Computer-assisted coding (CAC) workflow
- Front-end and back-end speech understanding-based documentation workflows
- Meaningful-use abstraction workflows to enable reporting on quality measures
- Meaningful-use list management including medication reconciliation (M*Modal 2014a)

Historically, narrative dictation has been preferred by providers to capture the complete patient scenario. Narratives also offer the best option for communication between providers resulting in improved patient care. Today's automated NLP options offer electronic alerts to prompt the physician when additional information is necessary (M*Modal 2014a). Prompts ensure the physician captures structured data elements for improved documentation and clinical analytics. For example, if the provider documents congestive heart failure (CHF), a prompt might appear asking if the patient has acute, acute-on-chronic, chronic, systolic, or diastolic CHF. This is not only important for patient care, but also provides the necessary detail for coding major complications and comorbidities (MCCs), and complications and comorbidities (CCs) for accurate reimbursement.

Using the functionality of collaborative intelligence, NLP captures the complete dataset required for using CAC and abstracting for Core Measures. Applications, similar to Siri for the iPhone, are available to assist physicians in navigating the EHR using Clinical Language Understanding (CLU) (Dreyer 2013). Overall, NLP improves physician productivity, quality of documentation, and acceleration of revenue cycle activities (M*Modal 2014a). Figure 16.1 provides a glimpse of collaborative intelligence at work using a content server to capture data for a variety of sources.

Using the collaborative intelligence model in conjunction with NLP, hospitals can facilitate the CDI process with automated narrative dictation, provider prompts for increased document detail, and data capture for improved CDI program analytics.

Computer-Assisted Coding

Health information management (HIM) and health informatics professionals have various views on the value-add for CAC. Some see CAC as "the savior

Figure 16.1 Collaborative intelligence

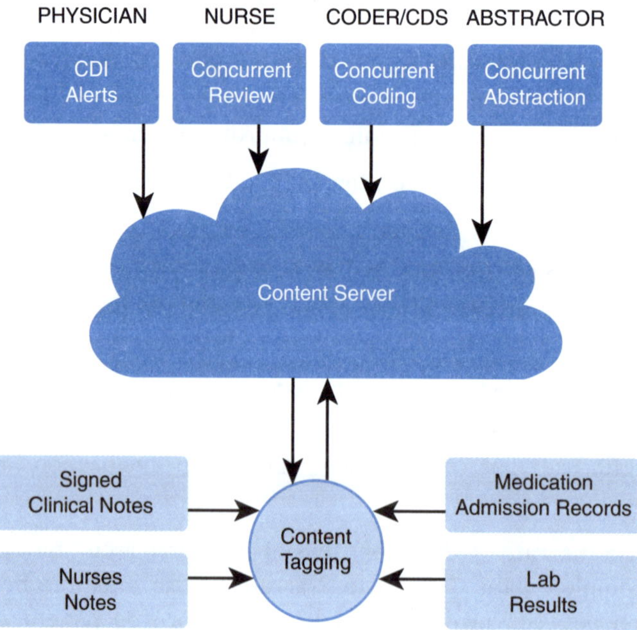

Used with permission from M*Model.

of coding-based bottom lines," while others consider it the "automated destroyer of human coding jobs" (Crawford 2013). Initially, HIM professionals viewed this technology as the future of HIM, but now it is a common plan for supporting International Classification of Diseases, Tenth Revision, Clinical Modification and Procedure Classification System (ICD-10-CM/PCS) implementation in HIM departments. The advantages of CAC include cost reduction and productivity enhancement. With an industry-projected ICD-10-CM/PCS productivity decrease of 50 percent and a professional coder shortage, HIM directors are turning to CAC for the answer to future resource needs (Crawford 2013).

CAC uses an NLP engine that scans the EHR for key terms. The NLP engine processes the key using encoder-like software to suggest applicable codes. A coding professional then reviews these recommendations and selects the final code. An advantage to CAC is that the clinical documentation required for coding is visible within the CAC. This saves the coder from having to view multiple systems. The process speeds up the clinical record review and encoding process. This is especially helpful in the EHR environment where the amount of clinical information has greatly increased compared to paper records. With both productivity issues (ICD-10-CM/PCS and EHR documentation) occurring in a short time frame, HIM directors are focused on a reasonable means to maintain production levels.

CAC offers an altered career path for the HIM production coder. Potentially, the new role is coding auditor. The coding auditor reviews the CAC-selected codes and determines whether they are accurate. The coder functions at a higher level, using technology to enhance skill set requirements. Industry leaders suggest that CAC will not decrease coding jobs, but will assist HIM departments to maintain current workload volumes under dramatic changes in government regulation and changes in technology. Many industry leaders believe that CAC may improve productivity by 20 to 40 percent, and additional improvements may follow shortly after implementation. Recently, the American Health Information Management Association (AHIMA) Foundation and the Cleveland Clinic conducted a study on CAC, verifying up to 50 percent gains in productivity when coders functioned as auditors. The productivity increase resulted from CAC allowing the coder to focus on one system to view the documentation required for coding (Crawford 2013).

CAC solutions are often paired by technology companies with CDI software technology. In these cases, there has been a dramatic increase in MCC/CC capture rates. This multi-use system assists the coder or CDI specialist to identify symptoms, signs, and clinical indicators that prompt a concurrent or retrospective query. This solution also assists in training new coders and CDI specialists by suggesting coding paths and query opportunities perhaps not apparent to a less seasoned professional.

Though the jury is still out, preliminary data supports a positive outcome for CAC in the healthcare industry. Many considerations influence its success including facility complexity, available resources, and effective implementation strategies by both the facility and the CAC vendor. Facilities that have experienced a successful CAC software implementation report a measurable and consistent improvement (Crawford 2013).

CDI Software

CDI programs have historically used manual workflows and tedious data-capture techniques to complete daily tasks and monitor program success. The last decade offered innovative technology solutions to improve these processes. Technology has now reached the next level using NLP. However, the basic tasks of a CDI specialist are still the same:

- Review the complete clinical record concurrently as the provider makes entries
- Identify signs, symptoms, and diagnostic test results needing further clarification for a more specific diagnosis
- Identify missing diagnostic or procedure detail that affects patient care, quality indicators, justification of medical necessity, and final coding of the record
- Document case detail for use during the next concurrent review and for retrospective coding and final billing
- Query the provider where documentation is inadequate
- Monitor the query submission and ensure the provider responds
- Track query activity and response times to use for program analytics and to support program success

Typically, two software modules are available to support these CDI program tasks. The first is a module that supports tracking case review activities that are part of the CDI workflow. The second supports analytics required to monitor areas of focus and program success. The tracking module may include the analytics module, or they may be separate modules specifically designed for data analytics. Refer to chapter 5 for more information and examples of analytics necessary to support CDI.

CDI Tracking Software Features

CDI tracking software collects data on the review activity by the CDI specialist. The software also accumulates productivity information on the number of reviews, queries, and responses. NLP applications enhance tracking software. Tracking software with an NLP application should include these basic features:

- CDI work list
- Concept search
- Concept dashboard
- Deficiency abstract (electronic CDI worksheet)

Screenshot examples in figures 16.2 through 16.5 correspond to the tracking software functionality listed above.

CDI Work List

The CDI work list (figure 16.2) is a daily list of cases specific to the CDI specialist's assigned location (nursing unit), focused DRG, diagnosis, or procedure. The CDI specialist can use the work list to ensure he or she reviews all cases within a designated time frame. The example screenshot below includes a snapshot of the cases the CDI specialist needs to review for the current date. The system allows for an initial review upon admission and a subsequent review after a specified number of days. Column headings from left to right include encounter number, patient name, location (nursing unit), payer, date of last CDI specialist access, CDI specialist ID, type (focused diagnosis), and status (not visible in the screenshot) such as "new," "in progress," or "satisfied." This feature serves as a tickler list to notify the CDI specialist of the next concurrent review date. Cases may be assigned to another CDI specialist by the CDI manager if needed during time off. The "last access" column lists the most recent review date. The CDI specialist can enter nursing unit location and payer type if desired. This feature is helpful if CDI specialist assignments are established by the CDI manager based on patient location or payer type.

Concept Search

The concept search feature (figure 16.3) uses NLP to identify cases with specific key words and phrases. This is especially helpful if the CDI taskforce has identified a high-risk DRG or diagnosis that needs monitoring. Using this search feature, the CDI specialist can view all new occurrences of the key word and determine the need for a query based on the linked clinical documentation. The example below identifies two cases for the diagnosis of cerebrovascular accident (CVA). The NLP

Figure 16.2 CDI worklist

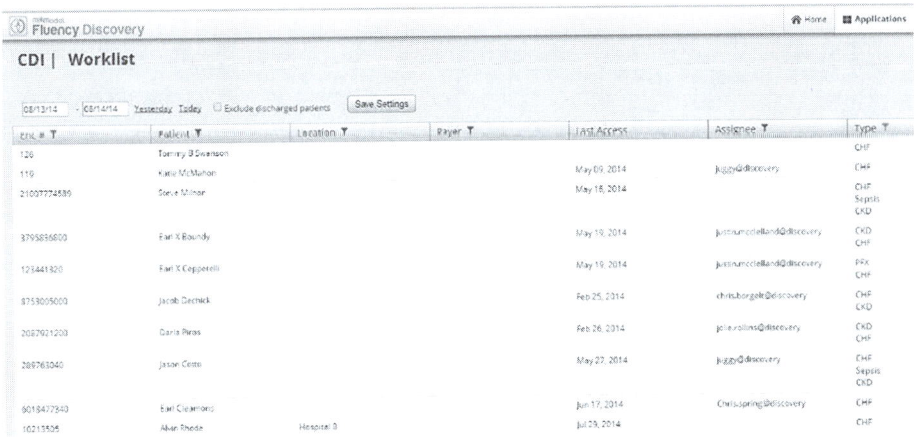

Fluency Discovery | Home | Applications

CDI | Worklist

08/13/14 - 08/14/14 Yesterday Today Exclude discharged patients Save Settings

Enc #	Patient	Location	Payer	Last Access	Assignee	Type
126	Tommy B Swanson					CHF
119	Katie McMahon			May 09, 2014	juggy@discovery	CHF
21007774589	Steve Milnor			May 18, 2014		CHF Sepsis CKD
3795836800	Earl X Boundy			May 19, 2014	justin.mcclelland@discovery	CKD CHF
123441320	Earl X Capperelli			May 19, 2014	justin.mcclelland@discovery	PFX CHF
8753005000	Jacob Dechick			Feb 25, 2014	chris.borgelt@discovery	CHF CKD
2087921200	Daria Piras			Feb 26, 2014	jolie.rollins@discovery	CKD CHF
289763040	Jason Cotto			May 27, 2014	juggy@discovery	CHF Sepsis CKD
6018477340	Earl Clearmons			Jun 17, 2014	Chris.spring@discovery	CHF
10213505	Alvin Rhode	Hospital B		Jul 29, 2014		CHF

Used with permission from M*Model.

Figure 16.3 Concept search

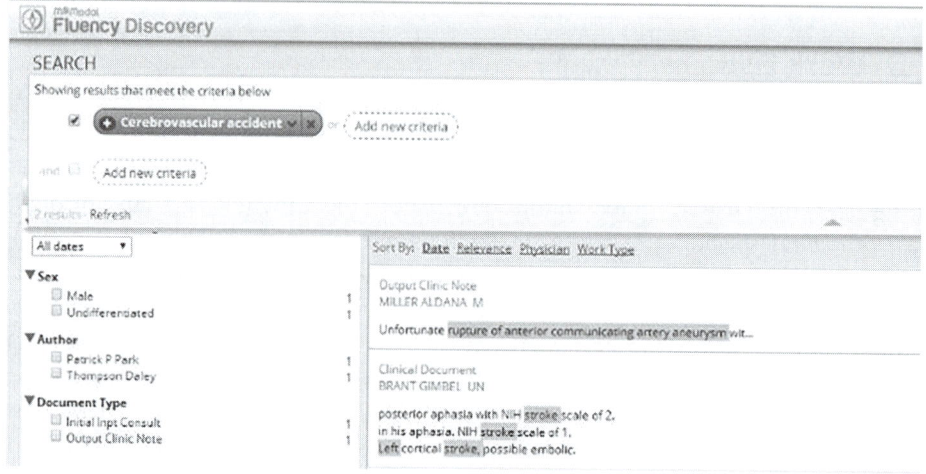

Used with permission from M*Model.

identified these potential CVA cases using a dictionary of associated terms such as ruptured artery and stroke. In addition, this screen also allows access to recent queries submitted for these cases. The CDI specialist can further narrow this search by document type, provider (author), and criteria type (CVA).

Concept Congestive Heart Failure Dashboard

The concept dashboard (figure16.4) offers a graphical depiction as well as a list of cases with specific key words. The example below includes a graph of CHF case volume over time. Also included is a list of cases where the provider mentions

Figure 16.4 Concept dashboard

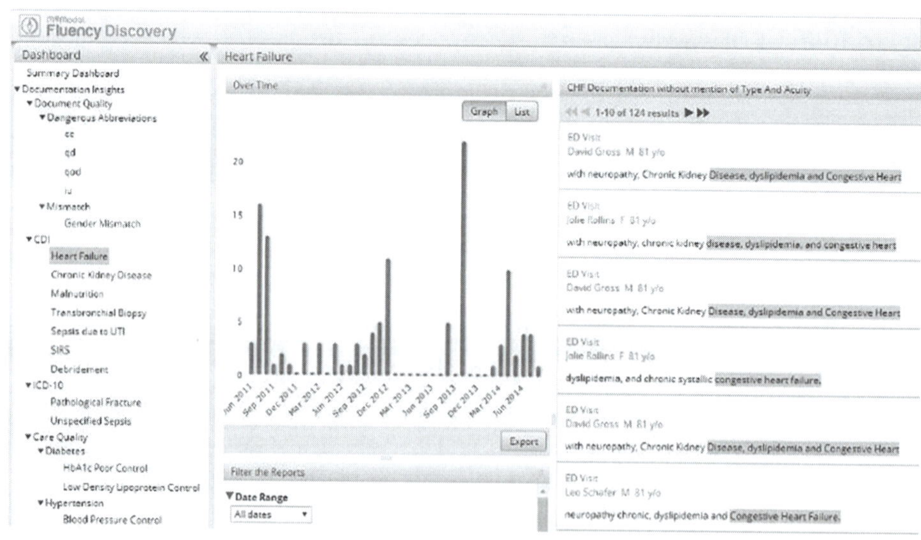

Used with permission from M*Model.

CHF but without the corresponding type and acuity. The concept dashboard is interactive and provides a window to select from a list of focused diagnoses. The CDI specialist may customize the dashboard by selecting date range, sex of patient, and provider name. The right hand window lists individual cases with insufficient documentation. The report type and author (provider) are associated with each case. The left hand window allows selection from a list of insufficient documentation types like documentation quality, CDI, ICD-10, care quality, abnormal lab findings, and abnormal imaging results. As an example, CDI professionals can use this screen to find instances of positive clinical indicators such as ejection fraction in CHF to determine whether the provider clearly documented the specificity of CHF.

Deficiency Abstract

The deficiency abstract (figure 16.5) is patient specific and supports the CDI specialist workflow. The left hand column includes patient demographic data, instances of unspecified documentation requiring CDI specialist intervention, query templates, CDI specialist comments, and disposition of the case (in progress, assigned to another CDI specialist, and so on). This screen takes the place of the manual CDI worksheet and uses NLP to identify clinical documentation issues. The example screen in figure 16.5 shows two cases of unacceptable documentation (malnutrition and chronic kidney disease [CKD]). The user can click the topic malnutrition in the left hand column, and the middle screen will show there are two discharge summaries with indicators for malnutrition. The first is an abnormal albumin value of 1.4. The next is documentation of chronic malnutrition post percutaneous endoscopic gastrostomy (PEG) tube placement. The provider did not document a specific type of malnutrition (mild, moderate, severe, or protein calorie) in either case. The right hand column documents the sequence of case assignments and the status of the assignment.

Figure 16.5 Deficiency abstract

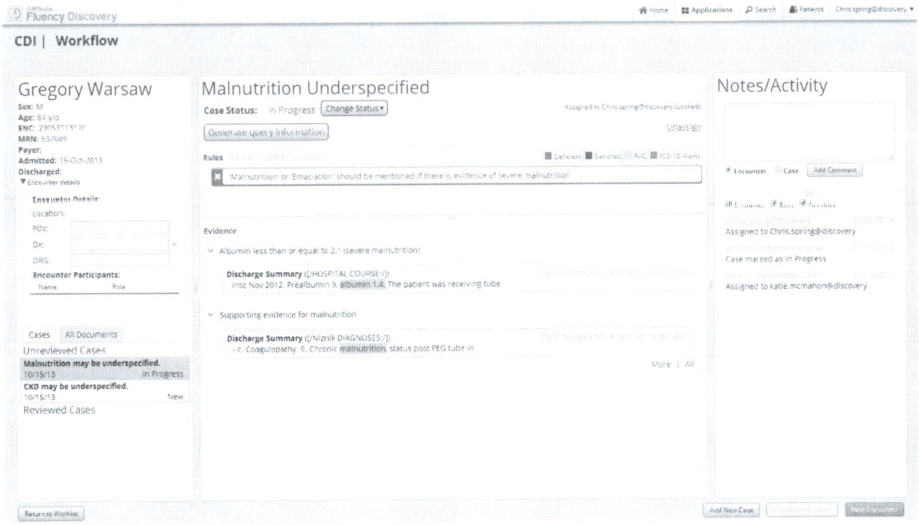

Used with permission from M*Model.

CDI tracking software is essential to an efficient program. Database applications allow the CDI specialist to collect case review activities and provides easy access for daily concurrent review. The success of any CDI program revolves around analytics, monitoring of productivity, provider response, and areas of focus (DRG, diagnosis, and procedures). The CDI staff can use the saved time for provider education, CDI team collaboration (CDI specialist or coder), and data analytics.

Conclusion

Healthcare organizations are faced with competing priorities related to meaningful use, ICD-10-CM/PCS implementation, government payer audits aimed at cost reduction, and accountable care organizations focused on improved quality and cost reduction. Technology offers solutions to these challenges using EHR-based NLP applications and work lists. Capturing structured data elements while using NLP improves provider efficiency, quality documentation for patient care, and compliance with meaningful use guidelines. Tracking CDI specialist activities through a work list is essential to showcase program success and ensure accurate reimbursement. CDI software in today's marketplace can not only track activities, but also enhance the clinical record review process using NLP. Efficiencies realized using NLP offer new ways of expanding the CDI program to all payers and increasing one-on-one provider communication. Innovation provides a way to complete old tasks using new technology.

Chapter Quiz

1. CDI teams can use the time saved by using NLP applications to:
   - A. Expand the program to include other payers
   - B. Improve core measure indicators
   - C. Decrease length of stay through discharge planning
   - D. Identify insufficient provider documentation retrospectively
2. The first phase in the history of NLP is known for which technology?
   - A. Artificial intelligence
   - B. Grammatico-logical
   - C. Machine translation
   - D. Statistical language processing
3. Which technology provides mined information from a narrative content that combines with structured EHR data to identify deficiencies in clinical documentation?
   - A. Machine learning algorithms
   - B. Natural language understanding
   - C. Real-time deficiency tracking
   - D. Speech-understanding technology

4. Collaborative intelligence offers solutions for improving clinical documentation such as:
   A. Manual data abstraction
   B. Handwritten provider documentation scanning
   C. Direct provider communication
   D. Real-time documentation improvement

5. Built-in EHR prompts such as "type and acuity" of CHF are an example of using____________ to improve the clinical record.
   A. Revenue cycle acceleration
   B. Structured data elements
   C. Alternate patient scenarios
   D. Provider decision making

6. A content server captures data from a variety of sources in collaborative intelligence software, including:
   A. Patient registration
   B. Back-end billing
   C. Ancillary department CPT codes
   D. Concurrent review (CDIP)

7. Industry projections suggest ICD-10-CM/PCS will initially reduce productivity by _____ percent.
   A. 20
   B. 30
   C. 50
   D. Yet to be determined

8. Computer-assisted-coding applications can be paired with _____________ software technology to increase MCC/CC capture rates.
   A. CDI
   B. CDM
   C. Inpatient code editor
   D. Semantic clinical reasoning

9. Typically, two software modules are available to support the CDI program tasks including analytics and:
   A. Tracking
   B. Clinical evidence support
   C. Medical decision database
   D. Online coding editors

10. The concept search feature uses NLP to identify:
    A. Key words and phrases
    B. High-risk MS-DRGs
    C. Case mix index
    D. SOI/ROM levels

REFERENCES

Crawford, M. 2013. Truth about computer-assisted coding: A consultant, HIM professional, and vendor weight in on the real CAC impact. *Journal of AHIMA* 84(7):24–27.

Dreyer, J. 2013. Humanizing healthcare with technology. *Health Management Technology* 34(5):14–15.

Friedman, C., T.C. Rindflesch, and M. Corn. 2013. Natural language processing: State of the Art and Prospects for significant progress, a workshop sponsored by the National Library of Medicine. *Journal of Biomedical Informatics* 46(5):765–773.

Jones, K. 2001. Natural Language Processing: A Historical Review. Retrieved from: http://www.cl.cam.ac.uk/archive/ksj21/histdw4.pdf.

M*Modal. 2014a. White paper: Collaborative intelligence. Retrieved from: http://mmodal.com/resources/white-papers/collaborative-intelligence/.

M*Modal. 2014b. White paper: Perfect storm. Retrieved from: http://mmodal.com/resources/white-papers/.

M*Modal. 2014c. White paper: Clinical reasoning. Retrieved from: http://mmodal.com/resources/white-papers/.

Chapter 17

Clinical Documentation Improvement: Multidisciplinary Team Approach

Introduction: Multidisciplinary Team

Multidisciplinary teams (MDT) examine complex issues and develop solutions. MDTs "offer a unique opportunity to examine synchronous collaboration through dynamic interaction, and the use of artefacts, among a number of different professional roles" (Kane 2009). This chapter provides a review of the team members and their collaborative roles in the clinical documentation improvement (CDI) process. The teams typically require a number of different professional disciplines to develop team goals and objectives, develop work plans, implement investigative activities, and coordinate solutions. Barriers to developing effective MDTs are often related to the lack of available team members to support governance, analytics, workflow design, information technology (IT), and provider, CDS, and coder education. It is unrealistic to delay team development until all identified team members are in place. Rather, facilities should establish a set of ideal members with sufficient commitment and vision to initialize the team (MHC 2006). The importance of the MDT relates to the critical success factors of the project at hand. In the context of CDI, the goal of the project at hand is to

- Support high-quality patient care
- Improve clinical documentation
- Ensure accurate reimbursement

The MDT goals are like a cog in a machine. Each cog works together with the others to create a functional machine. Figure 17.1 is a graphical depiction of a functional machine. Each member of the team represents a group of stakeholders that must meet these goals through an integrated team effort.

Figure 17.1 Interlocking MDT goals

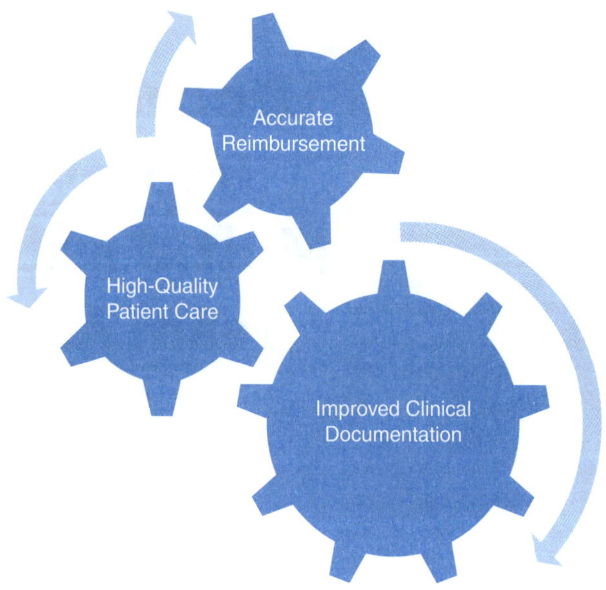

⊙ CDI Governance Team

The minimal MDT group make-up includes executive sponsors, medical staff leadership, and key department leaders. Leadership required for overseeing the CDI program include the health information management (HIM) department, CDI, care management, utilization review, revenue integrity, quality, compliance and IT. Figure 17.2 depicts the governance team and collaborating departments. These leaders are responsible for the governance of the CDI program by ensuring facility-wide visibility of the program, effective participation of each department within the group, monitoring of the program analytics, identifying root causes of issues, and implementing solutions. In other words, the governance group keeps the program on track. The CDI staff team should remind stakeholders at all levels within the facility of the importance of CDI, the positive impact of the CDI program, and the on-going successes achieved by the program. The CDI program ensures not only accurate reimbursement, but also accurate quality scores, accurate severity of illness and risk of mortality levels, enhanced patient care, and payment risk mitigation from payer denials. The governance group should showcase all of these improvements to motivate the MDT and continue the program's success and sustainability.

⊙ Core CDI Team

The daily CDI process requires a smaller group working closely together to ensure optimal clinical documentation that reflects the severity of the patient's condition and treatment. These are the core CDI team members:

- CDI manager
- HIM manager
- Physician (provider)
- CDI professional
- HIM coder

Developing group cohesiveness is challenging, especially when CDI and HIM report to different leaders within the organization. Two organization models are common: CDI reporting to care management, and CDI reporting to HIM. When the two groups are not within the same organizational structure, the two department leaders need to make a collaborative effort to ensure effective relationships among team members. The leaders can develop collaborative relationships with periodic weekly or monthly meetings including the two groups. The two teams should hold weekly meetings during the initial implementation or refresh of the CDI program. Suggested agenda items include the discussion of complex cases where diagnosis-related group (DRG) assignments vary between CDIP and coder, physician communication issues, proposed physician education sessions, and case mix index (CMI) targets by medicine, surgery, other specialties, and physicians.

A cohesive team results in improved overall performance. The CDI practitioner and coder can improve their performance by sharing their clinical and coding knowledge. Query workflow design is important to avoid duplication in provider communication and ensure queries are concise and consistent between the CDI

Figure 17.2 Multidisciplinary oversight team integration

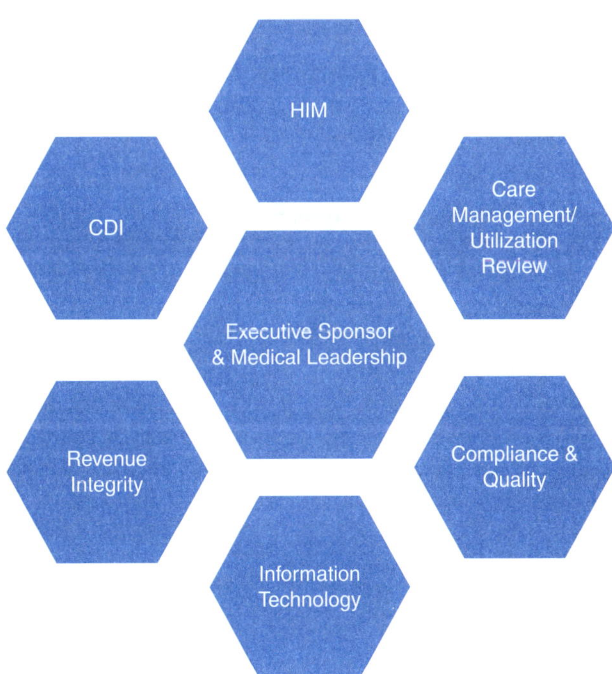

practitioner and coder. Knowledge transfer, effective workflow design, and proper oversight help the facility reach its CMI targets.

Essential goals and objectives of cohesive team members include

- Effective transfer of knowledge between CDI practitioner and coder
  - Clinical indicators
  - Coding guidelines
  - Principal diagnosis assignment
- Effective query submission ensuring enhanced clinical documentation and prevention of multiple queries to the same physician
- Prevention of conflicting information communicated to the physician
- Achievement of CMI targets

Each member of the core team brings a valuable skill set to the table. Managers bring effective oversight to the project, while CDI practitioners bring clinical knowledge to identify potential clarifications. Coders bring an understanding of clinical coding guidelines, and physicians bring quality documentation. Each member should focus on the additional knowledge they need for an effective CDI process. The establishment of a core team taskforce is an effective way to ensure each of these core groups meets the functional requirements needed for success. The taskforce should initially consider the positive attributes of each group and then determine deficiencies that require mitigation. For example, Table 17.1 lists important knowledge requirements for each core team member. The taskforce should provide adequate training so each group can master these skill sets.

Team Dynamics—Collective Team Identification

The MDT approach provides the beneficial impact of increased knowledge and exposure to different disciplines. Through this exposure, team members gain insight into how their daily operations affect other key department operations.

Table 17.1 Core team knowledge requirements

Physician	CDIP	Coder
Trigger words and phrases that will accurately reflect the severity of the patient's condition and treatment	How to identify missing trigger words and phrases	Understand additional clinical information that can result in a code or MS-DRG change
How to use EHR templates to improve clinical documentation	How to write an effective query and encourage a rapid response	Detailed coding guidelines and annual regulatory changes
How to respond to a query	Basic coding concepts and MS-DRG assignment guidelines	Clinical criteria to determine signs and symptoms that may lead to a query and subsequent MS-DRG change

Essential in this understanding are the basic goals, objectives, and tasks of each department. The following departments should be considered as team members based on their integral role in clinical documentation, reimbursement, and quality patient care.

Medical staff leadership plays an important role on the MDT. Most facilities have a physician advisor (PA) specifically assigned to the CDI program. The PA should report directly to medical staff leadership. This provides the visibility and accountability required for the PA to function properly. The organization's chief medical officer (CMO) should also be part of the MDT. The CMO's support is one of the most important factors for a sustainable program. Without this support, the medical staff may lose focus on the program and previous ineffective clinical documentation practices may emerge. The CMO and PA team offers great insight into best practices for physician education, dealing with difficult physicians, and identifying informal physician leaders beneficial to high-risk specialty areas such as cardiology and high-volume surgical specialties.

Revenue integrity is the key to achieving the facility's financial goals. This department is responsible for

- coordinating the hospital charge master functionality,
- billing inpatient and outpatient services,
- ensuring compliant charge capture processes (automated and manual),
- coordinating payer contracts,
- conducting billing audits (external and internal),
- coordinating payment denial and appeal activities, and
- ensuring accurate reimbursement through modeling, analytics, and measurement.

Revenue integrity is also responsible for providing the CDI MDT with analytics around CMI and DRG payments, monitoring and notifying the team of DRG-based denial and appeal trends, and notifying the team of changes in payer payment systems, that is, conversion from a per diem-based plan to APR-DRG payments.

HIM provides services related to maintaining and using health records for reimbursement, patient care, release of patient information, and public health statistics. HIM coders assign International Classification of Diseases, Ninth Revision (ICD-9) / International Classification of Diseases, Tenth Revision (ICD-10) and Current Procedural Terminology (CPT) codes to each diagnosis and procedure for billing, statistics, medical research, and epidemiologic purposes. They are responsible for understanding dynamic government and industry standards related to coding and reimbursement guidelines. Each coder is individually responsible for the work product produced during the coding assignment. The HIM department may be responsible for overseeing the CDI program. HIM managers are integral in the functionality of the core CDI team. The HIM team representative interprets analytics related to DRG assignment by specialty and physician, conducts root cause assessments, and creates action plans to mitigate errant practices.

Care management is responsible for comparing industry standard admissions, continued stay, and discharge criteria against the circumstances of inpatient and observation patient visits. They communicate with the payers to request preauthorization for admission and authorizations for continued stays. This process is known as utilization review. The care management staff also assists with the post-discharge planning activities when needed, reviewing medical necessity denials from payers, and developing written appeals. Payer denials are on the increase. An effective care management and utilization review process is essential to the financial health of the facility. The care management department may also be responsible for overseeing CDI program staff. The department plays an important role on the CDI team, providing insight into areas needing improved clinical documentation for patient care and reimbursement.

The revenue cycle includes several departments such as patient access, financial assistance, HIM, patient financial services, and revenue integrity. A vice president, who provides high visibility for the CDI program, typically leads this department. Many of the day-to-day activities related to CDI and reimbursement may be under the purview of the revenue cycle including coding, CDI, DRG reimbursement, billing, and denials management. The revenue cycle vice president can provide support and necessary resources for new tasks required for the CDI program.

Quality management is responsible for an increasingly complex "quality" patient-care delivery process. Quality management has evolved into a broad, hospital-wide program that requires communicating and assessing of hospital departments. The quality management director is in charge of garnering top management commitment for on-going departmental self-assessment and creative solutions to quality issues. The department oversees risk management, quality improvement, and patient safety. With the advent of governmental pay-for-performance programs, the quality department is integrally involved in the area of facility reimbursement. The quality management director provides important data on quality measurements such as hospital-acquired conditions. The quality indicators are identified in part through ICD-9/ICD-10 codes requiring the collaboration of the quality management and HIM directors. Improved clinical documentation increases quality scores for the facility.

IT is integral not only for the functionality of the electronic health record (EHR), but also for developing system enhancements that can be used by the CDI department and providers to improve clinical documentation. The IT director or chief information officer is responsible for understanding how the CDI-related systems function, and how they interrelate and interface with each other. The IT director can assist with assessing DRG-based analytic and CDI tracking software used to monitor and collect data on the daily activities of the CDIP. Health information systems, such as EPIC, now have templates to guide physicians entering clinical documentation. Within the templates, the IT team can build prompts for additional information to capture clinical information needed for further code specificity and DRG assignment. The CDI MDT should provide oversight and monitor the progress of these IT enhancements.

Team Dynamics

Working within a team is often harder than it appears given the variety of personalities, skill sets, and age groups. Many dynamics affect proper team function. Unconscious psychological forces influence team direction, behavior, and performance. In addition, "there are problems of cooperation and coordination; of time, space and place; roles and information; the kind of knowledge used and kind of technology employed" to effectively present information (Kane et. al. 2011).

Once the MDT is formed by the CDI team leader, it is important to build team cohesiveness. There is a wide variety of team-building methods to help the team to get to know each other on a level based on trust and common goals. The CDI team should take time in the early stages to use these team-building tools, creating a strong, long-term bond vital to their ultimate success. These activities help break down natural barriers and create an environment rich in cooperation and a sense of unity.

The culture of the facility also affects team dynamics. A culture of acceptance, collective decision-making, and accountability creates a positive group dynamic with improved creativity. The team leader is responsible for creating an open and respectful environment among members. He or she can do this by conducting an initial team development workshop that integrates the team and increases cohesiveness with a series of steps:

1. Create team goals and objectives
2. Understand the wider perspective and understand each other's roles in CDI
3. Develop a facility-wide communication plan
4. Generate a work plan for CDI program implementation
5. Determine other departments needed for collaboration on use of the clinical record
6. Determine the frequency of meetings, conference calls, and virtual communications
7. Plan for ongoing monitoring of program success (Yardley 2014)

Table 17.2 provides an example MDT CDI program plan. The team can use this sample plan as a high-level work plan to begin team integration activities for a new CDI program and to establish responsible parties and task due dates. The plan provides suggested tasks beginning with assessing DRG-based payer volumes, and running the governance and initial MDT workshop mentioned above. Additional tasks include hiring a PA and a CDI manager, establishing a comprehensive CDI work plan, assessing available software, identifying analytics for tracking, conducting CDI training, and monitoring the program.

Table 17.2 Multidisciplinary team CDI program plan

Task #	Task	Responsible Department(s)	Due Date	Completion Date	Status
1	Conduct assessment of DRG-based reimbursement	Revenue Cycle	Nov 2014	Nov 2014	Complete
2	Determine need and high-level plan for CDI program implementation	CFO, Revenue Cycle, CMO, HIM	Dec 2014	Dec 2014	Complete
3	Establish multidisciplinary CDI governance team and develop CDI work plan	CFO, Revenue Cycle, CMO, HIM, Care Management, Quality, IT	Dec 2014	Dec 2014	Complete
4	Conduct multidisciplinary team workshop	CFO, Revenue Cycle, CMO, HIM, Care Management, Quality, IT	Jan 2014		
5	Identify and hire Physician Advisor (PA)	CFO, CMO	Jan 2014		In Progress
6	Identify and hire CDI manager	Revenue Cycle, HIM	Jan 2014		In Progress
7	Develop CDI work plan	Revenue Cycle, PA, HIM, CDI Manager, Care Management, Quality, IT	Feb 2014		In Progress
8	Assess CDI software requirements	HIM, CDI Manager, IT	Feb 2014		In Progress
9	Identify and establish standard analytics required for program monitoring	HIM, CDI Manager, IT	Feb 2014		In Progress
10	Develop plan and conduct physician, CDI, coder training	Revenue Cycle, CMO, HIM, PA, CDI Manager	Jun 2014		In Progress
11	Begin monitoring CDI program through monthly analytics	CDI Manager	Jul 2014		In Progress
12	Develop focused DRGs and physician specialties for on-going coder, CDI, physician education (requires monthly update)	PA, CDI Manager	Jul 2014		In Progress

Figure 17.3 Multidisciplinary team (MDT) model

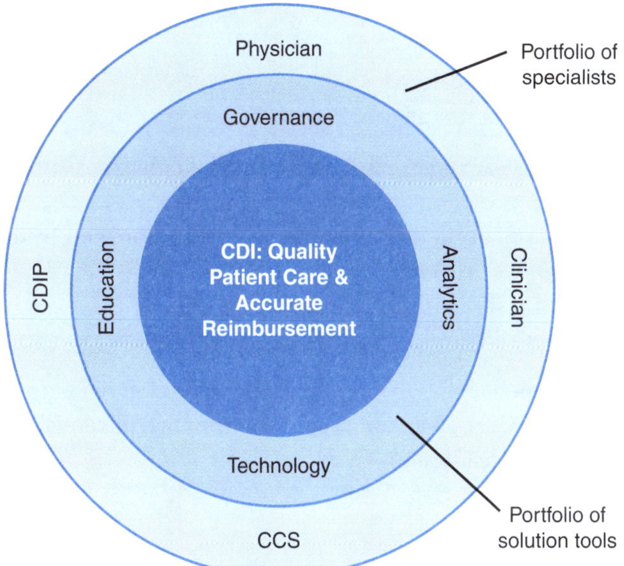

Reprinted with permission by the Financial Planning Association, *Journal of Financial Planning*, March 2014, Kirk Loury and Kevin Forbush, Achieving Higher Growth with Multidisciplinary Teams. For more information on the Financial Planning Association, please visit www.onefpa.org or call 1-800-322-4237.

Conclusion

Many organizations have used the MDT model to implement complex projects requiring a coordinated team of executives, physicians, registered nurses, clinicians, HIM, and other allied health professionals. Figure 17.3 shows an example of the MDT model. The insight and exposure to different healthcare-related disciplines can help the organization achieve the CDI program's goals: quality patient care, improved clinical documentation, and accurate reimbursement. The initial kick-off meeting for the MDT is important for the future collaboration and cohesion of the group. A culture of acceptance, collective decision-making, and accountability improve the positive impact for this important facility-wide project.

Chapter Quiz

1. Why are MDTs formed by the CDI team leader?
   A. To improve clinical documentation
   B. To advance departmental interconnectivity
   C. To examine complex issues and develop solutions
   D. To develop revenue cycle integrity

2. Which item below is one of the goals of a CDI project?
   A. Provide revenue cycle history
   B. Determine average daily encounters
   C. Analyze inpatient departmental integrity
   D. Ensure accurate reimbursement

3. The departmental leadership team designated to oversee the CDI program includes:
   A. Emergency room techs
   B. Revenue integrity
   C. Billing department leads
   D. Case management staff
4. Which of the following performance improvements result from a cohesive core CDI team?
   A. Prevention of conflicting information communicated to the physicians
   B. Improvement of revenue cycle integrity
   C. Decrease in risk management claims
   D. Advancement in clinical technology
5. The establishment of _________ is an effective way to ensure that all members of the CDI program meet functional requirements for success.
   A. Departmental leadership
   B. A resident team
   C. A core team taskforce
   D. HIM leadership
6. The MDT approach provides a beneficial advantage of _____________.
   A. Advanced improvements in revenue recognition
   B. Increased versatility of the core team
   C. Diverse schedules
   D. Increased exposure to different disciplines
7. Which member of the medical staff is usually assigned to the CDI program and reports directly to the medical staff leadership?
   A. HIM director
   B. Physician advisor
   C. Head nurse
   D. Departmental chief
8. Which department of the hospital is responsible for providing the CDI team with CMI and DRG payment analytics?
   A. Medical staff leadership
   B. Care management
   C. Revenue integrity
   D. Quality management
9. The utilization review process gathers authorizations for continued stays and is provided by which department?
   A. Quality management
   B. Case management
   C. Revenue integrity
   D. Care management

10. What activity can help break down natural barriers and create a rich cooperative environment in which CDI thrives?
    A. Building team cohesiveness
    B. Reporting directly to taskforce
    C. Coordinating of hospital charge master
    D. Assisting in post-discharge planning

REFERENCES

Kane, B. and L. Santurnino. 2009. Information Sharing at Multidisciplinary Medical Team Meetings. Group Decision and Negotiation, p. 437–464. Retrieved from: http://link.springer.com/article/10.1007/s10726-009-9175-9#page-1.

Kane, B., K. Groth, and D. Randall. 2011. Medical Team Meetings: utilizing technology to enhance communication, collaboration and decision making, Behavior and Information Technology. 437–442.

Yardley, J. 2014. Nursing & Residential Care. 16(5):284–286. (journal article - pictorial) ISSN: 1465–9301, Database: CINAHL Plus with Full Text.

Yardley, J. 2014. Team dynamics: The role it plays in shaping service delivery. Management. Retrieved from: http://connection.ebscohost.com/c/articles/95610974/team-dynamics-role-plays-shaping-service-delivery.

Chapter 18

Growing the Clinical Documentation Improvement Program in All Patient-Care Areas

Applying the Criteria for High-Quality Clinical Documentation to All Settings

Both the CAMP Method (coaching, asking, mastering, and peer learning) and the seven criteria for high-quality clinical documentation addressed in chapters 1 through 3 apply to all documentation by all clinicians in every patient setting. The CAMP Method and the criteria standardize the practice of clinical documentation. However, organizations still need to design training programs that contain examples specific to each outpatient setting and allow trainees to master clinical documentation in each setting. As seen in chapter 15 on electronic health record (EHR) system implementation, there is an opportunity to use EHR synergies to expand clinical documentation improvement (CDI) into all patient settings. The EHR can contain templates and alerts for documentation in every care area. However, the CDI team still needs to create an efficient review process that achieves the goals of CDI in the context of each patient setting.

Most organizations are in the beginning phases of expanding CDI to settings outside of acute care. Outpatient CDI programs apply to the emergency department (ED), outpatient surgery, outpatient testing, and the physician's office. While there are some common components to them, no two programs are exactly alike. This chapter will discuss examples of CDI training and reviews that have been successfully implemented in healthcare systems. Because outpatient CDI is still in its infancy, the programs will evolve over time. For this reason, this book only includes examples and practices that are more likely to stand the test of time because of their efficiency or added value to the organization. Most sections include CDI training and review principles that are common concerns for every organization.

As readers progress through the examples and recommendations, they should keep the unique aspects and needs of their own organizations in mind. In particular, they should note which activities they might need to implement differently in the organization because of those unique qualities.

Because the most significant amount of clinical documentation per patient occurs in the inpatient setting, many organizations focus their CDI program on inpatient records. However, clinical documentation and its impact permeates every patient-care setting. Most healthcare services in the United States occur in the outpatient setting. In 2010, there were 1.009 billion physician office visits, 100.7 million visits to hospital outpatient departments, and 129.8 million ED visits (NAMCS 2010). That same year, there were 35.1 million inpatient hospital discharges (excluding normal newborns). Therefore, there were approximately 1.239 billion outpatient visits in the United States compared to approximately 35.1 million inpatient visits to acute care hospitals (NHDS 2010). Because physician visits are responsible for 80 percent of all outpatient visits, especially if the healthcare system employs or owns physician groups, the importance of high-quality clinical documentation is clear.

Because of the complexity, most organizations implement CDI initiatives in the inpatient arena. However, others, depending on the organization, its structure, and strategic approach, may begin their CDI program across several different patient-care settings. For example, if structured by product line, the organization may decide to first focus on the cardiology product line. This strategy would involve quality initiatives for documentation in the inpatient cardiac units, the cardiac catheterization laboratory, cardiac rehabilitation programs, and the cardiology groups employed by the organization. The initial investment in this process is much higher than rolling out a program by setting. However, once the organization implements the program across one product line, the ease of implementation across others increases. Although this strategy is not the most common, the ability to build strong physician alliances is greater than when implementing a program by patient setting.

Tailoring CDI Training for the Outpatient Setting

The primary difference between CDI training in the acute care setting and other settings is the examples used to teach physicians the mastery part of the documentation process. Most organizations have created CDI training tailored to the inpatient setting using inpatient examples. It is possible, but not optimal, for physicians to learn from inpatient examples and apply the concepts in every setting. Creating examples from each outpatient setting is best. When constructing examples for use in outpatient CDI training programs, organizations must consider issues such as those discussed in the following sections.

Identify the Most Significant Documentation Challenges for Each Setting

There are some common documentation problems specific to each patient-care setting. However, each organization should assess documentation by setting and identifying documentation issues specific to its facility and practitioners. For example, one common documentation problem in the ED is using differential diagnoses documenting possible causes or diagnoses to be ruled out by the provider in addition to the symptoms. Documenting possible and probable diagnosis is especially important for patients admitted through the ED into the inpatient setting. For short-stay patients admitted through the ED, emergency room physician documentation is key to patient care (NACHRI 2007).

Not all ED physicians admit patients to the inpatient setting. Therefore, the ED record needs to stand on its own from a documentation perspective. Some ED documentation challenges may include documenting reasons for tests and medication orders. If a provider admits a patient to the ED who is already on a medication, the provider should document this as well. If the provider evaluates that patient for the condition, although it may not be the main reason for admission, the provider should document it so the coding staff can capture it.

In addition, the Office of the Inspector General (OIG) has identified medical necessity as a significant issue in most nonacute patient-care areas. The OIG has conducted medical necessity audits that link documentation or lack of documentation as the cause for many payment denials. According to the Centers for Medicare and Medicaid Services (CMS), a claim that requests payment for medically unnecessary services intentionally seeks reimbursement for a service the patient's current and documented medical condition does not warrant (CMS and NCHS 2006; HHS 1998). This official statement about medical necessity directly links the physician's documentation as the primary indicator of whether a patient's service is medically necessary. The OIG goes on to state that the failure of hospital staff to document items and services rendered is a major area of potential fraud and abuse in federal healthcare programs. The Department of Health and Human Services (HHS) statement goes on to say, "Upon request, a hospital should be able to provide documentation, such as patients' health records and physicians' orders, to support the medical necessity of a service that the hospital has provided" (HHS 1999). These statements continue to justify the need to train all staff in all patient-care settings on high-quality clinical documentation practices.

Utilize Unique Documentation Examples for Each Setting

It is most important in the training to use actual examples from each setting. The CDI trainers should obtain cases that emphasize the uniqueness and the particular documentation challenges of the setting so the physicians and clinicians can recognize the records as their own. All identifiers, especially for the providers, should be deleted by the CDI trainers from the training materials to avoid embarrassment. Providers should perceive training as positive, not as a punishment. The trainers should share a few examples of documentation problems and apply the criteria for high-quality clinical documentation to the cases during the lecture. Then, they should give the trainees sample cases, ask them to identify any documentation problems, and discuss how they would document the cases differently. This process of applying the concepts learned is important to the sustainability of the training.

Include Template Documentation in Examples

CDI programs use document templates in most outpatient settings. The templates have advantages and disadvantages. Trainers should use examples that identify cases that make good use of the template and those where documentation is less than optimal. The OIG in particular looks for templates where documentation for multiple patients is the same. Usually this involves using check boxes where the same boxes are checked off by providers for several consecutive patients. The likelihood of identical patient documentation is low. When templates contain the same information, it can point to a problem either with the physician's documentation practices or with the template design (Khoury et al. 1998). Trainers should address physician documentation practices during the educational settings.

Find 10 Problematic Documentation Examples for Each Setting

The CAMP Method study used 10 case studies when training physicians in the basic principles of high-quality clinical documentation. Because of the study outcome, this number is a best practice for physician documentation training. A CDI program may not be able to work the use of ten case studies into every physician training session, but over the first year, the trainers should expose physicians and clinicians in nonacute settings to ten example cases in subsequent training sessions. As an added tool, trainers may design web-based programs for outpatient CDI training. The training team can scan documentation examples into the training modules so physicians receive the benefit of applying or mastering the CDI process.

Prepare the CDI Staff or Train Locally

Most organizations that have extended clinical documentation functions into the outpatient areas rely on their CDI team, who likely began the program in the inpatient setting, to perform the work in the outpatient arena. This is especially true for clinical documentation training for physicians and clinicians. CDI program staff who are already experts in training physicians on the criteria for high-quality clinical documentation are generally the best individuals to conduct this training in all settings. The CDI program staff can also perform the query and data collection process in each outpatient area. On the other hand, if it is more geographically convenient, the training team can train local staff in each outpatient department to review documentation when and where possible. In each case, additional training in CDI documentation review and data collection (similar to that addressed in earlier chapters) should be provided to the outpatient staff.

Designing the CDI Review for the Outpatient Setting

The methodology for CDI concurrent review in the acute care setting is consistent and standardized throughout the healthcare industry. However, the same cannot be said for CDI reviews in the outpatient setting. Clinical documentation teams have developed the process for concurrent inpatient reviews using the structure and staffing in the hospital setting as the venue for the work. Reviewers must do the same in outpatient settings. The following are suggestions for creating an effective review process in alternative patient-care settings. In each setting, the issues have been addressed by the CDI manager of who should perform the review, when and where the review should be performed, how that person should perform it, and how he or she should provide feedback to physicians. The CDI practitioner should collect the same core key metrics for outpatient CDI as those discussed in earlier chapters. As with all CDI interventions, the key pieces of information are how often the CDI practitioner identifies documentation that does not meet the criteria for high-quality clinical documentation, who are the physician authors of that documentation, and whether they responded to inquiries to correct their documentation. The CDI practitioner may also collect other measures, depending on the organization. However, these core key metrics should be the minimum measurements for every CDI program regardless of the setting.

Emergency Department

Because providers admit many patients from the ED to the inpatient setting, the ED often is the second patient location where an organization implements the CDI program. The CDI staff members have had regular opportunities to review ED documentation during their concurrent review of inpatient records (for patients who providers admitted through the ED). Therefore, there usually is a good sense for the specific documentation issues the CDI program staff needs to address. Even in this case, the organization should perform a CDI assessment for ED records to ensure the CDI program staff identifies all relevant issues.

In the ED, physician intervention for CDI should occur prior to discharge. However, every ED will vary in terms of how and if this intervention can occur. The documentation process needs to work around the emergent needs of the patient. The ED is a good location for using templates, documentation tools, and EHR documentation alerts. In many hospitals, a case manager controls patient flow in the ED. Therefore, in some instances, the case manager's existing duties can include outpatient-CDI functions in the ED. Specific tools can be designed by the CDI staff in collaboration with the outpatient department manager for use with physicians in the ED to guide their documentation for both facility-based and physician professional fee coding and billing.

Figure 18.1 shows a summary report from a preliminary ED CDI assessment. The report shows the activities that occurred during the assessment as well as recommendations for implementing a CDI program for the ED. The summary provides some ideas as to the specific activities that might be included in an initial CDI assessment in the ED setting.

Ambulatory Surgery and Specialized Procedures

Outpatient surgery and procedures performed in specialized units such as interventional radiology and the cardiac catheterization laboratory each need to be assessed by the CDI manager to identify the most effective CDI process based

Figure 18.1 Emergency medicine CDI assessment summary

Emergency Medicine CDI Assessment Summary

Interviews:

1. Medical director of the ED, ED administrator, triage manager

Other activities:

1. General observation of the ED process
2. Extensive review of T-sheets and the facility's leveling process for ED care
3. Concurrent review of ED record documentation and content
4. Shadowing residents during the documentation process
5. Shadowing attending ED physicians during the documentation process

Observations:

1. Facility guidelines require ED physicians to be very specific in documenting a diagnosis for a patient in need of acute care admission. Specificity is lacking in almost one-third of ED patients who require admission. As a result, these patients must remain in the ED until they have a definitive diagnosis, possibly having a less than optimal impact on patient care.
2. Patients in need of consult have an average wait time of one hour.
3. One interviewee stated that residents are reluctant to write secondary diagnoses on the patient ED record because they do not want to be criticized by the attending physicians if the diagnosis is wrong when patient is admitted to the floor.
4. Specific inpatient CDI documentation issues:
   a. Symptoms as principal diagnosis without rule out or differential diagnoses
   b. Medications documented but no documentation of the reason for those medications
   c. Lack of clarity of a diagnosis or reason for patients on ventilators for brief periods

Preliminary recommendations:

1. Conduct ED-specific CDI training for residents, attending physicians, and nurses using ED record examples
2. Design and distribute an ED-specific documentation tool for use by clinicians
3. Consider redesigning templates to include prompters or locations requiring the documentation of diagnoses for medications and rule out or differential diagnoses for symptoms

on the structure of each unit. Similar to the initial ED assessment previously mentioned, it is necessary to understand the flow of patients and information to determine where the CDI function might be placed within the ED documentation, billing, and coding workflow. Since time is limited in the outpatient setting, CDI needs to accommodate the patient and the practitioner to create a workable process. Some issues to consider in assessing each outpatient setting include the following:

- Amount of documentation on the record at the time of patient's admission
- Specific times when the physician generally documents in the patient's record during the stay
- How many times the physician documents in the patient's record during the stay
- Availability of the health record during the patient-care process and location of the physician at those times
- Activities directly following patient discharge that may provide an opportunity to query the physician
- In an EHR setting, the location of data is less important. However, the availability of the physician is paramount.

Laboratory Outpatient Testing

In the diagnostic laboratory setting, the challenge for the healthcare organization is ensuring accurate detailed documentation by the physician in the physician order so that medical necessity for the test is documented in the clinical record prior to the patient having the test. Because effective physician intervention in the laboratory must take place in the physician's office, the healthcare organization must include specific strategies for interacting with physicians and their staff. These interventions may consist of having educational sessions, creating a virtual private network (VPN) or computerized "tunnel" from the physician's office to the hospital registration team, including the physicians in the design of the laboratory order form, and creating specific tools or cue cards to move behavior in the right direction.

Outpatient Testing that Involves a Physician Diagnostician

Outpatient testing involving a physician diagnostician's interpretation of the test results should be differentiated from laboratory testing where results are documented in the EHR without a physician interpretation. Examples of these types of tests include radiology, magnetic resonance imaging (MRI), nuclear medicine, electroencephalograms (EEGs), and electrocardiograms (EKGs). In each of these examples, a physician reviews the test results and documents the assessment of the results. There is an opportunity in non-laboratory diagnostic testing to create two interventions. The first intervention is similar to the intervention for laboratory testing where the ordering physician is educated by the CDI staff and provided with tools, such as order forms, to ensure the necessary information is documented by the provider. The second intervention is with the interpreting physician. Again, the intervention is likely to be with education and documentation tools that the physician can use to document an assessment of the test results.

In some diagnostic test areas, it may be possible for a concurrent reviewer to be available to the physician diagnosticians, particularly if multiple physicians are in one location while reviewing films. The reviewer would be available to answer documentation questions and ask questions (queries) based on information the physicians are dictating in the reports. This scenario may not be possible in many organizations due to the physicians' location and time constraints for review. Productivity for radiologists is intense. The number of tests a radiologist can evaluate is tied directly to the relative value units (RVUs) assigned by CMS to each Current Procedural Terminology (CPT) code for the test. The range of films reviewed per day is estimated by the Austin Radiological Association (ARA) to be anywhere from 40 to 175 depending on the level of complexity or RVUs for the test (ARA 2004). CDI program managers should be aware of the structure and process flow of work in the organization's non-laboratory diagnostic-testing areas. The CDI task force can use this information to design the optimal CDI intervention for radiology and other diagnostic test documentation.

Physician Office and Clinic Visits

With over one billion visits per year, physician office and clinic visits present the greatest opportunity, in terms of volume, to make a documentation impact (NAMCS 2010). The CDI program should employ a combination of physician education, templates, and other tools in these settings. Office and clinic visits present an excellent opportunity for physician one-on-one education, if physicians and their patients are willing to participate. This process, often referred to as physician shadowing, involves a CDI specialist with expertise in professional fee documentation and coding. The CDI specialist observes the physician treat the patient. The CDI specialist then documents the encounter concurrently and compares notes with the physician's documentation in the patient record. The CDI specialist and the physician later meet to discuss several patient cases. In the author's experience, the physician practices most conducive to the shadowing process are primary care practices, which may include family practice, internal medicine, or pediatric specialties.

The process works best when the healthcare system employs the physicians. Physicians whom the system does not employ may also be interested in having the CDI specialist perform shadowing and provide feedback about their documentation practices. To avoid any antitrust violations, when the healthcare system provides documentation review services to physicians who are not employees, the healthcare system must charge fair market value for the CDI specialist's services. A primary benefit of physician shadowing in the office setting is that it often engages physicians more strongly in the documentation process than a review of their hospital documentation. Physicians perceive the shadowing process as more of a personal benefit to them. It is likely they will carry over the habits they learn from the shadowing process into all of their documentation practices, including the hospital documentation. The physician-shadowing process is both a relationship-building activity and a CDI activity. Figure 18.2 presents a list of frequently asked questions about the physician-shadowing process. This page can be distributed by the CDI staff to physicians via e-mail or hard copy to provide them with a solid understanding of the shadowing process.

Figure 18.3 presents an executive summary of findings from physician shadowing performed for a three-member ED physician group. This reporting format can

Figure 18.2 FAQ fact sheet for shadowing physicians during a CDI assessment and education session

Physician Shadowing FAQs

What is the purpose of the program?

Physician shadowing is part of the hospital's initiative to improve clinical documentation to ensure accurate reimbursement and data quality reporting. The purpose of physician shadowing is to provide feedback to the physician regarding the quality and completeness of documentation for physician professional fee billing purposes. Improved documentation in the inpatient record will result in benefits to both the hospital and the physician. The physician-shadowing process is educational in nature.

How does physician shadowing work?

The physician-shadowing encounter involves a physician documentation and coding expert "shadowing" or observing the physician during a patient encounter, usually in the office or clinic setting. During the encounter, the coding expert records all of the physician's activities. At the conclusion of the visit, the coding expert shares the extent of the physician's activities, how they would appropriately be recorded, and the level of visit supported by this encounter and subsequent documentation with the physician. There is usually a comparison between the actual results recorded by the expert and the results recorded by the physician. This comparison allows for the physician to identify where the documentation practices could be improved to accurately reflect the care provided.

Who performs the shadowing?

Senior level, credentialed, physician coding experts with the clinical documentation improvement (CDI) team perform the physician shadowing. These professionals have a significant amount of experience working with physician documentation, coding, and billing processes.

What is the objective of the program?

To provide instructional feedback to the physician to improve the quality of the physician's documentation in the patient record as well as to ensure that the physician's documentation accurately reflects the care provided to the patient.

Figure 18.3 Sample summary of results for a physician office CDI review

Physician Shadowing Executive Summary	
ED Group: Sample Hospital	
Physicians: Dr. James; Dr. Smith; Dr. Henry	
1. Time period of review	May 1 & 2, 2006
2. Total patients shadowed	21
a. Dr. James	7
b. Dr. Smith	7
c. Dr. Henry	7
3. Records with differences between physician & shadower documentation	16
4. Impact of differences in #3 for facility E/M billing	**+6,083.00**
a. Positive impact	+7,300.00
b. Negative impact	–1,383.00
5. Differences: physician activity not documented	
a. Physician performed a "service" not documented	5
b. Physician identified a diagnosis not documented	3
c. Physician performed a procedure not documented	4
d. Physician provided a drug not documented	2
e. Physician provided a supply not documented	2
f. Other	0
6. Differences: physician documentation not supported	
a. Physician documented a service not performed	1
b. Physician documented a procedure not performed	1
c. Physician documented a drug not provided	0
d. Physician documented a supply not provided	1
e. Other	0
7. Differences: physician E/M documentation	6
a. History	2
b. Physical	3
c. Medical decision-making	1
d. Other	0
8. Impact in #7 of differences for professional fee billing	**267.00**

be used in an office or clinic setting. The summary shows both documentation inconsistencies between what the CDI specialist saw and heard during the patient visit and how the physician documented the visit. The most common finding in the example was that the physician performed services and discussed diagnoses but did not document them. While shadowing works best in the office and clinic setting, CDI specialists can also perform it in the hospital.

Service Line-Based CDI Implementation

A service line-based CDI strategy involves documentation initiatives for all patient settings for a particular service line. The primary reason for implementing a service-line strategy is the belief that it can increase quality of patient care for the organization. There may also be a focus on increased efficiency. Common examples of service-line management include cancer care, cardiology, neuroscience, pulmonary medicine, and gastroenterology. Managing a service line means consolidating all patient care within these specialties and reporting to the same manager. Organizations cannot compress all care into a service line. Organizations that use the service-line model may have 65 or 70 percent of patient care managed through a service-line director, and the remainder managed by functional managers, like diagnostic radiology and laboratory and pathology services, which treat patients from all different service lines.

An example of service-line management for cardiology consolidates the following services: cardiology diagnostic testing, chest pain clinic, cardiac catheterization laboratory, cardiac outpatient surgery, cardiology inpatient care, and cardiac rehabilitation. The organization can present these activities to the community as an intense expertise in cardiac care the hospital can offer to potential patients. From a clinical documentation perspective, implementation by service line has advantages and disadvantages. The two primary advantages are increased support from the physicians in the service line and the ability to seamlessly develop CDI in both inpatient and outpatient settings. Physicians are likely to align with the CDI program because, as with everything else in a service-line approach, the clinical focus is the guiding principle. As a result, physicians are more likely to perceive CDI as a patient-care initiative than a financial initiative. Second, physician and manager support is likely to make transitioning the CDI review process from the inpatient to the outpatient setting smoother as well.

The disadvantages of the service-line management approach for CDI are increased cost and time to implement the program. Specialization, at least initially, increases the number of staff members that need training since they must be trained in both the inpatient and outpatient review processes. In addition, specialization creates challenges for coverage during staff vacancies. Finally, service-line CDI implementation can generally only be implemented one service line at a time to be effective. Therefore, the timeframe for overall implementation may be two to three times as long as CDI implementation that an organization implements initially in the inpatient setting and then rolls out to outpatient and other settings. However, service-line implementations may be more likely to stick over time because of physician and clinician support. Since so few programs have been implemented using the service-line approach, it is only possible to hypothesize about outcomes at this point.

Conclusion

Clinical documentation principles are the same regardless of the practitioner or the patient setting. However, for the most effective CDI program, the organization must customize some training components and the review process for each patient setting. Training should include examples from patient records in each setting with the ability for the physician trainee to identify documentation problems in the examples and make suggestions about how to improve the documentation. The record review process must be specific to both the patient setting and the organization. The outpatient CDI programs most likely to succeed are those that mold the record review process to the existing flow and structure and those that continue to obtain feedback from physicians and clinicians in the setting.

Chapter Quiz

1. Why do most organizations implement CDI in inpatient areas first?
   A. The HHS mandates it
   B. The amount of documentation per patient
   C. The greatest number of patients
   D. The lower cost of implementation
2. What is the fundamental difference in the CDI implementation process between inpatient and outpatient settings?
   A. Amount of documentation
   B. Examples used to teach physicians
   C. Use of retrospective review
   D. Physician level of expertise
3. Which of the following does documentation for services rendered, such as patient health records and physician orders, support?
   A. Best of practice
   B. Present on admission
   C. Medical necessity
   D. High-quality clinical documentation
4. Which of the following is a standardized methodology for the inpatient setting but not for the outpatient setting?
   A. Concurrent review
   B. Prospective review
   C. Consecutive review
   D. Retrospective review
5. What is an excellent tool for outpatient CDI training?
   A. Having residents learn ICD-10 coding
   B. Providing 10 case studies in the same training session
   C. Web-based training
   D. Having physicians shadow CDI specialists during audits

6. In the diagnostic laboratory setting, what is the challenge for physicians ordering tests prior to rendering services?
   A. Availability of patient record
   B. Accurate detailed documentation
   C. Complexity of cases
   D. Physician level of expertise
7. Outpatient CDI functions in the ED can be woven into which position's duties?
   A. Receptionist
   B. Resident
   C. Case manager
   D. Department chief
8. Which type of medical visit presents the highest level of volume?
   A. Office or clinical visits
   B. ED visits
   C. Ambulatory surgery visits
   D. Acute care visits
9. What is the primary reason for implementing a service-based CDI strategy?
   A. Patient appreciation
   B. Medicare funding
   C. Lower cost of implementation
   D. Quality of care
10. What aspect of CDI remains the same regardless of the practitioner or patient setting involved?
    A. Strategy
    B. Principles
    C. Training
    D. Process

REFERENCES

Austin Radiological Association (ARA). 2004. Radiologist Productivity and Workflow. Retrieved from: http://www.imagingbiz.com/topics/imaging-informatics/ara%E2%80%99s-box-workflow-redefines-practice-productivity-platform.

Centers for Medicare and Medicaid Services (CMS) and the National Center for Health Statistics (NCHS). 2006. ICD-9-CM Official Guidelines for Coding and Reporting. http://www.cdc.gov/nchs/icd.htm.

Department of Health and Human Services (HHS). 1998. OIG Compliance Program Guidance for Clinical Laboratories. Vol. 63, No. 163. http://www.oig.hhs.gov/authorities/docs/cpglab.pdf.

Department of Health and Human Services (HHS). 1999. OIG Compliance Program Guidance for Hospitals. Vol. 63, No. 35. http://www.oig.hhs.gov/authorities/docs/cpghosp.pdf.

Khoury, A.T., H.L. Chin, and M.A. Krall. 1998. Successful implementation of a comprehensive computer-based patient record system in Kaiser Permanente Northwest: Strategy and experience. *Effective Clinical Practice* 1(2):51–60. http://www.acponline.org/clinical_information/journals_publications/ecp/octnov98/patient-record.html.

NAMCS. 2010. National Ambulatory Medical Care Survey: 2010 http://www.cdc.gov/nchs/data/ahcd/namcs_summary/2010_namcs_web_tables.pdf and http://www.cdc.gov/nchs/data/nhsr/nhsr004.pdf.

NACHRI. 2007. National Association of Children's Hospitals and Related Institutions Emergency Department Documentation Peer Review: Charting Improvements.

NHDS. 2010. National Hospital Discharge Data Survey—2006. National Health Statistics Reports. No. 5. http://www.cdc.gov/nchs/data/nhds/1general/2010gen1_agesexalos.pdf.

Chapter 19 Critical Thinking

What is Critical Thinking?

Critical thinking involves focusing thought to get results needed for various situations. "Critical thinking is the ability to apply intelligent problem-solving techniques to a particular situation" (Kokemuller 2014). Critical thinking means giving consideration to the questions to ask, who to ask them of, what is being said, and approach development based on goals and objectives. In other words determine "the best way of doing things" (Kokemuller 2014). Mastering this thought process could mean the difference between success and failure relating to the clinical documentation improvement (CDI) process. The primary difference between thinking and thinking critically is the added dynamic of having a purpose and control for the thought process (Elsevier 2014). During the thought process, one forms the thought about a specific situation. The application of critical thinking to this process involves being open to considerations, assumptions, and details prior to coming to a conclusion. It involves increased time, additional questions, and thoughtful contemplation of various considerations related to the situation at hand (Celine 2014).

An example of critical thinking in the CDI workplace is a CDI practitioner who reviews case documentation for a patient who has recently lost weight. The physician does not provide explanation for the weight loss. The CDI practitioner gives no further attention to the weight loss. The critical thinker further reviews the record for signs and symptoms causing the weight loss, such as peripheral edema, muscle wasting, subcutaneous fat loss, amount of weight loss, change in body mass index (BMI), nutrition notes describing changes in dietary habits and ideal body weight, and lab work providing indicators such as serum albumin. The critical thinker responds to the above scenario by querying the physician regarding the patient's nutritional status and possible malnutrition.

Critical thinking may be used by the CDI manager to improve communication with difficult staff members, determine a facility-specific best practice for CDI workflow, or develop an effective plan to meet the facility case mix index (CMI) target. Thinking critically requires knowledge of the topic at hand, and specific skill sets such as analysis, process improvement, experience in the areas of focus, and on-going practice using enhanced thought processes (Alfaro-LeFevre 2003).

Bloom's taxonomy delineating the six cognitive levels of knowledge, comprehension, application, analysis, synthesis, and evaluation helps to depict the higher order of thinking seen in the critical-thinking process. Figure 19.1 provides a graphical depiction of critical thinking using the six levels of Bloom's taxonomy. The CDI practitioner uses all levels to complete the CDI process:

- Evaluation by making conclusions related to data and by acting on those conclusions by developing education programs and future CDI program goals
- Synthesis by compiling data to present in a different more meaningful way to CDI stakeholders
- Analysis of CDI-related data to determine areas of future focus and physician and coder education
- Application by using knowledge to discern potential missing or incomplete diagnostic detail
- Comprehension of the facts previously learned and expression through organization of knowledge, translation, and interpretation during review of the clinical record for incomplete or inconsistent documentation
- Knowledge of pathophysiology, anatomy, clinical indicators, coding guidelines, and physician communication

Thinking critically requires more than criticism of the current state. Rather than a negative activity, it is a positive process developed to identify effective

Figure 19.1 Graphical depiction of higher level complex thinking

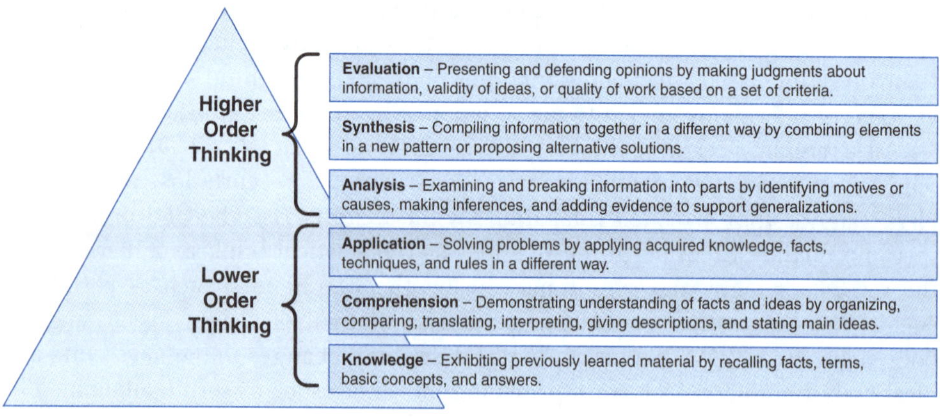

Used with permission from *The Learning Assistance Review*.

solutions to complex issues. Steps for critically considering a positive solution to a complex problem might be

- Gather and analyze information
- Develop a set of assumptions for a basis of the thought process
- Use scientific methods to develop conclusions
- Discern the validity of knowledge sources using questions and judgment
- Apply a creative thought process to develop possible solutions
- Analyze feasibility, pros, and cons of possible solutions
- Determine necessary action
- Positively communicate proposal to stakeholders
- Implement best practice solutions

Critical thinking allows confidence to grow through success, independent action, collaboration when needed, and effective, creative solutions that improve job satisfaction (Elsevier 2014).

Why is Critical Thinking Needed in the Healthcare Setting?

Healthcare delivery has changed dramatically over the past several decades. The transition from manual to electronic data processing and clinical record management is just an example of the dynamic healthcare environment. The skill sets required for clinicians and providers in the healthcare setting have changed from a more straightforward requirement to an exponential increase in technology skills needed to navigate the complex environment.

The recording of a clinical progress note has evolved from a written entry in a manual paper record at the nurse's station, to an electronic entry requiring a high-level skill set for navigating the electronic health record (EHR). As this relates to clinical documentation improvement, historically, improving the quality of the record required communication with the physician and a free text manual entry by the physician. This relatively simple process has changed to a complex process potentially requiring revised specialty templates, drop-down menus, and data analytics used to track complex clinical information.

This evolution translates into the need for providers and clinicians with a working understanding of medicine and patient care, health information systems, analytics, and project management for developing solutions to on-going complex problems. Clinicians and providers must now take additional responsibility, have a better understanding of work performed by colleagues in a wide variety of disciplines, and make decisions more quickly and independently (Alfaro-LeFevre 2003).

The role of the CDI practitioner has also evolved from a review of the clinical record for missing information to a partner in the development of new workflows, education programs, and technology applications. The CDI practitioner must not only review the clinical record and submit queries to the provider, but also identify patterns of lacking documentation by service line and provider. CDI practitioners can evaluate these patterns using the critical thinking process to develop new EHR templates with provider prompts to improve specificity of the clinical record. CDI practitioners can study the same patterns and develop improved educational sessions, either via standard one-on-one or group sessions, or online webinars and individually paced web-based classes. Critical thinking offers a way to work smarter without working extra hours. Using analytics and identifying problem-focused diagnosis-related groups (DRGs) and diagnoses allow for reduced reviews but better results. CDI practitioners can incorporate other payers into the CDI review process using more efficient and effective redesigned workflows.

Critical thinking in the healthcare setting not only allows for creative solutions to workplace challenges, but also and more importantly, the prevention of the problem. This becomes more important as the workplace becomes increasingly complex. An example of this is the evolution of the query process and resulting workflow challenges. Originally, queries were placed by the CDI specialist on the manual record typically at the nursing station during the patient stay. With the evolution of the paper health record into the EHR format, the query process is more complex allowing for break down in the workflow. The CDI practitioner may no longer go to the nursing unit to conduct reviews because the paper record is not there. This has changed provider habits with less time spent by the physicians at the nursing station. New ways of communicating with the physician are required because physicians now have less time to communicate with their peers and CDI specialists. The CDI practitioner must now review a clinical record that is much larger with duplicated portions and increased navigation challenges. On a positive note, the CDI practitioner may use the search feature to identify key words and terms that need further clarification. Overall, there is more information available in the new electronic patient record and critical thinking is necessary to navigate the new landscape effectively.

In Figure 19.2, the query process is relatively straightforward. The CDI practitioner identifies a need for specificity, creates a document, and places it on the chart at the nursing station. The CDI practitioner then flags the document using a tab or specific color paper to get the physician's attention. The physician responds to the query either on the form itself (if it is maintained as part of the permanent record), or in the clinical record if the query form is not part of the permanent record. The CDI practitioner can easily track the physician responses by checking the hard copy clinical record during daily rounds at the nursing station.

Figure 19.3 reflects the increased complexity of the query process based on the transition to the EHR. The initial process is virtually the same except that the CDI practitioner may review the record at any location and is not required to view the record at the nursing station. Because the physician may update the electronic record at any location, they do not spend as much time at the nursing unit. It is now more difficult to communicate with them in person.

There are barriers that prevent CDI practitioners from effectively using the critical-thinking process. They need specific skill sets to overcome these barriers to success. Table 19.1 offers a list of barriers with corresponding skill

Figure 19.2 Original query process

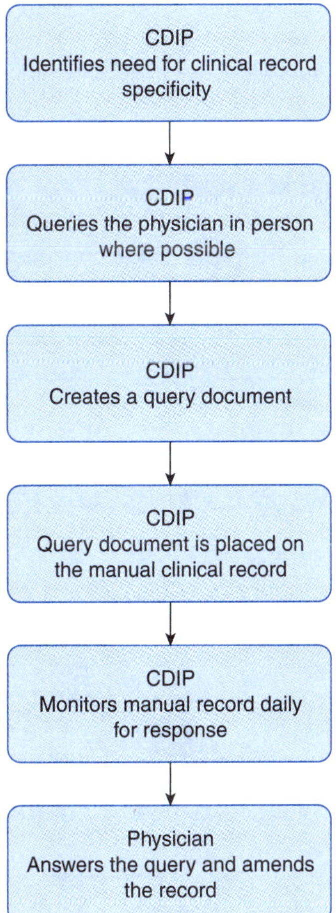

set requirements. Creative communication with the providers is one of the most important requirements for an effective CDI program. The ability to create an effective business relationship that garners respect and trust is important to ensuring a quick response form the physician. Technology skills are also essential for communicating with the physician and navigating the functionality of the EHR. Data analytical skills are crucial for not only reading and interpreting reports but also for creating effective presentations to stakeholders. The discussion below provides additional insight into the breaking down of these barriers utilizing new skill sets.

The first barrier to the new, more complex process is the lack of one-on-one communication. This lack of one-on-one communication is a special challenge to the query process. There are a number of possibilities based on the health information system (HIS) functionality. CDI practitioners may send queries via e-mail, the delinquent chart module, or electronic messages within the HIS. These variables, though seen as improved technology, include inherent problems. Organizations

Figure 19.3 EMR query process

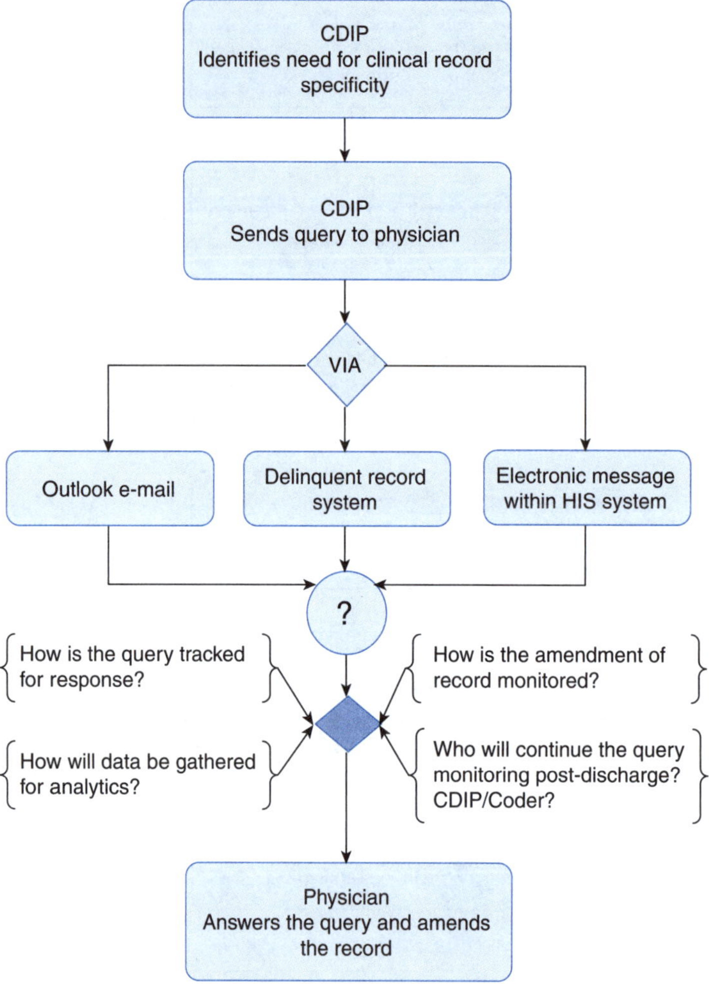

Table 19.1 Barriers and skill set requirements

Barrier	Skill Set Requirements
Lack of one-on-one communication with the physician	Creative communication skills in electronic environment without personal interaction and relationship building
Complex process without personal interaction with the provider is used to notify the physician of pending query	Technology skills for communicating with physician using multiple system functionality (e-mail, delinquent chart module, HIS system in-box message)
Analytic HIS system reports required for creation of CDI scorecard	Analytic and technology skills required to create and utilize HIS reports for daily work flow

should consider the following questions when developing a new query process using current EHR technology:

1. How will the query response be tracked by the CDI manager?
2. How will the amendment of the clinical record be tracked by the CDI manager?
3. How will data be gathered for analytical reporting by the CDI manager?
4. Who will monitor the unanswered query post-discharge (CDI practitioner or coder)?

Because the CDI practitioner does not see the paper record during rounds on the nursing unit, he or she must track the query response and perform the record amendment electronically. In addition, both the query and amendment processes pose a high compliance risk if done incorrectly. If CDI practitioners use the e-mail solution, physicians must carefully monitor their daily e-mail for a query notification. In this case, queries are often overlooked, requiring the CDI practitioner to resend the query. When the CDI practitioner uses the HIS delinquent record system to notify the physician, timeliness is often an issue. The physician may not complete delinquent records daily and this delays the query response past the discharge date. When this happens, the CDI practitioner or coder must continue to track the responses using some type of electronic list, prompt, or notification. The same issues arise when the HIS system notifies the physician of a query.

The second barrier is the complex EHR-based query process. CDI practitioners need extensive computer-based skill sets for daily communication with the physician. The lack of personal interaction creates a challenge to effective physician response. The manual query process allowed for easy tabulation of timeliness and type of query responses by provider. The new process requires a more complex methodology for developing analytics. The CDI practitioner must use the HIS to first develop the reports and then to track and analyze the data.

The third barrier is the requirement of complex data-gathering methodologies for tracking the program. Specific technology driven analytics skills are necessary to create standard reports. These skills include an understanding of databases and how they are used by the CDI manager to create reports, and a proficiency in the use of CDI software tools that provide analytics but require an in-depth understanding of report generation and creation. Most important is the skill set needed to analyze data and turn it into an understandable and meaningful presentation for all stakeholders including executives, management, medical staff, CDI practitioners, and coding professionals.

The AHIMA Clinical Documentation Improvement toolkit offers guidance for data strategy development:

> There are many different strategies for measuring clinical documentation improvement success. Organizations should ensure that goals are clarified and that both quick wins and long-term success are measured. There are many complex disease processes that need to be carefully considered when determining if the opportunity for documentation clarification exists and its potential impact (AHIMA 2014).

The healthcare setting requires critical thinking to prevent and resolve problems. Those without the required skill sets can become the problem. The CDI team (physician, CDI practitioner, and coder) must become more thought-oriented rather than task-oriented. This requires an on-going learning process focused on new technology, best practices, web-based and formal education, derived content knowledge, and the pursuit of credentials and certifications demonstrating team qualifications. Today's healthcare setting requires an expanded skill set including initiative, ownership, responsibility, independent thinking, group collaboration, effective use of resources, and development of interpersonal relationships. Also needed is organization, analytical thinking, performance improvement, technology solutions, reason, problem solving, judgment, and effective decision making (Alfaro-LeFevre 2003).

Importance of Effective Communication

Interpersonal communication is an essential part of the critical thinking process and requires a broad range of skills and attitudes. Effective communication should be person focused and include listening, curiosity, gentle inquiry, and open mindedness to the perspectives of others. Communication is not a one-way process, therefore, just as important is the ability, not only to receive information, but also to deliver it in a thoughtful, clear, culturally attuned, and respectful way. Skillful communication enlists and accommodates the other person's needs (Cavanaugh 2012, 294).

Each member of the CDI team should consider the following steps when communicating with a team member:

1. Consider the relationship between communicating parties. How can they improve the relationship?
2. Establish an attitude that there is benefit to working together. What action can the parties take to improve attitudes?
3. What is the main point the parties need to communicate?
4. What is the historical and current perspective of the other party?
5. How will this communication affect the other party?
6. What are the needs of the other party in relationship to the main point?
7. How can the parties meet each other's needs? Is a compromise possible? Show how each party will benefit.

These steps can be used by the CDI team to improve communication based on a sincere desire to work together and understand a coworker's diversities and needs. The following quote offers thoughts on working together to create a person-centered communication:

> The ideal thing in all health care—whether it's a doctor, the nurses, or the hospital executive—is to ask, 'How can I best communicate with you?' That's what I want to hear. We're all a little different...one thing is not going to work for everybody. So they should ask me, what do I need? (Cavanaugh 2012, 294).

Injecting both parties' perspectives into the communication process results in an effective person-centered communication that enhances the CDI team success.

Problem-Focused versus Outcome-Focused Critical Thinking

Problem-focused critical thinking and outcome-focused critical thinking are closely related. People tend to resolve problems in one of two ways. One way is to determine the reason for the problem and believe that understanding it will help resolve it even though it may continue. Another way is to develop a solution to the problem, which can eliminate it from happening in the first place. If one's problem-solving skills are deficient, the problem may continue without resolution and the results will not meet the goals and objectives. Perhaps both ways can achieve the desired result (Alfaro-LeFevre 2003; Mueller 2011).

Problem-focused thinking can be helpful to avoid the same problem in the future. However, it does not assist in developing a solution. The extended focus of "the problem" requires extensive time and may not result in a resolution (Mueller 2011). Whether it is the resolution of a difficult situation or just daily work challenges, one tends to use a favorite approach (problem- or solution-oriented thinking). The case study below offers a scenario based on critical thinking skills needed for an effective CDI process.

Case Studies: Critical Thinking Skills in the CDI Process

Problem- and outcome-focused thinking are options for each CDIP. The starting point for effective solutions management is the realization of the current method being used. In other words, which method is currently used to solve most of the CDI issues encountered on a daily basis?

Case Study 1

Problem Definition:

The CMI for the internal medicine department is lower than the target. Several high-volume attending physicians have boycotted the CDI program and refuse to respond to queries. The organization identified this pattern when it implemented the new CDI program a year ago.

Strategy 1

Problem-Oriented Thinking (What does the CDI practitioner think about?)

The CDI practitioner focuses on the negative aspects of the low CMI such as

- Pressure from the CDI governance committee regarding the lower CMI for internal medicine
- Pressure from the revenue cycle vice president and chief financial officer regarding reimbursement-related peer benchmarking for internal medicine

- Refusal by the two top admitters to answer queries or discuss cases
- The challenge CDI specialists face when they communicate with difficult providers

Problem-Oriented Actions (What does the CDI practitioner do about the problem?)
To develop solutions to the problem, the CDI practitioner

- Focuses on excuses for low internal medicine CMI at the committee meeting
- Holds discussions with colleagues and supervisors related to the behavior by the two internal medicine physicians
- Avoids physicians due to the uncomfortable communication dynamics
- Feels anxiety, stress, and lack of motivation in the workplace and at home due to the irresolvable ongoing problem
- Demonstrates a lack of confidence and defensive behavior when asked about the problem

Strategy 2

Solution-Oriented Thinking (What does the CDI practitioner think about?)
The CDI practitioner focuses on the solutions to the low CMI such as

- The need for CDI governance structure to support solutions regarding the lower CMI for internal medicine
- Understanding the need for peer CMI benchmarking and how benchmarks can be used to discuss quality scores and professional fee reimbursement for Internal Medicine
- Reasons for the two top admitters' behavior in answering queries or discussing cases

Solution-Oriented Actions (What does the CDI practitioner do about the problem?)
The CDI practitioner develops solutions to the problem such as:

- Analyzes reasons and solutions for low internal medicine CMI and presents to the CDI governance committee
- Holds discussions with colleagues and supervisors to find out their best practices for physician communication (what has worked, what has not)
- Discusses physician communication dynamics with department chair, CMI, or physician advisor to gather suggestions on the best way to approach the two physicians
- Analyzes the quality scores and medical necessity denials to determine how these are impacted by poor quality clinical documentation
- Develops a plan to assist physicians through a physician-friendly query process customized as much as possible to their practice patterns

- Develops a plan to educate physicians on their specific high-risk clinical documentation topics by MS-DRG, MCC, and CC
- Meets with physicians and physician advisor one-on-one to discuss query process and physician-specific clinical documentation topics

Case Study 2

Problem Definition:

The standard practice in this CDI department is to review the cases retrospectively that do not have the same CDI and coder final DRG assignment. The case scenario included a 45-year-old patient who sustained injury in a house fire with third-degree burns of his feet after returning to the burning home for his dog. The patient was busy caring for his pet while in the animal hospital for burn and inhalation injuries and did not take care of his foot injury. After several days, the patient saw a physician, who admitted the patient with third-degree burns of the foot, cellulitis, and sepsis. CDI practitioner selected a third-degree burn as the principal diagnosis with an MS-DRG and weight of 934/1.5748. The coder selected septicemia as the principal diagnosis with an MCC of acute respiratory failure, MS-DRG, and weight 871/1.8072.

Strategy 1

Problem-Oriented Thinking (What does the CDI practitioner think about?)

The CDI practitioner focuses on the negative aspects of the principal diagnoses mismatch such as

- My manager will review this case mismatch and question my skill set
- I spoke with the physician about this case and encouraged him to document the reason for admission to be the burn case
- I entered my original codes in the DRG grouper and found that the MS-DRG 934 has a higher weight of 1.5748 vs. the sepsis with an MS-DRG of 872/1.0528
- Questions why the coders have the final determination of the final DRG, it should be the CDI department

Problem-Oriented Actions (What does the CDI practitioner do about the problem?)

The CDI practitioner develops solutions to the problem such as

- Meets with the manager and explains how the coder is incorrect and the final DRG should be 934
- Speaks with the physician and mentions that the final principal diagnosis selected by the coder was sepsis instead of the burn, but does not explain why, which leaves the physician to question what happened
- Demonstrates a lack of confidence in the coding staff related to principal diagnosis selection
- Feels frustration related to the on-going irresolvable issues between the coding and CDI staff

Strategy 2

Solution-Oriented Thinking (What does the CDI practitioner think about?)

The CDI practitioner focuses on the solutions to the principal diagnoses mismatch such as:

- The need for additional review of the entire record to determine what information may have been added by the provider after the last CDI review
- Reasons for the suggestion by the coder and considers further discussion with the coder to understand possible coding guidelines or identify additional clinical information

Solution-Oriented Actions (What does the CDI practitioner do about the problem?)

The CDI practitioner develops solutions to the problem such as

- Reviews the entire clinical record for additional information not identified prior to the final CDI case disposition
- Schedules and meets with the coder to discuss the case and finds out that the physician documented an addendum post-coder query identifying sepsis as the principal diagnosis with a secondary diagnosis of respiratory failure allowing for a higher weighted MS-DRG 871/1.8072
- Establishes an ongoing bimonthly CDI practitioner and coder team collaboration session to discuss mismatch cases
- Encourages open discussion with thoughtful and respectful consideration from all parties of the new information presented
- Celebrates the improved coding compliance and reimbursements identified by the group

CDI practitioners can avoid problem-focused thinking by practicing a few simple steps:

1. Know your own behavior and be aware of negative thinking
2. Take focus off negative questions and place it onto questions that assist in a solution
3. Take focus off the debate about why a task is required and onto getting the task done
4. Understand the reason for the task and how it will change the outcome
5. Focus on solving the problem through research, knowledge, creative thinking, and problem solving

CDI practitioners should remember that they can use the energy drained through problem-focused thinking to develop an effective solution (Mueller 2011).

Stress Management

Critical thinking becomes difficult during stress. Therefore, critical thinking and stress management go hand-in-hand. When stress levels go up, there are transient changes within the brain with effects on learning, memory, and cognitive function. Severe or long-term stress can result in "detrimental changes in the brain structure and function" (Alkadhi 2013). Impaired cognitive functioning can result in dysfunctional learning, memory, and poor decision making. The result may be the inability to engage in critical thinking.

A healthy control of one's emotions results in more effective critical thinking skills as well as improved relationships with colleagues in the workplace. A calm mindset provides a more professional image, prevents poor outcomes due to negative communication, and allows for a more open mind. Those with less control of emotions may react without thinking and do or say things that have negative consequences. Effective management of one's emotions is especially important in leadership roles and communications in high-stress patient-care settings. The CDI team members benefit by contemplating triggers that cause negative emotions (Kokemuller 2014).

Specifically, workplace cultures that foster effective communication, collaboration, effective decision-making, appropriate staffing, meaningful recognition, and authentic leadership are poised for a lower stress work environment. Another common thread in low-stress environments is a change in the way staff members and leaders view mistakes. Knowing that other staff members allow mistakes gives permission to the critical thinker to be creative and think outside the box.

In addition to the broader challenge of workplace culture, individuals can contribute to a low-stress environment with humor, a healthy lifestyle, time management skills, and common-sense decision making. Forward and reflective thinking is superior to thinking on-the-fly with a rapid response and a possible deficit of knowledge. Planning ahead using organization skills and research helps avert an inappropriate rapid response. Reflection after the fact is helpful to gain understanding, consider flaws in the plan, and develop improvements for a better solution next time (Alfaro-LeFevre 2003).

Conclusion

Critical thinking is the ability to focus on the thought process to get results needed for various situations. It is not simply criticism. It is not the process of accepting information at face value. Instead of answering the question, critical thinking suggests one should question the answers. Critical thinking is based on several key tasks related to validating information, identifying exceptions, and analyzing trends. One should strive to be unbiased and open to new evidence and alternatives. Most of all, one should consider what is not there, think outside the box, and be creative (Darlington 2013; Alfaro-LeFevre 2003).

Chapter Quiz

1. What can the CDI team do to improve communication with difficult staff members?
   A. Motivational speaking
   B. Case management strategies
   C. Critical analysis
   D. Critical thinking

2. The use of critical thinking allows for confidence through success, independent action, and which item below?
   A. Motivation
   B. Collaboration
   C. Communication
   D. Exploitation

3. Why is critical thinking necessary in the current healthcare setting?
   A. Determining CMI
   B. Increased DRG analysis
   C. Technological development
   D. Development in coding systems

4. Which item below increases complexity with the query process?
   A. Decreased face-to-face communication
   B. Increased nursing-unit exposure
   C. Increased guidelines
   D. Decreased networking capability

5. How have complex barriers burdened the query process?
   A. Decreased frequency
   B. Multi-network tracking
   C. Increased medical complexity
   D. Governing body guidelines

6. Workplace cultures that foster effective communication, collaboration, effective decision-making, appropriate staffing, meaningful recognition, and authentic leadership often have:
   A. Low productivity
   B. High turnover
   C. Less stress
   D. Leadership turnover

7. Problem-focused thinking can be helpful to:
   A. Extend the focus of the problem
   B. Assist in developing a solution
   C. Improve relationships
   D. Avoid the same problem in the future

8. One major change found when moving to a newer EHR health information management systems is:
   A. Improved post discharge query follow-up processes
   B. Lack of face-to-face communication
   C. Increased face time at the nursing stations
   D. Ease of communicating with the physician

9. Which causes a decrease in memory and other cognitive functions while causing the release of cortisol?
   A. Self-control
   B. Critical thinking
   C. Decision making
   D. Stress

10. A result of having a calm mind-set includes each of the following except:
   A. A more professional image
   B. Improved trend analysis
   C. Prevents poor outcomes due to negative communication
   D. Allows for a more open mind

REFERENCES

AHIMA. 2014. Clinical Documentation Improvement Toolkit. Retrieved from: http://library.ahima.org/xpedio/groups/secure/documents/ahima/bok1_050585.pdf.

Alfaro-LeFevre, R. 2003. Strategies Promoting for critical thinking. Alfaro TeachSmart.com. Retrieved from: http://www.alfaroteachsmart.com/handouts/2CTstrategies.pdf.

Alfaro-LeFevre, R. 2011. *Critical Thinking, Clinical Reasoning, and Clinical Judgment: A Practical Approach* Elsevier: Philadelphia

Alkadhi, K. 2013. Brain Physiology and Pathophysiology in Mental Street. *ISRN Physiology*. Retrieved from: http://www.hindawi.com/journals/isrn/2013/806104/.

Cavanaugh, J.T., and S.C. Konrad. 2012. Fostering the development of defective person-centered healthcare communication skills: An interprofessional shared learning model. *Work*. 41(3):293–301. Database: Business Source Complete

Celine. Difference between thinking and critical thinking. Retrieved from: DifferenceBetween.net. June 4, 2011 http://www.differencebetween.net/science/nature/difference-between-thinking-and-critical-thinking/.

Darlington, R. 2013. How to think critically. Retrieved from: http://www.rogerdarlington.me.uk/thinking.html.

Kokemuller, N. 2014. Critical thinking and managing your emotions in the workplace. *The Houston Chronicle*. Retrieved from: http://work.chron.com/critical-thinking-managing-emotions-workplace-6509.html.

Mueller, S. 2011. Problem vs. Solution Focused Thinking. Retrieved from: http://www.planetofsuccess.com/blog/2011/problem-vs-solution-focused-thinking/.

Shaw, C. and K. Holmes. 2014. Critical thinking and online supplemental construction: A case study. *Learning Assistance Review*. 19(1):99–119.

Appendix A: Case Study: Using Data Analytics to Drive Physician Education

Susan Schmitz, JD, RN, CCS, CCDS, CDI-P
Manager, Clinical Documentation Improvement

Susan Schmitz is a nationally recognized leader in the field of clinical documentation improvement (CDI). She brings a unique set of skills with her Juris Doctor (JD) degree, RN, CDIP, CCDS, and CCS. Susan has delivered Best-in-Class, CDI implementations for Navigant Consulting, Inc. and large acute-care academic medical centers.

Data analytics were utilized to drive documentation improvement at an approximately $1 billion dollar nonprofit regional healthcare delivery network in Orange County, California, which includes two acute-care hospitals.

Realizing that improving physician documentation would be critical for the successful implementation of ICD-10, the health system invested in analytical systems and tools that would support their CDI program by identifying potential gaps in physician documentation. Having these tools allowed the CDI Manager and her team to prioritize and tailor their educational efforts to focus resources where they would add the most value.

Planning

The tools were utilized to identify the top five service lines by volume. The service lines included

1. Emergency Medicine
2. Internal Medicine
3. Cardiology (Cardiovascular surgery)
4. Neurology (Neurosurgery)
5. Orthopedics (Orthopedic surgery)

Drilling down further into each service line, the top 10 principal diagnosis codes, secondary diagnosis codes, and procedure codes at risk for ICD-10 impact were identified.

The necessary ICD-10-CM/PCS documentation concepts were reviewed for each diagnosis and procedure in the service line. Once reviewed, the top 10 physicians documenting the diagnoses and procedures with the documentation changes were identified. For each ICD-9-CM code with ICD-10-CM/PCS documentation changes, a random sample of accounts was pulled from each of the identified physicians. Support from all CDI team members, each reviewing different accounts from selected service lines, was necessary to complete the audits.

Example:

Top Diagnosis	ICD-10 Concept	Top Physicians	Chart Review Findings
1. Respiratory Failure	Specify hypercapnic vs. hypoxic	1. Dr. Smith	100% Compliant
		2. Dr. Jones	95% Compliant
2. Atrial Fibrillation	Specify paroxysmal, persistent, or chronic	1. Dr. Smith	50% Compliant
		2. Dr. Jones	50% Compliant
3. CVA	Specify culprit artery	1. Dr. Smith	43% Compliant

Analysis

Once the audit was complete, the documentation gaps were identified and education was planned. Noting that the concepts for acute respiratory failure were being captured, we focused our education efforts on the concepts which were not well documented.

Education

Initial education was provided in a group setting. A short PowerPoint presentation was prepared which included the results of the audit and the documentation concepts necessary for ICD-10-CM code assignment. The PowerPoint presentations were delivered at service-line department meetings. In addition, all electronic queries were updated to include the necessary concepts. Physicians were being educated in ICD-10-CM without even knowing it. Another round of data analytics will be completed with a focus on individual education as necessary.

Outcomes

Overall, the physician documentation was found to be exceptional. With the improved understanding of how good documentation leads to improved patient outcomes, physicians have embraced CDI with a 95 percent response rate to a 30 percent query rate. Using data analytics to drive our physician education has proven to be a successful and efficient way to identify documentation gaps, improve our physician documentation, and be ready for ICD-10-CM/PCS changes.

Appendix B: Case Study: A Final Note for CDI Success

Kathleen Luther, RHIT, is a nationally recognized expert in Clinical Documentation Improvement (CDI). She has implemented numerous programs with CDI corporate leaders such as FTI Consulting, HP3, and Accretive Health, Inc. In her candid recommendations for a best-in class program, Ms. Luther offers compelling evidence from her impressive, real-world clinical documentation redesign programs.

Remember: "It's a people thing."

The inpatient prospective payment system (IPPS) began in 1983. Once hospitals knew reimbursement could be optimized under the IPPS system, based solely on the way a diagnosis was written, early renditions of current CDI programs began to sprout up.

A lesson from the past—chief financial officers (CFOs) blamed health information management (HIM) if case mix dropped, HIM blamed the physicians for poor documentation, and the physicians blamed government regulation. What has changed since 1983? Is the landscape we operate in today any different? Less government regulation, greater comradery between the C-Suite and HIM? Are doctors are now documentation wizards with their electronic health records (EHRs), working "smarter, not harder?"

An entire industry has now been created around CDI programs. Millions of dollars are spent hiring the best CDI consulting firm to assist you, let alone the software programs on the market that assist with reports and everyday processes. EHRs now have logic built in to automate parts of CDI. If the patient's glomerular filtration rate (GFR) is X, consider this. If the patient's body mass index (BMI) is less than 19, consider that. Organizations have developed credentials to show an individual is CDI certified. Who makes the best clinical documentation specialist? A nurse? A coder? A physician?

We have had over 35 years to observe, create, and implement CDI programs that stand the test of time. Programs that work, creating long-term sustainability and continued growth have figured it out. These programs know the secret: "it's a people thing."

Meticulous planning for CDI success needs to begin months before kick off or reinvention. Starting with the executive leadership, a vision must be created and committed to. Key leaders within the organization need to be brought to the table. The vision must be clear and concise; there can be no room for doubt that this is what we are going to do. Personality conflicts cannot be tolerated as the vision and CDI program are brought to life. No past blame, no pointing fingers, no territorial issues can come to the table. If world peace depended on these key people to work together, they would do it. It might not be world peace, but the hospital's future very well could depend on the clinical documentation leadership working united to create a successful and sustainable program.

The "people thing"

Executive leadership and support—The C-Suite must be actively involved during the first quarter of implementation. They will provide the vision and the commitment and send the message organization wide: this is what we are doing, this is why we are doing it, and this is why you will be an active participant. Accountability begins at the top. First and foremost, the C-Suite needs to get in front of the program, stand behind it, and clearly communicate updates, successes, and failures. They must hold their key leaders accountable to work together.

HIM, case management, quality—Where do successful programs sit within the organizational structure? White papers, book chapters, and online blogs have addressed this subject. Knowing it is a "people thing," the program should be housed where the leadership will be most committed to its success. Since documentation drives final coding of the record, inpatient or outpatient, many organizations have had improved results when housing the program under HIM. That being said, simply putting the program in HIM will not guarantee success. People make a program successful, not the department.

CDI Steering Committee (the "people" at the table)

C-Suite: Have the CEO, chief medical officer (CMO), chief financial officer (CFO), chief nursing officer (CNO), and the chief information officer (CIO) take turns attending the meetings so all senior leaders are on board, are kept abreast and committed to the CDI program, and are continually holding the team accountable for excellence.

Physician leaders: Twenty years ago when a hospital put pressure on physicians to better document diagnoses and procedures, physicians may have had the opportunity to overrule. Because many hospitals now have CDI programs, physicians are held accountable for CDI outcomes just like the nursing and HIM departments. Both Surgery and Medicine physician leadership representatives sit at the CDI steering committee table. They are ambassadors to all the facility physicians and instrumental in rolling out the program, setting clear expectations, establishing accountability, and delivering physician impact.

When kicking off a CDI program, sending the director of HIM or case management to physician departmental meetings, on their own, is not going to work. A member from the C-Suite along with the appropriate physician leader should attend the key "kick off" and initial departmental meetings. This step should be taken seriously and maintained on a regular basis.

Other Steering Committee Key Members: These members include Directors of HIM, nursing, case management, coding. They need to set clear goals, establish and accountability, and send the message from senior leadership that we will all work together. If one member exhibits bad behavior, the behavior breeds discontent and problems, and the member must be replaced with someone who is willing to work with the team to create a change.

Other CDI Steering Committee invitees, knowing it is "a people thing"

Make a rotational schedule with other departments within the hospital: IT, nursing leaders, physicians, CDI specialists, coders, respiratory and physical therapists, and nutritionists. Send out monthly updates organization wide and then invite questions, ideas, and comments. Make the meetings fun, hold people accountable, and encourage people to challenge the ordinary. Encourage and reward "out of the box" thinking. Utilize case examples of wins and losses, share metrics, and discuss what is working and what is not. What will we do to turn the problem or failure into success? Be willing to make mistakes and address failures head-on. Take risks and learn from them. Let the team know it is okay to fail as long as they learn from it and move forward. Do not place blame; focus on facts, results, key goals, metrics, and continued accountability.

Mandating change is never easy; CDI success depends on changing the current ways of doing everyday jobs. From physicians documenting in the medical record and utilizing the correct language, to clinical documentation specialists and coders doing their everyday tasks: every person on the CDI team brings their own personality to the table. Team work, joint goals, and accountability will make the "people thing" work.

Kathy Luther, RHIT
Director, Clinical Documentation Improvement Services
Accretive Health, Inc.

Appendix C: Case Study: Sioux Valley Hospital USD Medical Center

The Pursuit of Excellence in Medical Record Reviews[1]

by Mary Nelson, RHIA, and Shari Aman, RN, CPHQ

> This project was selected as a 2001 Best Practice Award winner. The Best Practice Awards are generously underwritten by a grant from founding sponsor Healthcare Management Advisors, Inc. (HMA) to the Foundation of Research and Education (FORE). Since 1990, HMA has provided compliance and clinical data quality services to more than 1,600 hospitals and 20,000 physicians, and now also provides online solutions via the Internet.

Is your ongoing medical record review (MRR) process producing meaningful results? Are you able to use the data collected to improve documentation and ultimately, patient care? Are your record reviewers comfortable making decisions and able to meet their deadlines? If not, it may be time to take another look at your facility's MRR process.

At Sioux Valley Hospital USD Medical Center, our ongoing MRR program was piecemeal and clumsy. As the largest medical facility in the region with approximately 476 beds, we had 22,438 inpatient discharges and outpatient activity that resulted in 81,002 actual outpatient medical records in 2001. Our MRR program involved members of the nursing performance improvement (PI) council with additional multidisciplinary members to review 30 to 50 closed records every other month with the Joint Commission surveyor's entire record review tool. This process had several shortcomings, including a lack of ownership and meaning to the results obtained. Results were not valued because participants felt that the sample size was too small. Further, tallying and aggregation of results required much validation and re-review of records by the coordinators of the process.

We had resisted establishing a new program because of the significant time required. Moreover, we weren't convinced that the new program would be more valuable. However, we recognized the need to change the process when the same problems were found repeatedly in the records, despite calls for action from all departments. Additional motivation came after our Joint Commission survey in 1999. The surveyor identified three issues we needed to address:

- develop our program to provide more trended information
- give more focus to clinical pertinence
- show more documented performance improvement

[1] **Article citation:** Nelson, Mary, and Shari Aman. "The Pursuit of Excellence in Medical Record Reviews." *Journal of AHIMA* 73, no. 6 (2002): 45–50.

We decided to design a new ongoing MRR that would be more meaningful to the reviewer and use a more representative sample of records closer to the point of care. The new program became an organizational priority, but no additional resources were available to make it happen. We had to capitalize on existing structures, functions, and resources.

Defining Our Goals

We began by conducting an in-depth review of the Joint Commission standards, scoring guidelines, and intent statements; Centers for Medicare and Medicaid Services conditions of participation; state regulations; and our facility's policies, rules, and regulations. Then, together with the vice president of clinical services and the HIM director, we established goals and objectives for an ongoing MRR process. The goals included

- define representative sample size for hospital (5 percent was ideal)
- include inpatient and outpatient records in monthly documentation reviews
- incorporate timeliness of documentation monitoring
- provide trended data for analysis and prioritization of improvement opportunities
- provide analysis of aggregate data using Joint Commission scoring guidelines as benchmark
- meet the Joint Commission requirement for a multidisciplinary approach by requiring those who provide the care to conduct the reviews
- shift the focus of reviews to the point of care: the open record
- use the entire Joint Commission review tool and incorporate hospital-specific items and the 19 required elements
- promote action plans and remonitoring to show achieved and sustained improvement

In addition to complete support from management and administration, it was clear that a full multidisciplinary team would be needed to carry out the new MRR process. Our new team consisted of nursing PI council members, representatives from all ancillary areas, physicians, HIM, and PI staff. Further, it was critical to be able to produce department-specific as well as aggregate results for the process to be meaningful and to provide desired outcomes. Timely, regular communication of results would be key to a comprehensive process. Finally, this program had to be efficient and simple to implement.

Steps Toward Implementation

Sample Size

Establishing the monthly review sample size to fit our organization was our first hurdle. We wanted to ensure that we reviewed a large enough sample twice a year to start some meaningful trend lines, so we chose to review five percent of records monthly, with each team member reviewing 10 records per month for a particular element of the record. Because using additional staff to conduct the reviews was not an option, we had to use existing staff in a more creative manner. We were given the autonomy to design a program that would fit into our existing clinical environment and established workflow.

Timeline

The initial timeline for the pilot study was July 2000 through December 2000. We would then test the data, evaluate the program, and survey reviewers for improvement suggestions. January 2001 through June 2001 completed the second cycle of this first-year phase. By July 2001 we considered our program fully implemented with trended data for comparison and reporting mechanisms established.

Review Tools

To review open and closed records, we downloaded the Joint Commission Hospital Surveyor Medical Record Review Tool. The tool is designed to allow the reviewer to check for the presence or absence of key elements in the medical record. To work effectively with a multidisciplinary group, we needed to reengineer the tool to be more user friendly. We divided it into four sections and assigned each section to two months:

- assessment of patients (January and July)
- documentation of care (February and August)
- education (March and September)
- operative and invasive procedures (April and October)

We knew that verbal orders (May and November) and nursing assessment documentation (June and December) were two important areas for our organization, so we developed a separate review tool for each. For the clinical **pertinence reviews**, we developed our own tools to cover the remaining elements on the 19 required elements. Legibility and HIM indicator (documentation timeliness) reviews are addressed outside this structure, and the results are then incorporated into the program.

Then, after a detailed analysis of the earlier MRR process, we created binders for the open-record review for each reviewer. Each binder included the assigned tool for each month, guidelines for each of the review elements, action plan forms to record any items found that required improvement, and pre-addressed envelopes to submit the original review tools. We initially prepared these binders for a six-month trial knowing that the Joint Commission web tool changes frequently and to determine which information would be important and valuable to our organization. The binder enabled the reviewers to review their 10 charts anytime during the month, instead of at one designated time.

The focus studies on clinical pertinence involved the members of our multidisciplinary team that didn't have specific outpatient visits, such as the pharmacy, HIM, and PI. This focus group reviews different report types for content on a regular basis and much of the review is done on closed records (the autopsy and donation sections on the required 19 elements by nature can't be reviewed on an open record). The MRR program captures the record as soon as possible after discharge to get as close to the open record as possible. This focus group has evolved as HIM students on their clinical rotations participate in this process.

Next, we established tools to monitor the MRR process. To increase the likelihood of getting solid, factual results, the reviewers needed education and guidelines to follow at every step, especially because there is turnover in PI positions every year. We met with each reviewer and established monthly information sessions and e-mail and phone "hot lines" for questions and changes.

Tallying the Results

The review tools incorporated a tallying component, which was a manual process throughout the development of the program. Now, we use a computerized tally component for easier data compilation. We learned an important lesson while developing this portion of the tool. Although we give the reviewers only three options for an answer ("N" means that the element did not apply to the record, "P" means that the element is present, and "A" means that the element is absent) and guidelines to make judgments, we initially received many written comments on the data collection tools. This made the tally process more time consuming, and we realized the reviewers needed to feel more empowered to make decisions.

At the monthly nursing PI council meetings, we reviewed the results and explored details of the reviewers' concerns. As the reviewers became more comfortable with the review process, they also became more comfortable making their own judgment calls and discussing them. They realized that this new program was an avenue for learning, not criticism. We no longer felt compelled to re-review records.

Tracking and Trending the Data

To make our statistics measurable and trackable, we decided to convert our data into percentages. Then, once the data was ready to be disseminated, we wanted to benchmark it. We also wanted to show the nursing departments how they were doing with documentation each month by giving them an overall score. We decided to "score" each review and compare it to the Joint Commission scoring guidelines as a benchmark (see "MRR Scoring Formula" below). This method proved quite successful, especially at the administrative level. By trending aggregate data, we were able to see the individual departmental improvement opportunities. Directors were encouraged to keep copies of their own department's review results in order to establish their own thresholds and monitor progress by comparing current results to their previous results and identify and address their own department-specific PI opportunities.

By viewing the aggregate data, reviewers could more easily determine if data collection done on their unit was accurate. Because of the open communication structure we established, reviewers were able to ask questions about whether their interpretation had been accurate.

The staff learned that some of the elements were outside their control, but because they affect everyone across the board, we are still comparing like scores. The reviewers and the directors could then also compare their scores to the scores of the other nursing departments. The next time these elements were reviewed, they could see their overall improvement.

An essential component in gathering and reporting statistics is our master review book that includes all record review activities. It incorporates our policy, review plan, the documentation of the percentage of records reviewed each month against that month's discharges, the listing of the members of the multidisciplinary team, the summary checklist for the 19 required components, the schedule for review including the draft for the year's focus reviews, review results, the reporting and action taken, and a final section for evaluation and success stories.

Maintaining Progress

Once we established the review program, we needed ways to maintain its effectiveness and keep reviewers motivated. When a department shows a gap between its actual performance score and the benchmarks, it is documented on an action plan. The action plan form identifies the problem, to whom the problem was referred, and the action taken. Then, a follow-up is planned before the next scheduled review. Additionally, the process enables the department to devise its own strategy and re-review missing elements prior to the next hospital-wide review in six months.

Occasionally, reviewers are too busy to complete their reviews and do not send them in. To address this complaint, we send e-mails to the directors of departments listing the non-reporting areas after each tally. The directors' follow-up sends a clear message to reviewers that this program is a priority. Equally effective is posting the results in each committee meeting. When a department fails to submit its results, "No Report" is listed next to its name on the results projected to the entire group. This is necessary to keep our representative sample size for the Joint Commission and to get a good cross section of our overall hospital performance.

Another way ongoing progress is ensured is through support from administration. Each month, we report the MRR findings to nursing senate and patient services directors in addition to our monthly hospital-wide nursing PI council meetings. Upper management leaves no doubt that this is an organizational priority now that we have the tools necessary to determine our PI opportunities. All results from the ongoing MRR process are also reported into the medical record committee. Physicians then review the aggregate results, and records are brought in for their detailed review. Action for the physician component of the review lies with this committee and the chief medical officer who sits on this committee.

Impact

Looking back, we feel fortunate that the Joint Commission prompted us to improve our MRR program. The benefits we have realized over the last two years with the new MRR program have gone beyond our expectations. One of the major benefits has been increased efficiency in the review process. Because documentation has improved at the point of care, it requires less monitoring. Now, reviewers spend approximately two hours per month resulting in a total review of 400 to 500 records per month. And because the records are reviewed by those who actually use them, there is a heightened awareness of documentation expectations.

Further, the unit-specific results enable staff to aggregate and track their own progress over time. The immediacy of the results promotes sustained performance improvement for a department and also for the entire organization.

The required action plans have increased the effectiveness of performance improvement measures. The best part of the action plan process is that it is easily incorporated into our existing PI program. Denial of problems has been replaced with the realization that there are opportunities for improvement. While it took some time for the action plans to be accepted at the facility, administrators realized the value of promoting the process. In fact, there were several requests to use the same format for other PI activities. Due to the information gained from these reviews and the resulting increased awareness and education, pain assessment documentation went from 84 percent to 96 percent.

We continue to update and revise the ongoing MRR program. Review tools are updated as the Joint Commission revises its tool. Guidelines are also updated as indicated and at the suggestion of some reviewers. Equally important, the results from this process are evaluated monthly, and the process itself is evaluated annually with an informal survey sent to all reviewers, Joint Commission chapter committee chairpersons, directors, and administrators. We want to ensure that we continue to provide valuable data and meaningful information. The individual department binders are considered innovative as a result of analyzing existing processes in such detail prior to implementation of this process. Another innovative component of the ongoing MRR process is the ease in developing focused studies. Clinical pertinence indicators are mostly reviewed within focus studies now.

The most exciting part of this process has been the education all of the stakeholders have received. We've heard several comments like, "I didn't know I was supposed to document that!" Complex performance improvement projects involving multiple stakeholders can only achieve success with small, incremental changes. We believe the continuous monitoring and frequent evaluation of this process has been key to our success.

MRR scoring formula

150 (total number of review elements) – 50 (not applicable elements) = 100 (elements that apply)

100 – 10 (absent elements) = 90 (present elements)

$$\frac{90 \text{ (total present elements)}}{100 \text{ (elements that apply)}} = 90 \text{ percent (score)}$$

REFERENCES

Joint Commission on Accreditation of Healthcare Organizations. Comprehensive Accreditation Manual for Hospitals: The Official Handbook. Oakbrook Terrace, IL: Joint Commission, 1999.

The Joint Commission. www.jcaho.org.

Joint Commission Hospital Survey Medical Record Review Tool. www.jcaho.org/trkhco_frm.html.

Balanced Budget Act of 1997. Sec. 4317. www.hcfa.gov.

Mary Nelson *(nelsonm@siouxvalley.org) is the electronic medical record project manager and a supervisor in the HIM department and Shari Aman (amans@siouxvalley.org) is performance improvement coordinator in the quality resource management department at Sioux Valley Hospital USD Medical Center in Sioux Falls, SD. To view additional forms and resources from this best practice article, contact the authors via the e-mail addresses provided.*

Appendix D: Case Study: St. Vincent Catholic Medical Center

Clinical Documentation: The Saint Vincent Experience[1]

Ruthann Russo, JD, MPH, RHIT, and Maria Muscarella, RHIA

Hospitals throughout the country are conducting reviews on DRGs, case mix index (CMI), length of stay, carve-out days, and denials. St. Vincent Catholic Medical Center in New York City was no exception. Using "home grown" systems, the Case Management department worked collaboratively with the HIM department to measure the quality of clinical documentation and its impact on coding and the CMI. Without formal measurement tools to assist, collating the data was labor intensive. Despite this fact, a trend was identified—the clinical documentation did not always adequately reflect the severity of illness of the patient population and, in turn, did not support the HIM coders in their coding endeavors to achieve and sustain optimum quality and accuracy. Ultimately, an administrative decision was made to implement an independent clinical documentation improvement structure at St. Vincent's Hospital.

A multidisciplinary Clinical Document Improvement Steering Committee chaired by the senior vice president of Nursing Administration was developed. It included the medical director; chairperson of the Department of Medicine; vice president of Finance; vice president of case management; director of case management; vice president of HIM; director of HIM; coding manager; Information Technology; and HP3 personnel. The purpose of the group was to oversee the implementation, monitor the ongoing process, and address all identified issues.

The steering committee made two immediate decisions:

- Clinical documentation improvement (CDI) specialists would report to the director of Case Management
- Recruitment for the CDI specialists would be done internally

The rationale for internal recruitment was that staff members were already familiar with the medical staff and clinical documentation, and therefore would be several "steps ahead" of someone hired from the outside. This proved to be a wise decision, as the ideal candidates recruited came from Case Management and from the ICU and had significant experience reviewing clinical documentation in addition to established, positive working relationships with the medical staff.

[1] **Source**: Russo, Ruthann; Muscarella, Maria. "Clinical Documentation: The Saint Vincent Experience." AHIMA's 78th National Convention and Exhibit Proceedings, October 2006.

Role of the Medical Staff

A hospital's medical staff is the key to success of a clinical documentation improvement program. The physician's documentation ultimately will determine the coding; and, in turn, the coding is the data that will generate reimbursement, mortality and severity ratings, quality indicators, and research/planning information. A hospital should take a multi-tiered approach to involving the physician both individually and in groups in the clinical documentation initiative. First, physician champions or leaders should be involved with the initial creation of the hospital's specific CDI program. The physician CDI leaders will be most successful if they are involved managers or practicing members of the medical staff. Because of the differences in approach, it is best to secure the involvement of both a medicine physician and a surgeon. Other criteria that should be used to make the decision regarding who the organization's physician champions will be include likelihood of initial and ongoing support from the physician and how well respected the physician is by his/her peers.

A documented, structured communication plan should be created to ensure the physicians are informed about the clinical documentation program. The hospital needs to consider both content and methodology of communication in designing the CDI communication plan. For content, the communication plan should focus on why the physicians should be interested in participating in the hospital's CDI program and what value they personally will get from this program. The message may be structured differently for employed or house physicians than it is for voluntary physicians. For example, for employed physicians and house staff, there may be an interest in their own severity level curves for the patients they treat; whereas, voluntary physicians may be more likely to be interested in how improving their documentation will help to improve their own coding and reimbursement for their practices.

In structuring the communication plan, it is important to take both a top-down and bottom-up approach. Top-down approach strategies include starting with an announcement of the CDI program to the Medical Executive Committee. This is usually done through a presentation with handouts or take-aways. Each department head is then asked to communicate the information to their department members. The bottom-up approach is focused on identifying the most effective ways to get information into the hands of members of the medical staff. Depending on the organization, this may be through e-mail, hard copy mail, or announcements posted in the medical staff lounge.

Medical staff training and education in clinical documentation practices are the foundation for a successful and sustainable clinical documentation program. Again, the process must be approached with a multi-tiered strategy. Physicians should be educated in groups by specialty. They should also be educated one-on-one about the nursing units, when possible. Explaining the impact of improved clinical documentation to a physician is much more powerful when their own documentation and patients are used as examples. Physician-specific education can be provided on the units in the hospital, in the clinic, or in their offices. And, of course the most powerful education occurs when the physician sees a personal benefit in documenting better.

⊙ The Role of Concurrent Reviewers

The central catalyst in the clinical documentation program is the clinical documentation specialist, also known as the concurrent CDI reviewer. This individual is responsible for reviewing the inpatient record while the patient is still in-house and identifying opportunities to improve the documentation in the record. When an opportunity is found, the CDI specialist communicates with the physician to obtain necessary documentation in the patient record. Whatever your hospital decides to call these individuals, they are essential to the ongoing CDI process. The successful CDI specialist is likely to be a registered nurse with record review experience. In addition, CDI specialists who are already familiar with the hospital and the medical staff will have a higher degree of initial success than someone hired from outside of the organization.

Because CDI specialists are generally not in high supply, each hospital should plan to provide initial and ongoing training to the individuals hired to be the engine of the CDI program. The initial training must focus on an understanding of clinical documentation guidelines as described in Medicare Conditions of Participation, JCAHO regulations, UHDDS, and Coding Clinic guidelines. It is important for the CDI specialists to understand the need to obtain documentation from the physician or other practitioner that is legible, complete, accurate, reliable, precise, and clear. The CDI specialist should track and measure their review process and their physician interaction. This process is often omitted from a new CDI program. Omission of the tracking and measuring process, coupled with reporting of those results, is the greatest reason for lack of sustainability.

⊙ Role of the HIM Department

The HIM Department is integral to the success of a CDI project. From inception, CDI specialists must collaborate with the coding staff. A regularly scheduled meeting for the CDI specialists and the coding staff should be established. During the early phases of the project, a minimum of twice a month is recommended because there are numerous issues that can be identified and resolved early in the project. Some of the key issues that may arise are as follows:

- Are the communication tools effective?
- Are the coders able to identify all of the records reviewed by the CDI specialists?
- Is the information documented and collected by the CDI specialists useful?
- Is there additional information that the coders need?
- Are there any trends (diagnoses, procedures, physicians)?
- Do the records queried by the CDI specialists contain the documentation required by the coders to code the records accordingly?

These meetings will prove to be invaluable in identifying issues that otherwise go unnoticed.

In addition to the concurrent review conducted by the CDI specialists, it is imperative that the HIM Department also establish a retrospective query process. As the success of the concurrent queries ultimately rests with the coders, there must be specific guidelines in place. If a concurrent query remains unanswered by the physician at the time of discharge, the responsibility rests with the coder to conduct the necessary follow-up. Additionally, based upon CDI specialist staffing, if 100 percent concurrent review is not conducted, a formal retrospective query process should also be implemented. This process should be structured (with formal coding guidelines in place), tightly controlled, and measured for its success.

Queries should be precise and based on clinical documentation in the medical record that may be ambiguous, incomplete, or conflicting. As with the concurrent query process, communication tools for the retrospective queries, which are diagnosis/procedure specific, should be developed and used. To ensure consistency, accuracy, and pertinence of the queries conducted by the coders, it is recommended that the coding supervisor review all queries prior to physician contact. The coding supervisor should act as a liaison between the coders, the CDI specialists, and the medical staff.

Ongoing monitoring and tracking of queries with correlation to physicians, DRGs, coders, and quality outcomes should be conducted to measure success as well as identify trends and areas for improvement. Based on these findings, plans of corrective action and of education for both the medical staff and coders should be developed and implemented. The value of this education cannot be emphasized enough.

Role of Support Departments

In addition to the CDI specialists, other ancillary clinical staff can play an important role in the success of CDI. When ancillary staff members are tapped to participate in CDI, it makes the program more of a hospital-wide function than a traditional "silo" function. The value of a hospital-wide function is that everyone understands the process and its importance, and there is more likely to be an organizational attitude of joint responsibility. Organizations that embrace joint accountability are generally more productive and successful.

The following ancillary groups can be recruited to participate in the CDI program: case managers, nutritionists, nurse managers, unit secretaries, respiratory therapists, physical and speech therapists, wound care nurses, and other specialists. Each organization should design ancillary support based upon the strengths and resources in the organization and in each group. Generally, the case management group acts as a concurrent safety net for the CDI process. Case managers spend a lot of time interacting with physicians. And, if during their conversations, a physician has a question about a concurrent query, the case manager can provide basic information and direction. The same is true of therapists and specialists who may be trained as part of your clinical documentation program.

The key to cooperation from these groups is to provide communication, education, and feedback. First, communicate to the group or group's manager(s) that they have been tapped to participate in the new CDI initiative, which is designed to improve results throughout the organization. In the communication, be explicit about expectations. For example, you may want to state, "We will provide you with some basic training on CDI (may help with their CEUs) and will ask that you act as a 'resource' to the medical staff when questions arise." Education will vary based on the group trained. For example, the case managers may receive comprehensive training while the unit secretaries may receive general information sessions. Once the ancillary staff has been recruited and trained, it is important for them to receive updates about the progress of the program. If the program is doing well, they will feel part of the success. If the program is lagging, they may offer to contribute more with the physicians.

Maintaining Sustainability

Tracking, measuring, and reporting the impact of the CDI program is essential to ensuring a sustainable program. As noted above, many CDI programs have been shut down because the organization was unable to determine the value of the activities. The tracking and measuring process, generally driven by a computer program, will provide the ongoing assessment of the value of the questions to and responses from physicians. Objective measures of success that can be tracked with a good CDI tool include CMI, CMI by payer, query rate, and response rate. More importantly, these measures can be tracked by service, physician, time period, or CDI specialist. Generating reports by groups or individuals, if managed correctly, can increase accountability. For example, if the department of cardiology is identified as having only a 55 percent response rate to queries, this may trigger action by the chair and cardiologists to comply with queries moving forward. The reason for increased compliance can be as simple as the cardiologists' awareness that their response rate was much lower than other services in the medical staff.

Appendix E: Case Study: University of Michigan Health System

A Successful Clinical Documentation Improvement Program Using RHITs[1]

Gwen Blackford, RHIA, and Deborah Slater, RHIT

⊙ Introduction

The University of Michigan Health System (UMHS) is an award-winning healthcare system made up of University, Children's, and Women's Hospitals; 30 health centers; 120 outpatient clinics; the University of Michigan Medical School; faculty group practices; and the M-Care Health Plan System.

The task of obtaining clinical documentation at the point of care in a large teaching facility is challenging. The HIM Department at UMHS is using Registered Health Information Technologists (RHIT) to capture clinical documentation at the point of care to improve facility reimbursement, case mix, clinician communication, and severity and mortality reporting, and to decrease reimbursement denials.

The traditional model for a clinical documentation improvement program (CDIP) is to use nursing staff because of their clinical background. At UMHS, we believed that by using key coding staff, such as clinical documentation specialists (CDS), we were able to obtain necessary documentation in addition to meeting all coding guidelines.

Organizational leadership provided the stimulus for a CDIP, with the goals of accurately capturing inpatient reimbursement for services rendered and re-assessing internal coding operations.

⊙ Program Implementation

The need for a CDIP was identified based on the following:

- Ineffectual post discharge clinical query process
- Lack of clinician education in real time
- Need to obtain clinical documentation in real time
- Documentation needed to reflect the complexity/severity of patients at UMHS

[1] **Source**: Blackford, Gwen; Slater, Deborah. "Strengthening the HIM Profession: Implementing a Successful Clinical Documentation Improvement Program." AHIMA's 78th National Convention and Exhibit Proceedings, October 2006.

The deficiencies of the process prior to implementation of the CDIP were the lack of HIM staff visibility on the inpatient units, inadequate and delayed post-discharge clinician query process, querying of attending physicians' instead of documenting clinician, and missing the educational opportunities during querying.

A consultant performed an internal coding operation assessment and focused on capturing information to drive appropriate DRG assignments for facility reimbursement.

The consultant and the HIM director worked together on the following: rounding with clinical services to understand their documentation workflow process; developing a framework for the CDIP, which included a re-organization of the coding unit structure to create three clinical service teams (Mott, Maize, and Blue); creating new job descriptions for clinical documentation specialists (CDS) and coding compliance and education coordinators (CCEC); and developing a new salary scale. The coding staff was able to apply for all new positions.

The Clinical Information Decision Support Services (CIDSS) unit identified clinical services for potential documentation opportunities based on DRGs without CCs, such as cardiology, neurosurgery, orthopedics, and so on.

We used the P-D-C-A (Plan-Do-Check-Act) quality improvement tool to identify the following:

- Problems
- Root causes
- Improvement goals
- Mission statement

Problems: Incomplete and/or contradictory clinical documentation, incomplete documentation for facility reimbursement, severity and complexity of patient mix, and incomplete specificity of clinical documentation to support treatment rendered.

Root causes: Lack of clinician education regarding non-specific documentation, and the current clinician query process was post-discharge and missed opportunities for clinician interaction and education.

Improvement goals: Capture clinical documentation at the point of care, improve facility reimbursement and case mix, improve clinician communication, decrease reimbursement denials, and retain UMHS's reputation as a high-ranking hospital.

Mission statement: To improve continuity of high-quality patient care; to support appropriate facility reimbursement; to accurately reflect the severity and complexity of the patients treated at UMHS.

Clinical Documentation Improvement Program Process

The HIM manager and the CDS presented CDIP to clinical departments and identified who performed documentation for each service—for example, residents, physician assistants, or nurse practitioners. A clinical notification and education tools were developed for each clinical service. We identified a contact for clinical service resident rotation schedules and set up rounding times.

CDSs use wireless laptops with 3M/HDM and all clinical online information systems on the inpatient units.

A CDS admission work list was created in the 3M/HDM system for each clinical service team. The CDS performs case review 24 to 48 hours after admission to obtain the "working DRG." The CDS will determine cases for clinical intervention, such as documentation stating "troponin leak." The CDS will contact documenting clinician (resident, physician assistant, nurse practitioner, or attending physician) by either e-mail, page, or in person to ask for clarification if a patient has an MI (myocardial infarction) and if so, to please document diagnosis in progress note and/or discharge summary. CDS chapter was created in 3M/HDM to capture working and final DRGs, the question asked, clinician query response, the clinician response (yes/no), and the reimbursement difference between the working and final DRGs. The CDS will continue to review the cases to check for a clinician response, and if no response, the CDS will continue to contact the clinician up to discharge. The CDS will not follow cases after discharge. The CDS reviews all payers. At the time of coding, the coder will review the "communication" chapter in 3M/HDM to look for documentation of clinician response.

The CDSs round with each of their clinical services at least once a week. The rounding process allows for the CDS to interact with the clinicians, gain a basic understanding of the treatment plans, and make themselves visible to the clinical teams. The CDS for the Cardiology service was asked to participate in creating an online educational CD on clinical documentation, which is used on a monthly basis to orientate all new residents to the service. Also, clinical services have asked their CDSs to assist with the creation of online documentation templates.

The CDS works closely with the manager to prepare "Documentation Tip" pocket cards with commonly missed complications/comorbidities. We have worked with the clinical departments to meet their needs, such as placing the transcription directions on the back of the tip cards and adding core measure information on the cardiology cards.

Outcomes

Presentations were developed to provide feedback on the CDIP for each clinical service, which included the following: outlining high complexity DRGs, presenting opportunities for improved clinician documentation, providing case-specific examples of DRGs with and without CCs, and identifying clinician response rates and potential reimbursement. CDS staff members have been asked to present the CDIP at various department meetings. We have found that clinicians are receptive to the front-end query process. Also, there is a high level of support from the clinical division chiefs. We actually received applause from the clinical staff after one of our presentations. We created a Quality Improvement Story Board for Quality Improvement Month and received an award.

There is improved communication between the coder and the CDS staff. Documentation is available at the time of coding. We have seen a strong improvement in clinical documentation with the implementation of the CDIP. Our residents will rotate to other services, and they will take what they have learned and practice it on other services.

The physician query response rate is 90 percent, and the potential reimbursement identified through the physician query process is approximately $5 million.

Next Steps

Since the CDIP has been a great success, our plan is to create one to two additional CDS positions to cover the remaining clinical services. We will continue to monitor outcomes of the CDIP and make improvements, trend pre- and post-CDIP data, review documentation for All Payer Refined-Diagnosis Related Groups (APR-DRGs), work with clinicians on creating documentation templates, and create methods to improve clinician education, such as newsletters, website material, and presentations at resident grand rounds.

In a teaching institution, learning is a never-ending process, and our goal is to become a larger part of that process.

Getting Quality Clinical and Coded Data: How UMHS's CDIP Improved Clinical Coded Data and Clinical Staff Relationships

by Gwendolyn Blackford, BS, RHIA, and Rosanne Whitehouse, MPH[2]

Obtaining codeable clinical documentation at the point of care in a large teaching facility can be challenging. However, the HIM department at the University of Michigan Health System (UMHS) in Ann Arbor, MI, took on the task, implementing a clinical documentation improvement program (CDIP). As a result of UMHS's successful CDIP implementation, HIM staff and clinicians are well positioned to effectively code under the new MS-DRG system and capture present on admission reporting indicators.

This article details UMHS's program and how it has improved the organization's coding and reimbursement.

Improving the Bottom Line

UMHS decided to implement the program to improve its bottom line. Organizational leaders wanted to accurately capture inpatient facility reimbursement. The program also provided UMHS the opportunity to re-assess internal coding operations.

[2] **Article citation**: Blackford, Gwendolyn; Whitehouse, Rosanne. "Getting Quality Clinical and Coded Data: How UMHS's CDIP Improved Clinical Coded Data and Clinical Staff Relationships." *Journal of AHIMA* 78, no. 9 (October 2007).

UMHS identified four areas for improvement as part of its CDIP implementation:

- Improve the post-discharge query process
- Implement real-time clinician education
- Obtain complete clinical documentation at the point of care
- Ensure documentation reflects the complexity and severity of patients treated

Prior to implementation, UMHS experienced many of the same inefficiencies in its coding functions that other hospitals experience. There was a lack of HIM staff visibility on the inpatient units. Oftentimes, the only interaction coding professionals had with physicians was through an inefficient and delayed post-discharge query process.

Although documentation is done by attending physicians, fellows, residents, nurse practitioners, and physician assistants, the query process was geared toward attending physicians instead of documenting clinicians. Most important, UMHS felt that it was missing valuable educational opportunities for clinicians.

Program Implementation

With the support and strategic leadership of the chief administrator for HIM, a workgroup formed to identify a consultancy to develop and implement the program. UMHS used the consultancy to assess its internal coding operations and to identify opportunities for capturing information to drive appropriate DRG assignment for facility reimbursement.

The consultancy and the coding manager worked together to develop a framework for the CDIP. They rounded with clinical services to understand the documentation workflow process. They then reorganized the coding unit structure to create three clinical service teams, created a new job description for clinical documentation specialists (CDSs), and developed a new salary scale.

CDIPs often use nursing staff to capture clinical documentation at the point of care because of their clinical background, but UMHS decided to employ key coding staff (registered health information technicians) in the CDS role. This approach not only allows coders to obtain the documentation needed for coding and reimbursement, it also helps develop positive working relationships with medical staff.

The clinical information decision support services unit assisted the HIM Department in identifying clinical services for potential documentation opportunities based on DRGs without complications/comorbidities (CCs).

UMHS used the plan-do-check-act quality improvement process to identify the problems, root causes, and improvement goals. The problems included incomplete or contradictory clinical documentation that did not consistently support facility reimbursement, the severity and complexity of the patient mix, or treatment rendered. The root causes were found to be a lack of clinician education regarding nonspecific documentation and a post-discharge query process that resulted in missed opportunities for clinician interaction and education.

UMHS set the following improvement goals:

- Capture clinical documentation at the point of care
- Improve facility reimbursement and case mix
- Improve clinician communication
- Decrease reimbursement denials
- Retain UMHS's reputation as a high-ranking hospital

The CDIP Process

The coding manager and CDS staff presented the improvement program to clinical departments and identified who performed documentation for each service (for example, residents, physician assistants, or nurse practitioners). They also identified a contact for the clinical service resident rotation schedules and set up rounding times.

The CDSs use wireless laptops to capture clinical data at the point of care, and all online clinical information systems on the inpatient units facilitate baseline and working DRG assignment to determine if there are query opportunities.

A CDS admission work list was created for each clinical service team. The CDS performs a case review 24 to 48 hours after admission to obtain the baseline DRG. The CDS then selects cases for intervention. For example, if the documentation states "troponin leak," the CDS will contact the documenting clinician (resident, physician assistant, nurse practitioner, or attending) by e-mail, page, or face-to-face conversation to ask whether the patient also had a myocardial infarction. If the patient did, the CDS would then request the clinician document the diagnosis in a progress note and the discharge summary.

The CDS will continue to review the case to check for a clinician response. If no response is received, the CDS will continue to contact the clinician up to discharge. When the chart is coded, the coder has access to the CDS's notes in the abstract to alert the coder to look for documentation of a clinician response in the record.

UMHS modified the abstract to capture a baseline DRG and any potential working DRGs, the questions asked, and whether the clinician responded. If the clinician did respond, the CDS notes in the abstract if the requested information was documented in the chart. If the query resulted in a DRG change, the reimbursement difference between the baseline and working DRG is calculated.

The CDS staff rounds with each of their clinical services at least once a week. The rounding process allows the CDS to interact with the clinicians, gain a basic understanding of the treatment plans, and make themselves visible to the clinical teams. The CDSs also have been asked by clinical services to assist with the creation of online documentation templates.

In order to facilitate documentation for clinicians, pocket cards with documentation tips were developed, including commonly missed CCs and other documentation hints specific to the clinician's service. In addition, space on the back of the cards was dedicated for clinician requests, such as directions on how to use the dictation system and core measures information for the cardiology tip cards.

Reaping the Benefits

The CDIP team periodically presents the results of the program to each clinical service. The presentations outline the high-complexity DRGs and identify opportunities for improving clinician documentation. The team also provides case examples of DRGs with and without CCs to show the financial impact of accurate and complete documentation. The clinicians are presented with their query response rates. The CDS staff has also been asked to present the program's results at various department meetings.

UMHS has found that clinicians are very receptive to the front-end query process. There has also been greater collaboration between clinicians and the CDS staff.

Using RHITs in the CDS role has created positive communication between coders and the CDS staff. The coding team has benefited from documentation being available at the time of coding. UMHS has seen great improvement in clinical documentation with the implementation of the CDIP.

The physician query response rate is 82 percent. The CDIP team feels it is truly higher than this, as physicians will add documentation at discharge and the current process reports the rate while patients are still in-house. The post-discharge query process has decreased significantly from 819 queries in 2003 to 380 in 2006. The potential reimbursement identified through the physician query process from the point of the admitting DRG to the working DRG to date is more than $13 million.

Next Steps

Given the success of the program, UMHS plans to create additional CDS positions to cover the remaining clinical services. The organization will continue to monitor CDIP outcomes to make improvements to the program.

UMHS plans to continue to trend pre- and post-CDIP data and review documentation for present on admission indicators and MS-DRGs as part of its improvement goals. The CDIP team also will continue to work with clinicians on improving documentation, creating documentation templates, producing newsletters and a CDIP website, and presenting at resident grand rounds.

***Gwendolyn Blackford** (gmbford@umich.edu) is the coding manger and Rosanne Whitehouse is the chief administrator of HIM at the University of Michigan Health System in Ann Arbor, MI.*

Index

C

E

F

G

H

I

N

O

P

Q

R

T

U

V

W